tres

The Clinician's Handbook of Natural Medicine

To Dr John Bastyr and all the other physicians of natural medicine who kept the hope of natural healing alive during the dark ages of the Twentieth Century.

For Churchill Livingstone:
Publishing Manager, Health Professions: Inta Ozols
Project Development Manager: Katrina Mather
Project Manager: Ewan Halley
Design: George Ajayi

The Clinician's Handbook of Natural Medicine

Joseph E Pizzorno Jr ND
President Emeritus and faculty member, Bastyr University, Kenmore, Washington, USA

Michael T Murray ND
Faculty member, Bastyr University, Kenmore, Washington, USA
Leading author and educator in naturopathic medicine

Herb Joiner-Bey ND
Faculty member, Bastyr University, Kenmore, Washington, USA

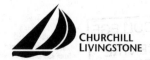

CHURCHILL
LIVINGSTONE

EDINBURGH LONDON NEW YORK OXFORD PHILADELPHIA ST LOUIS SYDNEY TORONTO 2002

CHURCHILL LIVINGSTONE
An imprint of Elsevier Science Limited

First published 2002
    Reprinted 2002, 2003

ISBN 0443 07080 6

British Library Cataloguing in Publication Data
A catalogue record for this book is available from the British Library.

Library of Congress Cataloging in Publication Data
A catalog record for this book is available from the Library of Congress.

Note
Medical knowledge is constantly changing. As new information becomes available, changes in treatment, procedures, equipment and the use of drugs become necessary. The authors and the publishers have, as far as it is possible, taken care to ensure that the information given in this text is accurate and up to date. However, readers are strongly advised to confirm that the information, especially with regard to drug usage, complies with the latest legislation and standards of practice.

ELSEVIER SCIENCE

your source for books,
journals and multimedia
in the health sciences

www.elsevierhealth.com

Printed in China
P/03

The publisher's policy is to use paper manufactured from sustainable forests

Preface

The Clinician's Handbook of Natural Medicine has been created as a companion to the *Textbook of Natural Medicine*. It was written to provide the busy clinician with concise guidance for the care of patients who may suffer from one or more of 80 of the most common diseases effectively treated with natural medicine. While Sections IV and VI of the *Textbook* provide in-depth discussion of the pathophysiology, causes, documented natural medicine interventions, and full references for these diseases, the *Handbook* provides only the most pertinent information needed for intervention for the typical patient. Working together, these works provide the clinician with the best of both worlds: easily accessible advice for quick guidance for the less complicated patient and in-depth understanding when needed. Of course, the *Textbook* also contains considerable additional information in its other four sections.

The astute reader may notice a few inconsistencies between the recommendations found in the *Handbook* and *Textbook*. As the *Handbook* was written approximately three years after the *Textbook*, we have worked to ensure that the latest research has been incorporated.

Each chapter of the *Handbook* is composed of several components: Diagnostic Summary, General Considerations, Therapeutic Considerations, Flowchart, and Therapeutic Approach. We believe this a unique work and are aware of no other textbook providing the flowchart approach to providing guidance for natural medicine care.

The flowchart separates the diagnostic/therapeutic deliberation into three phases: Determine need for conventional intervention; Minimize obstacles to healing; and Tailor natural interventions to patient needs. The first phase is provided to assist the clinician in understanding which patients may immediately require a more conventional intervention. The other phases present the most relevant diagnostic and therapeutic differentiations needed to determine which cause(s) must be controlled and which interventions are needed to provide each patient with highly personalized natural medicine care. Carefully following this thoughtfully constructed logic chain will efficiently provide key therapeutic insights.

We are excited to provide the clinician with this special resource, which we believe will substantially aid their efforts to provide their patients with the best care possible.

Acknowledgements

Most of all I would like to acknowledge that inner voice that has guided me in my life, providing me with inspiration, strength, and humility at the most appropriate times. My motivation has been largely the good that I know can come from using natural medicine appropriately. It can literally change people's lives. I know it changed mine.

There are many things that I am thankful for. I am especially thankful for my wife and best friend, Gina. I have also been blessed by having wonderful parents whose support and faith have never waned. I now have the opportunity to carry on their legacy of love with my own children, Alexa and Zachary.

In addition to my family, those people who have truly inspired me include Dr Ralph Weiss, Dr Ed Madison, Dr Bill Mitchell, Dr Gaetano Morello, my classmates and the entire Bastyr University community, and all of the special people I am lucky enough to call friends who have helped me on my life's journey.

And finally, I am deeply honored to have Dr Joe Pizzorno and Dr Herb Joiner-Bey, not only as my co-authors, but also as truly valued friends.

Michael T. Murray ND

First, I would like to acknowledge our new co-author, Dr Herb Joiner-Bey. His conversion of the much more complex *Textbook of Natural Medicine* into this concise, insightful, and extremely accessible resource is very impressive.

As ever, this work would not have been possible without the love and care of my family: Lara, my dear wife, and Galen and Raven, my beloved children. Thank you for bringing such joy and fullness to my life.

Joseph E. Pizzorno Jr ND

I would like to acknowledge Dr Joseph Pizzorno and Dr Michael Murray for the privilege of being the one to prepare the initial draft of this companion to their monumental *Textbook of Natural Medicine*. I greatly appreciate their confidence in my ability to do justice to this extremely worthwhile project.

In addition, I acknowledge the spiritual inner guidance that has directed me to take bold risks, purely on faith, in order for my soul to grow and heal from these experiences. I have been blessed along the way by the unshakable love and support by my unconditionally loving Divine Mother, Roberta, my Divine Brother, Michael, and the most thoughtful and resilient friends a person could have – Dr Judy Christianson, Dr Patrick Donovan, and Mr Peter Kaiser.

May God eternally bless all the gifted and generous teachers and mentors who prepared and inspired me to meet the daunting challenges of modern naturopathic medicine. This group includes, among many others, Drs John Bastyr, Bill Mitchell, Ed Madison, Robin Murphy, Stephen King, Bob Ullman, Steve Austin, Jim Koski, Marc Lappe, and George Bloch. I am indebted to my dedicated and diligent fellow students, at Pacific College of Naturopathic Medicine and Bastyr University, who catalyzed my learning and made medical school a much more bearable endeavor. I am also indebted to the people who planted within me, beginning three decades ago, the continually germinating seed of natural healing: Dean Rachau, Sandra Fresh Bey, and Dr Robert Hitchcock.

Even healers need healing and I am no exception. With the greatest appreciation, I honor the gracious spiritual healing facilitators who have allowed me to fulfill the most essential mission for my soul in this life. They are Dr Joyce Hawkes, Ingrid Dunki-Jacods, Michelle Phillips, Diana Urbas, and Ann Porter.

Herb Joiner-Bey ND

Finally, we would all like to acknowledge the outstanding professional staff at Harcourt Health Sciences/Churchill Livingstone, whose creative talents and expertise have been indispensable to the publishing of this book. In particular, thank you to Inta Ozols, Martina Paul, Katrina Mather and Ewan Halley.

Acne vulgaris and acne conglobata

DIAGNOSTIC SUMMARY

Open comedones (dilated follicles with central dark horny plugs – blackheads); closed comedones (small follicular papules with [red papules] or without [whiteheads] inflammation); superficial follicular pustules; nodules (deep collections of pus in dermis); cysts (nodules failing to discharge pus at surface); large deep pustules (nodules break down adjacent tissue, causing scars).

GENERAL CONSIDERATIONS

Most common skin problem; lesions are mainly on the face, but also back, chest, and shoulders; more common in males; onset during puberty, but later for conglobata; acne vulgaris onset from increased size of pilosebaceous glands and sebum secretion via androgenic stimulation; severity and progression – interaction among hormones, keratinization, sebum, and bacteria.

● **Progression:** hyperkeratinization of upper portion of follicle, blockage of canal, dilation and thinning, formation of comedones (open or closed based on degree of keratinization and blockage of duct), purulent exudate in pustules and cysts.

● **Bacteria:** normal skin species (*Propionibacterium acnes* [*Corynebacterium acnes*] and *Staphylococcus albus*); *P. acnes* releases lipases, hydrolyzing sebum triglycerides into free fatty acid lipoperoxides, promoting inflammation.

● **Inducing compounds:** corticosteroids, halogens, isonicotinic acid, diphenylhydantoin, lithium carbonate, machine oils, coal tar derivatives, chlorinated hydrocarbons, cosmetics, pomades, over-washing, and repetitive rubbing.

● **Endocrinological aspects:** androgen-dependent condition; androgens control sebaceous secretion and exacerbate follicular hyperkeratinization; endocrine disorders producing excess androgens induce acne development: idiopathic adrenal androgen excess, 21-hydroxylase, polycystic ovaries, free testosterone (T), DHEA, DHEA sulfate, deficient sex-hormone binding globulin; skin of acne patients had greater activity of 5-alpha-reductase, elevating more active DHT locally in skin tissue.

THERAPEUTIC CONSIDERATIONS

Nutrition

● **Diet:** high-protein diet (44% protein, 35% carbohydrate [CHO], 21% fat) decreases 5-alpha-reductase activity and increases cytochrome P-450 degradation of estradiol; high CHO diet (10% protein, 70% CHO, 20% fat) has opposite effect; limit foods high in iodine and milk (high hormone content); eliminate *trans* fatty acids and high-fat foods.

● **Sugar, insulin, and chromium:** insulin efficacy in treating acne suggests defective cutaneous tolerance and/or insulin insensitivity; acne patients' skin glucose tolerance is significantly impaired – acne may be called "skin diabetes"; eliminate concentrated CHOs to minimize immunosuppression; high-chromium yeast improves glucose tolerance and may help acne.

● **Vitamin A:** retinol reduces sebum production and hyperkeratinization of sebaceous follicles; effective at toxic dosage of 300,000–400,000 IU q.d. × 5–6 months. *Toxicity:* cheilitis (chapped lips) and xerosis (dry skin), especially in dry weather; headache (HA) then fatigue, emotional lability, and muscle and joint pain; lab tests are unreliable to monitor toxicity – serum vitamin A correlates poorly with toxicity, while SGOT and SGPT are elevated only in symptomatic patients; massive doses are teratogenic – women of child-bearing age must use birth control during and for at least 1 month after treatment; reserve massive doses for intractable cases and it should not be used alone.

● **Zinc:** involved in production of local hormones and retinol binding protein; wound healing, tissue regeneration, and immune function; absorption characteristics of Zn salts may affect results; requires 12 weeks to show good results; prefer Zn picolinate or monomethionine; Zn is essential to normal skin function (e.g. Zn-deficient syndrome acrodermatitis enteropathica); Zn is essential for retinol-binding protein and serum retinol levels; low Zn levels increase 5-alpha reduction of T and high Zn inhibits this reaction; serum Zn is lower in 13- and 14-year-old males than in any other age group.

● **Vitamin E and selenium:** vitamin E regulates retinol levels in humans; male acne patients have decreased RBC glutathione peroxidase, which normalizes with vitamin E and selenium; acne of men and women improves with this treatment – inhibits lipid peroxide formation – suggesting other free-radical quenchers.

● **Pyridoxine:** helpful for women with premenstrual acne due to effect on steroid hormone metabolism; B_6 deficiency causes increased uptake and sensitivity to T; in some patients, thyroid therapy markedly improves.

● **Pantothenic acid (PA):** active in synthesis of cholesterol and steroids; high dosages (10 g q.d. in four divided doses × 1–2 weeks) induce regression of lesions without side-effects.

● **Miscellaneous factors:** acne patients have elevated circulating endotoxins, which can elevate copper:zinc ratio and enhance tissue destruction via alternate complement pathway and fibrin formation.

Topical treatments

Goal is to reduce bacteria and inflammation.

● **Tea tree oil (*Melaleuca alternifolia*):** from leaves of small trees in New South Wales, Australia; antiseptic properties; ideal skin disinfectant: effective against wide range of organisms (including 27 of 32 strains of *P. acnes*); good penetration without skin irritation; therapeutic uses are based on antiseptic and antifungal properties; 5% tea tree oil solution is as beneficial as 5% benzoyl peroxide with substantially fewer side-effects; however, 5% tea tree oil solution is not strong enough for moderate to severe acne; stronger solutions (up to 15%) offer better results; occasionally produces contact dermatitis.

● **Azelaic acid:** natural 9-carbon dicarboxylic antibiotic against *P. acnes*; 20% azelaic acid creams are as effective as benzoyl peroxide cream or oral tetracycline; has an effect in all forms of acne; must be applied b.i.d. to affected areas × 4 weeks and must be continued × 6 months; 20% azelaic acid cream is as effective as 5% benzoyl peroxide, 4% hydroquinone cream, 0.05% tretinoin, 2% erythromycin and 0.5–1 g/day oral tetracycline at ameliorating comedonal, papulopustular and nodulocystic acne, but less effective than oral isotretinoin 0.5–1 mg/kg q.d. at reducing conglobate acne; few side-effects, no overt systemic toxicity, plus lower incidence of allergic sensitization, exogenous ochronosis, and residual hypopigmentation – better clinical choice.

THERAPEUTIC APPROACH

Rule out treatable underlying causes and hormonal abnormalities; consider consequences of long-term antibiotics – candidiasis (*Textbook*, Ch. 48).

● **Diet:** eliminate refined and/or concentrated CHOs and foods containing *trans* fatty acids and iodine.

● **Supplements:**
  — vitamin A: 100,000 IU q.d. × 3 months
  — vitamin E: 400 IU q.d.
  — vitamin C: 1,000 mg q.d.
  — zinc: 50 mg q.d. (picolinate or monomethionine)
  — selenium: 200 μg q.d.
  — brewer's yeast: 1 tbsp b.i.d. (gout patients – use chromium instead).

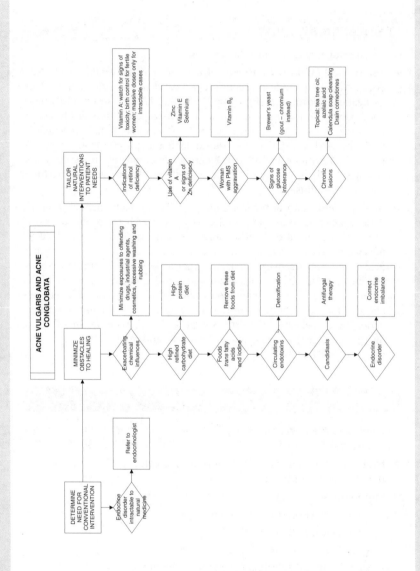

ACNE VULGARIS AND ACNE CONGLOBATA

DETERMINE NEED FOR CONVENTIONAL INTERVENTION

Endocrine disorder intractable to natural medicine → Refer to endocrinologist

MINIMIZE OBSTACLES TO HEALING

Exacerbating chemical influences → Minimize exposures to offending drugs, industrial agents, cosmetics, excessive washing and rubbing

High refined carbohydrate diet → High-protein diet

Foods *trans* fatty acids and iodine → Remove these foods from diet

Circulating endotoxins → Detoxification

Candidiasis → Antifungal therapy

Endocrine disorder → Correct endocrine imbalance

TAILOR NATURAL INTERVENTIONS TO PATIENT NEEDS

Indications of retinol deficiency → Vitamin A: watch for signs of toxicity; birth control for fertile women; massive doses only for intractable cases

Use of vitamin A or signs of Zn deficiency → Zinc, Vitamin E, Selenium

Woman with PMS aggravation → Vitamin B₆

Signs of glucose intolerance → Brewer's yeast (gout – chromium instead)

Chronic lesions → Topical: tea tree oil; azelaic acid, Calendula soap cleansing, Drain comedones

- **Physical medicine:** sun or UV lamp.
- **Topical medicine:**
  - tea tree oil (5–15%) preparations
  - azelaic acid (20%) preparations
  - cleansing daily with calendula soap
  - drain comedones with comedo extractor.

Affective disorders

DIAGNOSTIC SUMMARY

● **Depression** (DSM-IV criteria): poor appetite with weight loss, or increased appetite with weight gain; insomnia or hypersomnia; physical hyperactivity or inactivity; loss of interest or pleasure in usual activities, or decrease in sexual drive; loss of energy and feelings of fatigue; feelings of worthlessness, self-reproach or inappropriate guilt; diminished ability to think or concentrate; recurrent thoughts of death or suicide. *Diagnosis:* presence of five of these eight symptoms = definite clinical depression; four symptoms = probably depressed; symptoms must be present at least 1 month to be called depression; clinical depression is also termed major depression or unipolar depression.

● **Dysthymia:** patient depressed most of the time × at least 2 years (1 year for children or adolescents) plus at least three of following – low self-esteem or lack of self-confidence; pessimism, hopelessness, or despair; lack of interest in ordinary pleasures and activities; withdrawal from social activities; fatigue or lethargy; guilt or ruminating about past; irritability or excessive anger; lessened productivity; difficulty in concentrating or making decisions.

● **Manic phase:** mood typically elation, but irritability and hostility not uncommon; inflated self-esteem, grandiose delusions, boasting, racing thoughts, decreased need for sleep, psychomotor acceleration, weight loss due to increased activity and lack of attention to dietary habits.

● **Seasonal affective disorder:** regularly occurring winter depression frequently associated with summer hypomania.

Introduction: Affective disorders = mood disturbances; mood = prolonged emotional tone dominating one's outlook; transient moods (sadness, grief, elation, etc.) part of daily life – demarcation of "pathological" difficult to determine; depression and mania, alone or in alternation, are the most common disorders and depression alone is much more common; "unipolar" = depression alone; "bipolar" = either mania alone or mania alternating with depression.

● **Eight factors modify functional state of brain and affect mood and behavior:** genetic inheritance; age of neuronal development (age-specific variability); functional plasticity of brain during development; motivational state affected by biological drives, channeling behavior toward goals via priorities or prejudicing context of incoming information; memory-stored information and processing strategies; environment that adjusts incoming input according to momentary significance; brain disease or lesion causing aberrant function; metabolic/hormonal system or biochemical environment of central nervous system (CNS).

Chapter focus = nutritional, environmental, and lifestyle factors affecting mood and therapies to alter brain neurotransmitter levels.

DEPRESSION

GENERAL CONSIDERATIONS

Seventeen million Americans are depressed; 28+ million take antidepressants or anxiolytics.

● **Five theoretical models:** "aggression turned inward" (apparent in many cases but no substantial proof); "loss model" (depression = reaction to loss of person, thing, status, self-esteem, or habit pattern); "interpersonal relationship" (depressed person uses depression to control other people, including doctors, via pouting, silence, or ignoring something or someone); "learned helplessness" (habitual feelings of pessimism and hopelessness); "biogenic amine" hypothesis (biochemical derangement of biogenic amines).

● **Biogenic amine model:** the dominant medical conception of depression; counseling is valuable, especially with clear psychological etiology; learned helplessness model (Martin Seligman PhD) most useful to the authors – animals can be trained to be helpless. The learned helplessness model.

● **Learned helplessness (Seligman):** animals can be experimentally conditioned to feel helpless and many humans react in identical fashion to similar conditioning; this model revolutionized psychopharmacology – effective test for antidepressive drugs: animals conditioned to be helpless and then given antidepressant drugs unlearn helplessness and exercise control over environment; animals conditioned to be helpless experienced alteration of brain monoamine content; antidepressants restore monoamine balance and alter behavior; animals with conditioned helplessness taught how to gain environmental control experienced brain chemistry normalization; altered brain monoamines in animals with learned helplessness mirrors altered monoamines in human depression; helping patients to gain control over their lives produces greater biochemical changes than drugs; powerful techniques = teach optimism; determining factor for person's reaction to uncontrollable events = explanatory style (how events are explained); optimistic people are immune to helplessness and depression; pessimists are susceptible to depression when "bad" things happen; there is a direct correlation between level of optimism and risk for depression and other illnesses.

THERAPEUTIC CONSIDERATIONS

Psychiatry focuses on manipulating neurotransmitters rather than identifying and eliminating psychological factors.

- **Organic/physiological causes:** pre-existing physical condition, diabetes, heart disease, lung disease, rheumatoid arthritis, chronic inflammation, chronic pain, cancer, liver disease, multiple sclerosis, prescription drugs, antihypertensives, anti-inflammatories, birth control pills, antihistamines, corticosteroids, tranquilizers and sedatives, PMS, stress/low adrenal function, heavy metals, food allergies, hypothyroidism, hypoglycemia, nutritional deficiencies, sleep disturbances.

- **Conduct comprehensive clinical evaluation:** ascertain nutritional, environmental, social, and psychological factors; rule out organic factors: nutrient deficiency or excess, drugs (prescription, illicit, alcohol, caffeine, nicotine), hypoglycemia, consumption, hormonal derangement, allergy, environmental factors, microbes; counseling recommended regardless of underlying organic cause.

- **Counseling:** most merit and support in medical literature – *cognitive therapy* – as effective as antidepressants for moderate depression with lower rate of relapse; patient taught new skills to change the way he or she consciously thinks about failure, defeat, loss, and helplessness; *five basic tactics*: (1) recognize negative automatic thoughts when patient feels worst, (2) dispute negative thoughts by focusing on contrary evidence, (3) generate different explanation to dispute negative thoughts, (4) avoid rumination (constant churning of negative thoughts in mind) by consciously controlling thoughts, (5) question negative thoughts/beliefs and replace with empowering positive thoughts/beliefs; does not involve long psychoanalysis – solution-oriented.

Hormonal factors

The focus of this text is on thyroid and adrenal hormones.

- **Thyroid:** depression = early manifestation of thyroid disease: subtle decreases in thyroid hormone can be symptomatic; whether hypothyroidism results from depression-induced hypothalamic–pituitary–thyroid (HPT) dysfunction or from thyroid hypofunction is uncertain, but it may be a combination; screen for hypothyroidism, particularly with suggestive symptoms (e.g. fatigue).

- **Stress and adrenal function:** adrenal dysfunction associated with depression can result from stress; adrenal stress index measures cortisol and DHEA in saliva; depression signs: elevated morning cortisol and decreased DHEA; cortisol elevation reflects disturbed hypothalamic–pituitary–adrenal (HPA) axis and is the basis of the dexamethasone suppression test (DST); HPA dysregulation affecting mood = excessive cortisol independent of stress responses, abnormal nocturnal cortisol release of cortisol, and inadequate suppression by dexamethasone; CNS effects of increased endogenous cortisol = depression, mania, nervousness, insomnia, and schizophrenia (high levels); glucocorticoid effects on mood related to induction of tryptophan oxygenase, shunting tryptophan to kynurenine pathway at the expense of serotonin and melatonin synthesis.

● **Tests of hypothalamic–pituitary function:** DST and thyroid stimulation test – determine if mood is caused by hypothalamic dysfunction and categorize psychiatric illness (e.g. severe major affective disorders vs. severe psychotic disorders); DST – little clinical value for screening and not better than urinary free cortisol; thyroid hormone assays do not detect all cases of hypothyroidism – not an effective screening procedure; thyroid stimulation test (TRH) is more sensitive, diagnosing "subclinical hypothyroidism"; TRH grading system for hypothyroidism is as follows:

— *grade 3* (subclinical hypothyroidism – 4%): patients without classic hypothyroid signs; normal T_3RU, T_4, and TSH; abnormal TSH response to TRH test;

— *grade 2* (mild hypothyroidism – 3.6%): mild isolated clinical signs or symptoms; normal T_3RU and T_4; baseline TSH elevated; abnormal TRH test;

— *grade 1* (overt hypothyroidism – 1%): classic hypothyroid signs and symptoms; abnormal lab values (reduced T_3RU and T_4, increased TSH, abnormal TRH response).

Environmental toxins

● **Heavy metals** (Pb, Hg, Cd, As, Ni, Al), solvents (cleaning materials, formaldehyde, toluene, benzene, etc.), pesticides, herbicides – affinity for nervous tissue; associated symptoms = depression, HA, mental confusion, mental illness, tingling in extremities, abnormal nerve reflexes, other signs of impaired nervous function (*Textbook*, Chs 18 and 37);

● **Detailed medical history and hair mineral analysis** screen for environmental toxins; if hair mineral analysis is inconclusive, a more sensitive test is the 8-h lead mobilization test – chelating agent EDTA (edetate calcium - disodium) – measure lead excreted in urine for 8 h after injection of EDTA.

Lifestyle factors

Eliminate smoking, excess ETOH, caffeine; add regular exercise and healthful diet – better clinical results than antidepressants with no side-effects or monetary cost.

● **Smoking:** major factor contributing to premature death; nicotine stimulates adrenal secretion (cortisol) = feature of depression; cortisol (and stress) activates tryptophan oxygenase, reducing tryptophan delivery to the brain; brain serotonin is dependent upon amount of tryptophan delivered – cortisol reduces levels of serotonin and melatonin; cortisol "downregulates" brain serotonin receptors, reducing sensitivity to available serotonin; smoking induces relative vitamin C deficiency – vitamin C utilized to detoxify smoke; low levels of brain vitamin C can cause depression and hysteria.

● **Alcohol:** brain depressant; increases adrenal hormone output; interferes with brain cell processes; disrupts sleep cycles; leads to hypoglycemia and craving for sugar, which aggravates hypoglycemia and mental and emotional problems.

● **Caffeine:** stimulant; intensity of response varies greatly – people prone to depression or anxiety are sensitive to caffeine; "caffeinism" = clinical syndrome – nervousness, palpitations, irritability, and recurrent HA; students with moderate/high coffee intake score higher on depression scale and have lower academic performance than low users; depressed patients have high caffeine intake (> 700 mg/day); caffeine intake is positively correlated with degree of mental illness in psychiatric patients; caffeine plus refined sugar is worse than either alone – association between combination and depression has been confirmed by several studies; average American intake = 150–225 mg caffeine q.d. = 1–2 cups coffee; some people are more sensitive to effects than others – even the small amount in decaf; patients with psychological disorder should avoid caffeine completely.

● **Exercise:** natural antidepressant; benefit in heart health may be related as much to improved mood as to cardiovascular function; profound antidepressive effects – decreased anxiety, depression, and malaise plus higher self-esteem and more happiness; increases endorphins – directly correlated with mood; sedentary men are more depressed, perceive greater life stress, have higher cortisol and lower beta-endorphins than joggers; depression is very sensitive to exercise and helps firm up biochemical link between physical activity and depression; relieves depression and improves self-esteem and work behavior – can be as effective as antidepressant drugs and psychotherapy; best exercises = strength training (weight-lifting) or aerobics (walking briskly, jogging, bicycling, cross-country skiing, swimming, aerobic dance, and racquet sports).

Nutrition

Any single nutrient deficiency can alter brain function, inducing depression, anxiety, etc. (*Textbook*, Table 126.2); nutrition powerfully influences cognition, emotion, and behavior; full-range high-potency multiple = foundation; nutrient deficiencies are common in depressed individuals: most common = folate, B_{12}, and B_6.

- **Diet:** brain requires constant sugar supply: hypoglycemia must be avoided; hypoglycemia symptoms: psychological disturbances (depression, anxiety, irritability, etc.), fatigue, HA, blurred vision, excessive sweating, mental confusion, incoherent speech, bizarre behavior, convulsions; hypoglycemia is common in depressed individuals; eliminate refined carbohydrates; health-promoting rich in whole "natural", unprocessed foods, especially high in plant foods (fruits, vegetables, grains, beans, seeds, nuts).

- **Folate and B_{12}:** function together in many pathways; folate deficiency is the most common nutrient deficiency worldwide; 31–35% of depressed patients are folate-deficient, 35–92.6% being among the elderly; depression is the most common symptom of folate deficiency; B_{12} deficiency is less common, but can also cause depression, especially in the elderly; folate, B_{12}, and SAM (S-adenosyl-methionine) are "methyl donors"; SAM is the major methyl donor in the body; antidepressant effects of folate = increasing brain SAM; the key brain compound dependent on methylation is tetrahydrobiopterin (BH_4), a coenzyme in the manufacture of monoamine neurotransmitters (e.g. serotonin and dopamine) from respective amino acids; patients with recurrent depression have reduced BH_4 synthesis probably from low SAM levels; BH_4 synthesis is stimulated by folate, B_{12}, and C – supplementation can increase BH_4 and serotonin content; folate dosages as antidepressant – very high: 15–50 mg is safe (except in epilepsy) and is as effective as antidepressant drugs; dosages of 800 μg folate and 800 μg B_{12} are sufficient to prevent deficiencies; folate supplement should always be accompanied by B_{12} to prevent masking B_{12} deficiency.

- **Vitamin B_6:** low in depressed patients, especially women on birth control pills or Premarin; essential to manufacture of all monoamines; dosage = 50–100 mg q.d.

- **Omega-3 fatty acids:** insufficiency linked to depression; affect phospholipid composition of neurological cell membranes; brain is the richest source of phospholipids in the body; lack of essential fatty acids (EFAs) (omega-3 oils) and excess saturated fats induce formation of cell membranes less fluid than optimal and impair membrane regulation of passage of molecules into and out of cell, disrupting homeostasis and proper nerve cell function – impact on behavior, mood, and mental function; biophysical properties, including fluidity, of brain cell membranes, influence neurotransmitter synthesis, signal transmission, neurotransmitter binding and uptake, and activity of monoamine oxidase – factors implicated in depression; omega-3 EFAs may inhibit development of depression as they do cardiovascular disease: lowering plasma cholesterol by diet and medications increases suicide, homicide, and depression; the quantity and type of dietary fats consumed alter biophysical and biochemical properties of cell membranes; dietary efforts to lower cholesterol tend to increase the omega-6:omega-3 ratio and decrease docosahexanoic acid (DHA); decreased consumption of omega-3 EFAs correlates with increasing rates of depression; there is a consistent association between depression and coronary artery disease.

● **Food allergies:** depression and fatigue linked to food allergies; "allergic toxemia" (coined by Rowe) is a syndrome with symptoms of depression, fatigue, muscle and joint aches, drowsiness, difficulty concentrating, and nervousness.

Monoamine metabolism and precursor therapy

Monoamine (MA) precursors (tryptophan, 5-hydroxytryptophan [5-HTP], and tyrosine) offer natural alternative to monoamine oxidase (MAO) inhibitors and tricyclics for influencing MA metabolism.

● **Tryptophan catastrophe:** For > 30 years, L-tryptophan has been used by millions in the US and around the world safely and effectively for insomnia and depression; in October 1989, one Japanese manufacturer, Showa Denko, the largest supplier to the US (50–60%), produced batches contaminated with substances now linked to EMS (eosinophilia-myalgia syndrome) due to changes in the bacteria used to produce L-tryptophan and the filtration process; EMS patients have these signs and symptoms: eosinophils > 1,000/mm^3 (2 × normal); allergic and inflammatory symptoms from release of histamine by eosinophils – severe muscle and joint pain, high fever, weakness, swelling of arms and legs, skin rashes, and shortness of breath; EMS affected 144 of every 50,000 men and 268 of every 50,000 women or 1 in 250 people taking contaminated L-tryptophan; only those with an abnormal activation of kynurenine pathway reacted to the contaminant; kynurenine and its metabolites (quinolic acid) are linked to other EMS-related illnesses (e.g. Spain's 1991 toxic oil syndrome, one of the largest food-related epidemics ever); people who took multiple vitamin preparation were somewhat protected against EMS – vitamins (B$_6$ and niacin) shunted tryptophan away from the kynurenine pathway or contaminants were somehow metabolized by vitamin-dependent enzymes.

● **L-Tryptophan:** increases brain serotonin and melatonin; many depressed individuals have low tryptophan and serotonin; supplementation provides mixed clinical results: only two of eight studies indicated superiority compared with placebo, but nine of 11 studies indicated equivalence to antidepressant drugs; factors to consider – study size, severity of depression, duration, and dosage; hormones (estrogen and cortisol) and tryptophan itself stimulate tryptophan oxygenase, converting to kynurenine with less tryptophan delivered to brain. *Summary*: L-tryptophan is only modestly effective when used alone; must be used with B$_6$ and niacinamide to block kynurenine pathway; better results with 5-HTP.

● **5-Hydroxytryptophan (5-HTP):** 5-HTP cannot be converted to kynurenine and easily crosses the blood–brain barrier; only 3% of oral L-tryptophan is converted to serotonin, while over 70% of oral 5-HTP is converted; 5-HTP causes increased endorphins and catecholamine; "equipotency" with serotonin reuptake inhibitors (SRIs) and tricyclics; advantages: less expensive, better tolerated, fewer and milder side-effects.

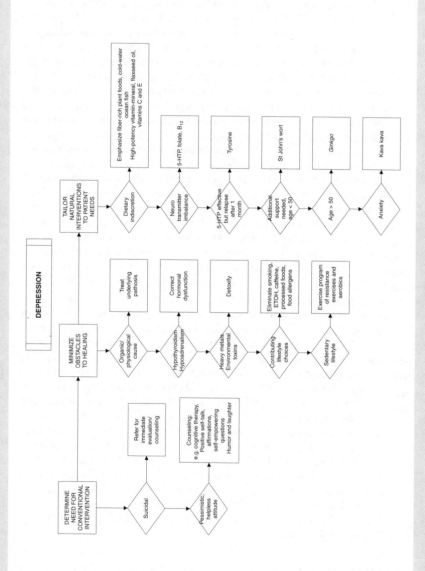

DEPRESSION

DETERMINE NEED FOR CONVENTIONAL INTERVENTION

Suicidal → Refer for immediate evaluation/counseling

Pessimistic, helpless attitude → Counseling: e.g. cognitive therapy, Positive self-talk, affirmations, self-empowering questions Humor and laughter

MINIMIZE OBSTACLES TO HEALING

Organic/physiological cause → Treat underlying pathosis

Hypothyroidism/Hypoadrenalism → Correct hormonal dysfunction

Heavy metals Environmental toxins → Detoxify

Contributing lifestyle choices → Eliminate smoking, ETOH, caffeine, processed foods, food allergens

Sedentary lifestyle → Exercise program of resistance exercises and aerobics

TAILOR NATURAL INTERVENTIONS TO PATIENT NEEDS

Dietary indiscretion → Emphasize fiber-rich plant foods, cold-water ocean fish High-potency vitamin-mineral, flaxseed oil, vitamins C and E

Neurotransmitter imbalance → 5-HTP, folate, B$_{12}$

5-HTP effective but relapse after 1 month → Tyrosine

Additional support needed, age < 50 → St John's wort

Age > 50 → Ginkgo

Anxiety → Kava kava

● **Phenylalanine and tyrosine:** *phenylalanine* is hydroxylated to tyrosine and degraded to phenylketonic acids, but also decarboxylated to phenylethylamine (PEA); PEA is an amphetamine-like endogenous stimulatory/antidepressive substance in humans (PEA = biogenic amine in high concentrations in chocolate); low urinary PEA in depressed patients, high levels are in schizophrenics; D- and L-phenylalanine increase urinary and CNS PEA; phenylalanine is a tyrosine hydroxylase inhibitor – shunting phenylalanine to PEA synthesis occurs with supplementation; *tyrosine* increases "trace amines" (octopamine, tyramine and PEA), enhances catecholamine synthesis, stimulates thyroid hormone synthesis; L-dopa alone is ineffectual in affective disorders; central norepinephrine turnover is decreased in depressed patients – may result from low serum tyrosine seen in some depressed individuals; brain tyrosine is best determined by ratio of serum tyrosine to sum of its brain-uptake competitors (i.e. leucine, isoleucine, valine, tryptophan, and phenylalanine); tyrosine ratios increased by high-protein meals; tyrosine supplements increase urine 3-methoxy-4-hydroxyphenethylene glycol (MHPG), the principal breakdown product of norepinephrine in CNS and a biochemical marker for determining which amino acid to supplement; phenylalanine and tyrosine are encouraging alternatives to tricyclics and MAO inhibitors; van Praag study: 20% of patients who responded well to 5-HTP relapsed after 1 month despite the fact that blood 5-HTP and presumably brain serotonin remained the same as when experiencing benefit – other monoamine neurotransmitters (dopamine and norepinephrine) declined; patients responded to supplemental tyrosine.

● **S-Adenosyl-methionine (SAM):** involved in methylation of monoamines, neurotransmitters, and phospholipids; brain manufactures SAM from methionine; SAM synthesis is impaired in depressed patients; SAM supplementation in depressed patients increases serotonin, dopamine, and phosphatides, and improves binding of neurotransmitters to receptors, increasing serotonin and dopamine activity and improving neuron membrane fluidity and clinical symptoms; SAM is a very effective natural antidepressant, but expensive; oral dosage 400 mg q.i.d. (1,600 mg total); better tolerated with quicker action than tricyclics; study comparing SAM to tricyclic desipramine: 62% of SAM patients and 50% of desipramine patients significantly improved – regardless of type of treatment, patients with 50% decrease in Hamilton Depression Scale (HAM-D) had significant increase in plasma SAM; no significant side-effects with oral SAM: nausea and vomiting (N&V) in some people; start dosage at 200 mg b.i.d. first day, 400 mg b.i.d. day 3, 400 mg t.i.d. day 10, and 400 mg q.i.d. after 20 days; bipolar (manic) patients should not take SAM – susceptible to hypomania or mania.

Botanical medicines

● *Hypericum perforatum* (St John's wort): extracts standardized for hypericin and hyperforin = most thoroughly researched natural antidepressants; improves many symptoms: depression, anxiety, apathy, sleep disturbances, insomnia, anorexia, feelings of worthlessness; advantage over antidepressant drugs are side-effects, cost and patient tolerance; beware of hyperforin's enhancement of drug degradation by liver cytochrome p450 enzymes. (*Textbook*, Ch. 93).

● *Piper mythisticum* **(Kava kava):** approved in Germany, UK, Switzerland, and Austria in treatment of nervous anxiety, insomnia, depression, and restlessness based on detailed pharmacological data and favorable clinical studies; efficacy compares quite favorably with benzodiazepines without drug side-effects (impaired mental acuity, addictiveness, etc.); prefer extracts standardized for kavalactones (30–70%); most useful for depression with severe anxiety (*Textbook*, Ch. 104).

● *Ginkgo biloba*: leaf extract standardized to 24% ginkgo flavonglycosides and 6% terpenoids; exerts good antidepressant effects, especially over age 50; improves mood in patients with cerebrovascular insufficiency; can be used with antidepressant drugs and may enhance their efficacy in patients over age 50; counteracts one of the major brain chemistry changes associated with aging – reduction in number of serotonin receptors; increases protein synthesis and acts as a potent antioxidant (*Textbook*, Ch. 88).

THERAPEUTIC APPROACH

Accurate determination of which factors contribute to patient's depression; balancing of errant neurotransmitter levels; and optimizing patient's nutrition, lifestyle, and psychological health.

● **Diet:** increase fiber-rich plant foods (fruits, vegetables, grains, legumes, raw nuts and seeds); avoid caffeine, nicotine, other stimulants, and ETOH; identify and control food allergies; increase cold water fish to at least twice per week.

● **Lifestyle:** refer to counselor or counsel patient to develop positive, optimistic mental attitude – help patient set goals, use positive self-talk and affirmations, identify self-empowering questions, and find ways to inject humor and laughter into life; exercise at least 30 min at least three times a week; relaxation/stress reduction technique 10–15 min q.d.

● **Supplements:** high-potency multiple vitamin-mineral; vitamin C (500–1,000 mg t.i.d.); vitamin E (200–400 IU q.d.); flaxseed oil (1 tbsp q.d.); 5-HTP (100–200 mg t.i.d.); folic acid and vitamin B_{12} (800 μg each q.d.).

● **Botanical medicines:** *under age 50* – St John's wort extract (0.3% hypericin, 4% hyperforin): 300 mg t.i.d.; severe cases – St John's wort in combination with 5-HTP; *over age 50* – *Ginkgo biloba* extract (24% ginkgo flavonglycosides, 6% terpenoids), 80 mg t.i.d.; severe cases – use in combination with St John's wort and/or 5-HTP; significant anxiety – kava extract (standardized to kavalactones): 45–70 mg kavalactones t.i.d.

BIPOLAR (MANIC) DEPRESSION AND HYPOMANIA

DIAGNOSTIC CRITERIA

Must have at least three of the following: excessive self-esteem/grandiosity; reduced need for sleep; extreme talkativeness, excessive telephoning; extremely rapid flight of thoughts plus feeling that mind is racing; inability to concentrate, easily distracted; increased social or work activities, with 60–80 h work week; poor judgment: spending sprees, sexual indiscretion, misguided financial decisions.

GENERAL CONSIDERATIONS

Bipolar depression – characterized by periods of major depression alternating with periods of elevated mood; if elevated mood is relatively mild and lasts 4 days or less, it is called hypomania; mania is longer and more intense; full-blown manic attack requires hospitalization – loss of self-control, may hurt themselves or others; standard treatment is lithium – stabilizes mood, prevents manic phase – used either alone or with antidepressant; antidepressant drugs can occasionally induce mania and hypomania – difficult to control lows in bipolar depressives with drugs.

THERAPEUTIC CONSIDERATIONS

Initially hospitalize × 2 weeks under sedation with antipsychotic drugs until blood lithium levels acceptable; refer for conventional therapy until mood stabilized; principles outlined for depression are applicable to mania; seriousness of condition – use nutritional therapy as adjunct rather than primary therapy; SRIs (Prozac, Zoloft, Paxil) helpful in combination with lithium suggests 5-HTP and St John's wort may be useful as adjuncts to lithium but without side-effects.

- **Tryptophan:** effective doses generally quite large: 12 g q.d. L-tryptophan; a better choice is 5-HTP, helpful in combination with lithium at much lower dosage (100 mg t.i.d.).
- **Phosphatidylcholine (PC):** large amounts of PC (15–30 g q.d. in both pure form and lecithin) – better results for mania than MA precursors; lithium promotes increased CNS cholinergic activity via inhibition of choline flux across the blood–brain barrier; mania is associated with reduced CNS cholinergic activity; using PC to increase CNS choline may improve symptoms in some patients.

BIPOLAR (MANIC) DEPRESSION

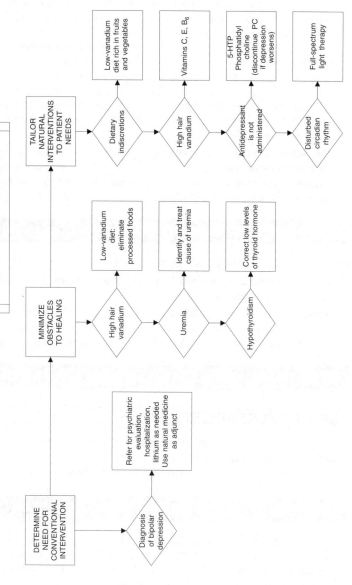

- **Vanadium:** increased vanadium found in hair of manic patients and levels normalize with recovery; depressed patients have normal hair vanadium, with whole blood and serum vanadium elevated and returning to normal upon recovery; vanadate ion is a strong inhibitor of Na^+,K^+-ATPase; lithium reduces this inhibition; therapies to reduce vanadate to less inhibitory vanadyl form include ascorbic acid, methylene blue, and EDTA separately and in combination; ascorbic acid (3 g q.d.) provides significant clinical improvement; "low-vanadium diet" advocated by Naylor not consistent with vanadium content of foods determined by flameless atomic absorption spectroscopy; other correctable factors known to inhibit Na^+,K^+-ATPase are uremia, hypothyroidism, and catecholamine insensitivity; vitamins E and B_6 increase Na^+,K^+-ATPase activity in vitro; vitamin E also stabilizes membranes.

- **Circadian rhythms:** manic depressive patients have disturbed circadian rhythms, seasonal patterns of exacerbations, and supersensitivity to light; alteration of circadian light–dark cycles via light therapy may help (see "Seasonal affective disorder" below).

THERAPEUTIC APPROACH

Same dietary and lifestyle guidelines as for depression.

- **Diet:** low-vanadium diet – eliminate all refined and processed foods; promote fresh fruits and vegetables.

- **Supplements:** Phosphatidylcholine (10–25 g q.d.) (PC may induce depression in some patients; if this occurs, discontinue immediately); vitamin C (3–5 g q.d.) in divided doses; vitamin E (400–800 IU q.d.); pyridoxine (100 mg q.d.).

SEASONAL AFFECTIVE DISORDER (SAD)

GENERAL CONSIDERATIONS

Associated with winter depression and summer hypomania. Typically, patients feel depressed, slow down, oversleep, overeat, and crave carbohydrates in winter. In summer, they feel elated, active, energetic.

THERAPEUTIC CONSIDERATIONS

- **Melatonin:** light exposure is the main contributing factor; key hormonal changes are reduced melatonin from pineal and increased cortisol from adrenals; melatonin supplementation may improve SAD – increases brain melatonin and suppresses cortisol secretion.

- **Light therapy:** full-spectrum light therapy has antidepressive effects in SAD and clinical depression, probably due to restoring proper pineal melatonin synthesis and secretion, re-establishing proper circadian rhythm; place full-spectrum fluorescent tubes in regular fluorescent fixtures (eight tubes total); patients sit 3 ft away from light 05.00–08.00 h (5–8 a.m.) and 17.30–20.30 h (5:30–8:30 p.m.); patients are free to engage in activities as long as they glance at the light at least once per minute; protocol restricts social life – replacing standard bulbs with full-spectrum light may help.

● ***Hypericum perforatum:*** St John's wort extract (standardized to 0.3% hypericin, 4% hyperforin) (*Textbook*, Ch. 93) at dosage of 300 mg t.i.d. improves SAD, but is more effective in combination with light therapy. Beware of enhanced drug degradation by liver cytochrome p450 enzymes.

THERAPEUTIC APPROACH

Extend light exposure on winter days – use full-spectrum lighting throughout indoor environment; night-time melatonin (3 mg 45 min before retiring): daytime St John's wort or 5-HTP.

Alcoholism

DIAGNOSTIC SUMMARY

ETOH dependence manifested when ETOH is withdrawn (tremulousness, convulsions, hallucinations, delirium); binges, benders (48+ h drinking with failure to meet usual obligations), or blackouts; ETOH-induced illnesses (cirrhosis, gastritis, pancreatitis, myopathy, polyneuropathy, cerebellar degeneration; physical signs of ETOH abuse (ETOH breath odor, flushed face, tremor, ecchymoses); psychosocial signs (depression, loss of friends, arrest for DWI, surreptitious drinking, drinking before breakfast, frequent accidents, unexplained work absences).

GENERAL CONSIDERATIONS

WHO definition = consumption exceeding limits accepted by culture or which injures health or social relationships.

- **Consequences:** increased mortality: 10–12 years lower life expectancy; 2 × death rate in men, 3 × in women; 6 × suicide rate; major factor in four leading causes of death in men aged 25–44 (accidents, homicides, suicides, cirrhosis); economic toll; health effects: metabolic damage to every cell; intoxication; abstinence and withdrawal syndromes; nutritional deficiency diseases; cerebellar degeneration; cerebral atrophy; psychiatric disorders; esophagitis, gastritis, ulcer; increased cancer of mouth, pharynx, larynx, esophagus; pancreatitis; liver fatty degeneration and cirrhosis; arrhythmias; myocardial degeneration; hypertension; angina; hypoglycemia; decreased protein synthesis; increased serum and liver triglycerides; decreased serum testosterone; myopathy; osteoporosis; rosacea, spiders; coagulation disorders.
- **Effects on fetus:** growth retardation; mental retardation; fetal alcohol syndrome; teratogenicity.
- 18 million alcoholics in US; often a "hidden" disease disguised by sympathetic family and friends.

The brief Michigan alcoholism screening test (MAST). Note: alcoholism is indicated by a score of greater than 5

1. Do you feel you are a normal drinker?	Yes (0)	No (2)
2. Do friends or relatives think you are a normal drinker?	Yes (0)	No (2)

The brief Michigan alcoholism screening test (MAST). Note: alcoholism is indicated by a score of greater than 5

3. Have you ever attended a meeting of Alcoholics Anonymous (AA)?	Yes (5)	No (0)
4. Have you ever lost friends or girlfriends or boyfriends because of drinking?	Yes (2)	No (0)
5. Have you ever gotten into trouble at work because of drinking?	Yes (2)	No (0)
6. Have you ever neglected your obligations, your family, or your work for 2 or more days in a row because you were drinking?	Yes (2)	No (0)
7. Have you ever had delirium tremens (DTs), severe shaking, heard voices, or seen things that weren't there after heavy drinking?	Yes (2)	No (0)
8. Have you ever gone to anyone for help about your drinking?	Yes (5)	No (0)
9. Have you ever been in a hospital because of drinking?	Yes (5)	No (0)
10. Have you ever been arrested for drunk driving or driving after drinking?	Yes (2)	No (0)

- **Etiology:** obscure; multifactorial, but genetic factors may be most important – genetic marker for alcoholism; incidence of alcoholism is four to five times more common in biological children of alcoholic than of non-alcoholic parents; associated with genetic markers: color vision, nonsecretor ABH, HLA-B$_{13}$, and low platelet MAO; biochemical studies show importance of alcohol dehydrogenase polymorphism in racial susceptibility to alcoholism.

Intoxication and withdrawal

- **Intoxication signs:** CNS depression – drowsiness, errors of commission, disinhibition, dysarthria, ataxia, and nystagmus; 15 ml pure ETOH (1 oz whiskey, 4 oz wine, or 10 oz beer) raises blood ETOH level by 25 mg/dl in 70 kg person; effects of varying levels of blood ETOH are as follows:

Blood level (mg/dl)	Effect
< 50	No significant motor dysfunction
100	Mild intoxication – decreased inhibitions, slight visual impairment, slight muscular incoordination, slowing of reaction time
	Legally intoxicated in most jurisdictions
150	Ataxia, dysarthria, slurring of speech, nausea and vomiting
350	Marked muscular incoordination, blurred vision, approaching stupor
500	Coma and death

- **Withdrawal symptoms:** 1–3 days after last drink; anxiety, tremulousness, mental confusion, tremor, sensory hyperactivity, visual hallucinations, autonomic hyperactivity, diaphoresis, dehydration, electrolyte disturbances, seizures, and cardiovascular abnormalities.

Metabolic effects of alcohol and alcoholism

- **Ethanol metabolism:** factors influencing ETOH catabolism = rate of ETOH absorption; concentration and activity of liver alcohol dehydrogenase (ADH) and aldehyde dehydrogenase (ALDH); NADH/NAD+ ratio in liver mitochondria; availability and regeneration of NAD+ = rate-limiting factors for ETOH oxidation; ETOH is converted to acetaldehyde by ADH, with cofactor NAD+; aldehyde is responsible for harmful effects and addictive process; high blood aldehyde found in alcoholics and relatives after ETOH consumption – either increased ADH activity or depressed ALDH activity in people susceptible to alcoholism; acetaldehyde is converted by ALDH to acetate with little entering Krebs cycle – most is converted to long-chain fatty acids.

- **Fatty liver:** in all alcoholics, even with minimal consumption; severity proportional to duration and degree of ETOH excess; pathogenesis = increased endogenous fatty acid synthesis, diminished triglyceride utilization, impaired lipoprotein excretion, direct damage to endoplasmic reticulum by free radicals produced by ethanol metabolism, high-fat diet of alcoholic.

- **Hypoglycemia:** ETOH induces reactive hypoglycemia, produces craving for foods that quickly elevate blood sugar (sugar and ETOH); sugar aggravates reactive hypoglycemia, particularly with ETOH-induced impairment of gluconeogenesis; hypoglycemia aggravates mental/emotional problems of alcoholics and withdrawal with sweating, tremor, tachycardia, anxiety, hunger, dizziness, HA, visual disturbance, decreased mental acuity, confusion, depression.

THERAPEUTIC CONSIDERATIONS

Nutrition

Problems related to ETOH and fact that alcoholics tend not to eat: ETOH = substitute.

- **Zinc:** ADH and ALDH are Zn-dependent enzymes, with ALDH more sensitive to deficiency; acute and chronic ETOH induces Zn deficiency – decreased dietary intake, decreased ileal absorption (interference with Zn-binding ligand, picolinic acid, and non-specific mucosal damage), hyperzincuria; low serum Zn is associated with impaired ETOH metabolism, risk of cirrhosis, and impaired testicular function; Zn supplementation, particularly with ascorbate, greatly increases ETOH detox and survival in rats.

- **Vitamin A:** deficiency is common in alcoholics and works with zinc deficiency to produce major complications of alcoholism – reduced intestinal absorption of A and Zn, with impaired liver function (reduced extraction of Zn, mobilization of retinol binding protein [RBP], and storage of vitamin A), results in reduced blood Zn, vitamin A, RBP, and transport proteins, and a shift to non-protein ligands; reduced tissue A and Zn, abnormal enzyme activities and glycoprotein synthesis, and impaired DNA/RNA metabolism with increased kidney Zn loss; resulting symptoms of alcoholism: night blindness, skin disorders, liver cirrhosis, reduced skin healing, decreased testicular function, impaired immunity; supplementation inhibits ETOH consumption in female, but not male, rats, and the effect is inhibited by exogenous testosterone; ovariectomized and adrenalectomized rats show decreased preference for ETOH; corticosterone injections increase preference; supplementation in alcoholic corrects A deficiency – improved night blindness and sexual function. *Caution*: excessive amounts are contraindicated – ETOH-damaged liver loses ability to store A; risk vitamin A toxicity at dosage > dietary allowance of 5,000 IU.

- **Antioxidants:** ETOH increases lipid peroxidation, causing increased lipoperoxide in liver and serum; alcoholics are deficient in antioxidants and nutrients: E, Se, and C; there is significant correlation between serum lipid peroxide, SGOT activity, and liver cell necrosis; antioxidants, prior to or simultaneous with ETOH intake, inhibit lipoperoxide formation and prevent fatty liver infiltration; effective antioxidants = C, E, Zn, Se, and cysteine.

- **Carnitine:** common lipotropic agents (choline, niacin, cysteine) are of little value; carnitine (Crn) significantly inhibits ETOH-induced fatty liver disease; chronic ETOH abuse causes functional Crn deficiency; Crn facilitates fatty acid transport and oxidation in mitochondria – high liver Crn needed for increased fatty acids produced by ETOH; Crn supplements reduce serum triglycerides and SGOT levels while elevating HDL.

- **Amino acids (AAs):** chromatography patterns are aberrant in alcoholics; normalization greatly assists alcoholics (liver is the primary site for AA metabolism); particularly indicated in hepatic cirrhosis and depression; branched-chain amino acids (BCAAs) (valine, isoleucine, leucine) inhibit hepatic encephalopathy and protein catabolism (sequelae of cirrhosis); deranged neurotransmitter profiles (very low plasma tryptophan) cause depression, encephalopathy, and coma – aggravated by low-protein diet in standard therapy for cirrhosis, avoided via free form amino acids without risk of hepatic encephalopathy; individual approach indicated due to differences in nutritional status, biochemistry, and amount of liver damage; amino acid chromatography is helpful for best results.

- **Vitamin C:** deficiency of ascorbate found in 91% of patients with alcohol-related diseases; helps ameliorate effects of ethanol toxicity in humans and guinea pigs (species unable to synthesize own ascorbate); there is a direct correlation between leukocyte ascorbate (good index of body ascorbate status), rate of ETOH blood clearance, and activity of hepatic ADH; strong reducing agent = electron donor similar to NAD in ETOH metabolism, increasing ETOH conversion to acetaldehyde and catabolism of acetaldehyde.

- **B vitamins:** alcoholics are deficient in most B vitamins; mechanisms: low dietary intake, deactivation of active form, impaired conversion to active form by ETOH or acetaldehyde, impaired absorption, decreased storage capacity; B_1 deficiency is the most common (55%) and most serious – beriberi and Wernicke–Korsakoff syndrome, and greater intake of ETOH (B_1 deficiency may predispose for alcoholism); functional B_6 deficiency is also common – impaired conversion to active form, pyridoxal-5-phosphate, and enhanced degradation; ETOH decreases absorption and utilization by liver, and/or increases urinary excretion of B vitamins (folate).

- **Magnesium:** deficiency common in alcoholics (60%), strongly linked to delirium tremens, and major reason for increased cardiovascular disease in alcoholics; deficiency due to reduced intake plus ETOH-induced renal hyperexcretion, which continues during withdrawal despite hypomagnesium; alcoholic cardiomyopathy is associated with B_1 deficiency, but may instead be due to Mg deficiency.

- **Essential fatty acids (EFAs):** ETOH interferes with EFA metabolism – ETOH abuse may produce symptoms of EFA deficiency.

- **Glutamine:** supplementation (1 g q.d.) reduces voluntary ETOH consumption in uncontrolled human studies and experimental animal studies; this preliminary research is 40+ years old, but there has been no follow-up despite efficacy, safety, and low cost.

Psychosocial aspects

Physicians must be non-judgmental, but not passive, in their attitude towards their patients; alcoholism is a chronic, progressive, addictive, and potentially fatal disease; social support for patient and family essential; success is often proportional to involvement of Alcoholics Anonymous (AA), counselors, and social agencies; maintain close working relationships with experienced counselors, AA, Al-Anon, and Ala-Teen. *Requirements for successful initiation of treatment:* patient realization that he/she has ETOH problem; education of patient and/or family about physical and psychosocial aspects of alcoholism; and immediate patient involvement in treatment program. *Elements of successful programs:* strict control of ETOH plus replacement with another addiction that is non-chemical, time-consuming, and heavily supported by family, friends, and peers; strict abstinence safest and most effective choice.

Depression: common in alcoholics, leads to high suicide rate; many depressed first then become alcoholic (primary depressives); others alcoholic first then develop depression in context of alcoholism (secondary depressives); alterations in serotonin metabolism and availability of precursor (tryptophan) are implicated in some forms of depression; other forms are linked to catecholamine metabolism and tyrosine availability; alcoholics have severely depleted tryptophan – depression and sleep disturbances; ETOH impairs tryptophan transport into brain; enzyme tryptophan pyrolase is rate-limiting in tryptophan catabolism and more active in rats during ETOH withdrawal; plasma tryptophan is depleted in withdrawing alcoholics but normalizes after 6 days of treatment and abstinence; brain tryptophan uptake is also influenced by competition from amino acids sharing the same transport (tyrosine, phenylalanine, valine, leucine, isoleucine, methionine) – elevated in malnourished alcoholics; depressed alcoholics have lowest ratios of tryptophan to these amino acids; amino acids that lower ratio are catecholamine precursors (tyrosine and phenylalanine); elevated plasma catecholamines are common in alcoholics and may contribute to depression; taurine is also low in depressed alcoholics, with lowest levels in psychotic alcoholics.

Miscellaneous factors

● **Intestinal flora:** severely deranged in alcoholics; endotoxin-producing bacteria induce malabsorption of fats, carbohydrates, protein, folate, and B_{12}; abnormalities of small intestine common in alcoholics; ETOH increases intestinal permeability to endotoxins and macromolecules – increased toxic and antigenic effects, contributing to complications of alcoholism; addictive tendency of food allergies may contribute to ETOH cravings.

● **Exercise:** graded, individually tailored fitness program improves likelihood of maintaining abstinence; regular exercise alleviates anxiety and depression and enables better response to stress and emotional upset.

● ***Silybum marianum* (milk thistle):** flavonoid complex (silymarin) effective in treatment of full spectrum of ETOH-related liver disease; extends life span of alcoholics; silymarin can improve immune function in patients with cirrhosis.

THERAPEUTIC APPROACH

Alcoholism is difficult to treat; little documented long-term success, except for Alcoholics Anonymous (overall success of AA highly controversial); requires integrated, whole-person, stage-oriented program; design for four stages: (1) active consumption, (2) withdrawal, (3) recovery, (4) recovered; recovery stage = period between withdrawal and full re-establishment of normal metabolism; complete diagnostic work-up required due to high risk for wide variety of clinical/subclinical diseases; therapeutic support needed in all stages.

● **Diet:** Stabilize blood sugar; eliminate simple sugars (sucrose, fructose, glucose; fruit juice; dried fruit; low-fiber fruits: grapes and citrus); limit processed carbohydrates (white flour, instant potatoes, white rice, etc.); increase unprocessed complex carbohydrates (whole grains, vegetables, beans, etc.).

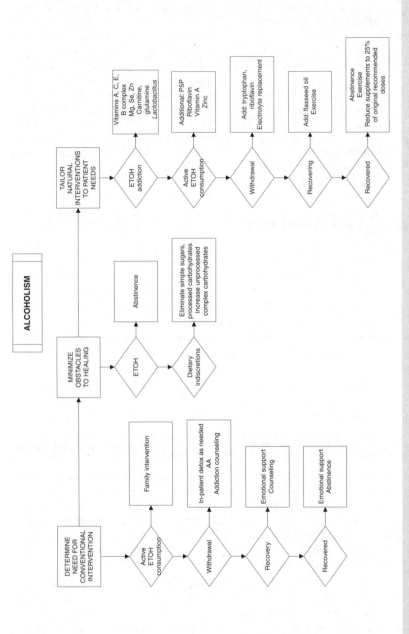

ALCOHOLISM

DETERMINE NEED FOR CONVENTIONAL INTERVENTION

Active ETOH consumption → Family intervention

Withdrawal → In-patient detox as needed
AA
Addiction counseling

Recovery → Emotional support
Counseling

Recovered → Emotional support
Abstinence

MINIMIZE OBSTACLES TO HEALING

ETOH → Abstinence

Dietary indiscretions → Eliminate simple sugars, processed carbohydrates
Increase unprocessed complex carbohydrates

TAILOR NATURAL INTERVENTIONS TO PATIENT NEEDS

ETOH addiction → Vitamins A, C, E, B complex
Mg, Se, Zn
Carnitine,
glutamine
Lactobacillus

Active ETOH consumption → Additional: P5P
Riboflavin
Vitamin A
Zinc

Withdrawal → Add: tryptophan, riboflavin
Electrolyte replacement

Recovering → Add: flaxseed oil
Exercise

Recovered → Abstinence
Exercise
Reduce supplements to 25% of original recommended doses

- **Supplements:**
  - vitamin A: 25,000 IU q.d.
  - B complex: 20 × RDA
  - vitamin C: 1 g b.i.d.
  - vitamin E: 400 IU q.d. D-alpha-tocopherol
  - magnesium: 250 mg b.i.d.
  - selenium: 200 μg q.d.
  - zinc: 30 mg q.d. picolenate
  - carnitine: 500 mg b.i.d. L-carnitine
  - glutamine: 1 g q.d.
  - *Lactobacillus acidophilus*: 1 tsp q.d.
- **Exercise:** graded program using heart rate response to determine intensity; 5–7 times weekly for 20–30 min at intensity, raising heart rate to 60–80% of age group maximum.
- **Counseling:** AA and experienced counselor with addiction expertise.
- **Additional recommendations for four stages:**
  - (1) *active ETOH consumption:* family, peers, social group support to elicit patient's recognition of ETOH problem and willingness to enter treatment program; additional supplements: pyridoxal-5-phosphate (20 mg q.d.); riboflavin (100 mg q.d.); vitamin A (50,000 IU q.d.); zinc (30 mg q.d.);
  - (2) *withdrawal:* symptom severity variable, proportional to degree of dependence and duration of disease; milder cases – within a few hours after cessation of drinking and resolves within 48 h; more severe cases – in patients over age 30 and develop after 48 h of abstinence – need inpatient facility; additional supplements (obtain institutional permission before admission): tryptophan (3 g q.d.); riboflavin (100 mg q.d.); electrolyte replacement as needed;
  - (3) *recovering:* strong emotional support network; involve patient in intense, people-oriented activities; help patient reject ETOH as destructive response to stress and develop more effective ways of handling adversity; additional supplement: flaxseed oil (1 tbsp t.i.d.);
  - (4) *recovered:* maintain emotional support network; continue total abstinence; slowly reduce supplement doses, after 6 months of abstinence, to 25% of above recommendations.

Alzheimer's disease (AD)

DIAGNOSTIC SUMMARY

Progressive mental deterioration, loss of memory and cognitive functions; inability to carry out activities of daily life; characteristic symmetrical, usually diffuse, EEG pattern; diagnosis usually made by exclusion; definitive diagnosis can be made only by postmortem biopsy of brain, demonstrating atrophy, senile plaques, and neurofibrillary tangles.

GENERAL CONSIDERATIONS

Alzheimer's disease is a neurodegenerative disorder – progressive deterioration of memory and cognition or dementia; 5% of US population over 65 have severe dementia, another 10% have mild/moderate dementia; frequency rises with increasing age; 50–60% of all cases of dementia (senile and presenile) are caused by AD; "the disease of the 20th century": 10-fold increase in AD in US population over age 65.

Neuropathology

Distinctive neuropathological features: plaque formation, amyloid deposition, neurofibrillary tangles, granulovascular degeneration, massive loss of telencephalic neurons; particularly evident in cerebral cortex and hippocampal formation; clinical features of AD believed to be from cholinergic dysfunction via reduced activity of enzyme choline acetyltransferase (which synthesizes acetylcholine) and neuronal transfer of choline.

Etiology

Genetic factors play a major role – amyloid precursor gene on chromosome #21 (close association between Down's syndrome and AD); presenilin genes on #14 and 1; apolipoprotein E (*ApoE*) gene on #19; mutations on #21, 14, and 1 – rare and associated with symptoms before age 50; most significant genetic finding is the link with *ApoE*; *ApoE* of e4-type is linked to much greater risk; e2-type is linked to greater protection.

Environmental factors also play a major role – traumatic head injury, chronic exposure to aluminum and/or silicon, neurotoxins, and free radical damage; oxidative damage plays central role in pathophysiology.

- **Aluminum (AL):** concentrated in neurofibrillary tangle (NFT) and contributes significantly to AD; strong affinity for and cofactor with paired helical filament tau (PHFt) involved in forming neurofibrillary tangles; AL selectively binds to PHFt, induces PHFt aggregation, and retards brain's ability to break down PHFt; increasing AL levels in brain – AD increases with age; serum AL increases as people age; AD patients have much higher AL than normal people and patients with other dementias (ETOH, atherosclerosis, stroke); efforts to remove AL help some, but probably too late, after disease is well established; even in those without mental disease, elevated AL is linked with poorer mental function; sources of AL are water supply (immediately enters brain tissue), food, antacids, antiperspirants.

DIAGNOSTIC CONSIDERATIONS

Only 50% of patients with dementia have AD – comprehensive diagnostic work-up paramount; diagnosis depends on clinical judgment. *Work-up:* detailed history; neurological and physical exam; psychological evaluation with particular attention to depression; general medical evaluation revealing subtle metabolic, toxic, or cardiopulmonary disorders inducing confusion in elderly; neurophysiology tests to document the type and severity of cognitive impairment; social worker mobilizing community resources; lab tests (EKG, EEG, CT scan).

- **Diagnostic process:** exclusion of other possible diagnoses: (1) diagnose dementia (10–50% error rate when diagnosis of dementia based only on first evaluation; misdiagnosis of pseudodementing functional illness; depression mimicking dementia in elderly is common; *Textbook*, Table 128.1); (2) careful neuro exam required whenever dementia is suspected, to reveal: (a) focal, circumscribed brain disease, (b) diffuse, bilateral brain dysfunction, or (c) no evidence of neurological dysfunction; "routine" neuro exam recognizes (a) and (c) but not diffuse brain dysfunction displaying subtle indications – patient's level of consciousness, attentiveness to examiner, comprehension, performance of tasks, facial expressions, quality of speech, posture, respiratory rhythm, and gait.

- **Signs of diffuse brain dysfunction:** persistent glabella-tap response (light tapping above bridge of nose produces blink which normally fatigues rapidly); corneomandibular reflex (ipsilateral strong blink and contralateral movement of chin from firm stimulus applied quickly to cornea); sucking reflex; snout reflex; palmomental reflex (ipsilateral contraction of mentalis muscle in response to stimulating thenar eminence); grasp reflex.

- **Recognizing reversible causes for diagnosed dementia:** drug toxicity, metabolic and nutritional disorders (hypoglycemia, thyroid disturbances, deficiencies of vitamin B_{12}, folate, or thiamine), neurosyphilis, disorders causing dementia (Huntington's chorea, cerebral vascular disease, normal pressure hydrocephalus, intracranial masses).

- **Recommended lab tests in dementia:** CBC (anemia, infection); VDRL (syphilis); electrolyte (metabolic dysfunction); liver function tests (hepatic dysfunction); BUN (renal dysfunction); TSH, T_4, T_3, T_3U (thyroid dysfunction); serum B_{12} and RBC folate (deficiency); urinalysis (renal/hepatic dysfunction); hair mineral analysis (heavy metal intoxication); EKG (heart function); EEG (focal vs. diffuse); CT scan (atrophy, intracranial mass).

- **EEG:** an important tool in differentiating dementias; normal EEG does not rule out dementia, particularly early stages, but provides valuable information; AD has characteristic symmetrical diffuse slowing of EEG; EEG differentiates focal (intracranial mass or vascular disease) and diffuse (metabolic disorders or normal pressure hydrocephalus) dysfunction.

- **CT scan:** high incidence (4–5%) of silent brain tumors/other lesions (e.g. subdural hematoma) in patients with dementia; limited use in AD – brain atrophy = "normal" part of aging process.

- **Fingerprint patterns:** abnormal in Alzheimer's and Down's; increased number of ulnar loops on fingertips, with concomitant decrease in whorls, radial loops, and arches; ulnar loops (pointing towards ulnar bone, away from thumb) frequently found on all 10 fingertips; radial loops (pointing towards thumb), when they occur, are shifted away from index and middle fingers – where they most commonly occur – to ring and little fingers; appearance of Alzheimer fingerprint pattern warrants immediate aggressive preventive approach.

THERAPEUTIC CONSIDERATIONS

(1) Prevention by addressing suspected pathophysiology and (2) using natural measures to improve mental function in early stages; advanced stages – natural measures are of only limited benefit.

- **Estrogen:** promoted to offer protection and therapeutic benefits, but epidemiological and clinical evidence is very weak – no major gender differences in rate or severity of AD.

- **Aluminum:** avoid all known sources of AL – antacids, antiperspirants, baking powder, cookware, foil food wrap, non-dairy creamers, table salt additives; citric acid and calcium citrate supplements increase AL absorption (but not Pb) from water and food; AL absorption decreased by Mg (competes for absorption at intestinal mucosa and blood–brain barrier); recommend Mg-rich diet: unprocessed foods (avoid milk and dairy), vegetables, whole grains, nuts and seeds.

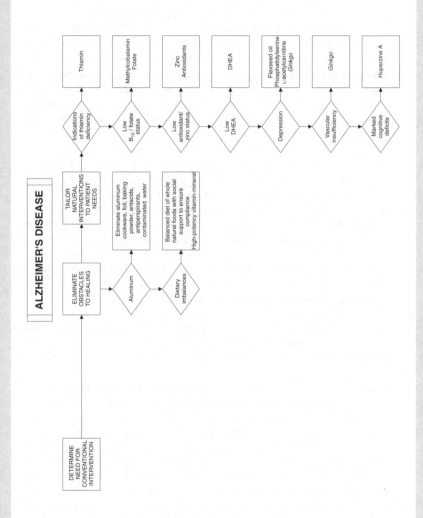

Nutrition

Directly related to cognition in the elderly – nutrient deficiency common.

- **Antioxidants:** oxidative damage plays a major role in AD; antioxidant nutrients offer significant protection; antioxidants like vitamins C and E slow progression of Parkinson's in patients not yet on medications; vitamin E (2,000 IU/day) provides some benefit for patients with moderately severe AD dementia; better results likely if antioxidants started earlier in disease process and by using antioxidant combinations.

- **Thiamin (vitamin B_1):** deficiency rather uncommon (except alcoholics) but many elderly do not get even RDA (1.5 mg); B_1 potentiates and mimics brain neurotransmitter of memory – acetylcholine; B_1 (3–8 g/day) improves mental function in AD and age-related impaired mental function (senility) without side-effects.

- **Vitamin B_{12}:** deficiency induces impaired nerve function causing numbness, paresthesiae, or burning feeling in feet, impaired mental function that mimics AD in the elderly; B_{12} deficiency is common in the elderly and a major cause of depression in this age group; best test = serum cobalamin or urine methylmalonic acid; plasma homocysteine indicates B_{12} and folate status; B_{12} declines with age and deficiency is found in 3–42% of persons aged 65 and over; untreated deficiency impairs neurological and cognitive function; B_{12} screening tests are indicated in elderly given positive cost–benefit ratio; urinary methylmalonic acid assay is the best – sensitive, non-invasive, and relatively convenient for patient; correcting B_{12} deficiency improves mental function and quality of life; low and deficient B_{12} levels are common in AD patients; B_{12} and/or folate supplements may completely reverse some patients, but generally there is little improvement in patients with AD symptoms > 6 months – irreversible changes; active forms in body: methylcobalamin and adenosylcobalamin.

- **Zinc:** common nutrient deficiency in the elderly and may be a major factor in AD development; enzymes involved in DNA replication, repair, and transcription are Zn-dependent; long-term Zn deficiency may cause cascading effects of error-prone/ineffective DNA-handling enzymes in nerve cells; Zn is required by antioxidant enzymes (superoxide dismutase); levels of Zn in brain and cerebrospinal fluid in AD patients are markedly decreased; there is a strong inverse correlation between serum Zn and senile plaque count; supplementation is beneficial in AD; Zn is neurotoxic at high concentrations and accumulates at sites of degeneration; total tissue Zn is markedly reduced in brains of AD patients; much higher concentration of copper-zinc superoxide dismutase in and around damaged brain tissue of AD patients – suggests increased Zn in damaged areas due to body's efforts to neutralize free radicals by increasing local production of dismutases; possible corollary – higher focal Zn results in increased amyloid formation when free radical scavenging is inadequate.

- **Phosphatidylcholine (PC):** dietary PC can increase brain acetylcholine (Ach) in normal patients; AD characterized by decreased cholinergic transmission; PC supplementation would seem beneficial in AD; basic defect in cholinergic transmission in AD = impaired enzyme acetylcholine transferase, which combines choline (provided by PC) with acetyl moiety to form neurotransmitter Ach; providing more choline (via PC) will not increase enzyme activity; mild to moderate dementia may be helped by high-quality PC (15–25 g q.d.) – discontinue if no noticeable improvement within 2 weeks.

- **Phosphatidylserine (PS):** the major phospholipid in the brain; helps in determining integrity and fluidity of cell membranes; deficiency of methyl donors (S-adenosyl-methionine [SAM], folate, B_{12}) or essential fatty acids may inhibit production of PS; low brain PS is linked to impaired mental function and depression in the elderly; useful in treating depression and/or impaired mental function in the elderly, including AD (100 mg t.i.d.).

- **L-Acetylcarnitine (LAC):** thought to be much more active than other forms of carnitine in brain disorders; close structural similarity to Ach; mimics Ach and benefits early-stage AD patients and elderly with depression or impaired memory; powerful antioxidant within neurons; stabilizes cell membranes; improves energy production within neurons; delays progression of AD (2 g b.i.d.); also beneficial for non-AD mild mental deterioration in the elderly (1,500 mg q.d.).

Other therapies

- **DHEA (dehydroepiandrosterone):** the most abundant hormone in the bloodstream, with extremely high brain levels; levels decline dramatically with aging – symptomatic including impaired mentality; DHEA itself has no known function, but is a source for all endogenous steroids (e.g. sex hormones and corticosteroids); declining DHEA is linked to diabetes, obesity, hypercholesterolemia, heart disease, and arthritis; DHEA may enhance memory and cognition; dosages: men over 50, 25–50 mg q.d., women, 15–25 mg, men and women aged 70+, 50–100 mg; excessive dosing causes acne and, in women, menstrual irregularities; use lab assessment before prescribing.

- ***Ginkgo biloba* extract (GBE):** standardized to 24% ginkgo flavonglycosides/6% terpenoids great benefit in senility and AD; increases brain functional capacity; normalizes Ach receptors in hippocampus of aged animals, increasing cholinergic transmission (*Textbook*, Ch. 88); GBE (240 mg q.d.) only helps reverse or delay mental deterioration in early stages of AD – may help patient maintain normal life, avoiding nursing home; improves Clinical Global Impressions (CGI) scale (120 mg q.d.), stabilizes AD, and significantly improves mental function without side-effects; reverses mental deficits due to vascular insufficiency or depression; must be taken consistently for at least 12 weeks to determine efficacy.

- **Huperzine A (HupA):** alkaloid isolated from moss *Huperzia serrata* – long used in China for fever and inflammation, but no antipyretic or anti-inflammatory properties in experimental models; potent inhibitor of acetylcholinesterase; more selective and much less toxic than conventional drugs (physostigmine, tacrine, donepezil); used by over 100,000 people since early 1990s with no serious adverse effects; considerable benefit for dementia; 200μg b.i.d. improves memory, cognition, and behavior in AD.

THERAPEUTIC APPROACH

Goal = prevention, or starting therapy as soon as dementia noted.

- **Dietary/lifestyle recommendations:** avoid aluminum; general healthful dietary and lifestyle plan.
- **Supplements:** high-potency multiple vitamin-mineral supplement:
  — vitamin C: 500–1,000 mg t.i.d.
  — vitamin E: 400–800 IU q.d.
  — flaxseed oil: 1 tbsp q.d.
  — thiamin: 3–8 g q.d.
  — phosphatidylserine: 100 mg t.i.d.
  — L-acetylcarnitine: 500 mg t.i.d.
  — methylcobalamin: 1,000 μg b.i.d.
- **Botanical medicine:** *Ginkgo biloba* extract (24% ginkgo flavonglycosides/6% terpenoids): 80 mg t.i.d.; Huperzine A: 200 μg b.i.d.

Angina pectoris

DIAGNOSTIC SUMMARY

Squeezing or pressure-like pain in chest immediately after exertion; other precipitating factors: emotional tension, cold weather, large meal; pain may radiate to left shoulder blade, left arm, or jaw; pain typically lasts 1–20 min; stress, anxiety, and hypertension typically present; many demonstrate abnormal EKG (transient ST-segment depression) in response to light exercise (stress test).

GENERAL CONSIDERATIONS

Results when oxygen supply, and occasionally other nutrients, is inadequate for metabolic needs of heart muscle; primary cause = atherosclerosis; also platelet aggregation, coronary artery spasm, non-vascular mechanisms (e.g. hypoglycemia) and increased metabolic need (e.g. hyperthyroidism); primary lesion of atherosclerosis = atheromatous plaque blocking coronary artery; symptomatic after major coronary artery > 50% blocked, transient platelet aggregation (*Textbook*, Ch. 133) and coronary artery spasm.

Prinzmetal's variant angina: most common form of coronary artery spasm, not due to plaque, occurs at rest or at odd times during day or night; more common in women under age 50.

Magnesium insufficiency-induced coronary artery spasm: more common in men than in women; important cause of MI and significant in angina pectoris.

DIAGNOSTIC CONSIDERATIONS

Diagnosis frequently made by history alone; work-up: 12-lead EKG at rest, chest X-ray, EKG stress test or 24–h Holter monitor (ambulatory EKG); EKG changes seen with angina provide evidence of previous MI, and ST-segment and T-wave changes occurring during attacks of pain – displacement of ST segment, with or without T-wave inversion; hypoglycemia-induced angina does not manifest with rate or ST-segment abnormalities.

THERAPEUTIC CONSIDERATIONS

Angina pectoris is a serious condition requiring careful treatment and monitoring; prescription medications may be necessary; condition controllable with help of natural measures; significant blockage of coronary artery: i.v. EDTA chelation, angioplasty or coronary artery bypass may be appropriate; two primary therapeutic goals: improve energy metabolism within heart and improve blood supply to heart; heart uses fats as major metabolic fuel: defects in fat metabolism in heart greatly increase risk of atherosclerosis, MI, and angina attacks; impaired utilization of fatty acids by heart results in accumulation of fatty acids within heart muscle – extreme susceptibility to cellular damage and MI; carnitine, pantethine and coenzyme Q_{10} are essential to fat metabolism and extremely beneficial in angina – prevent accumulation of fatty acids within heart muscle by improving conversion of fatty acids into energy.

Coronary angiogram, artery bypass surgery and angioplasty

Angiogram (cardiac catheterization) = X-ray procedure: dye injected into coronary arteries to highlight blockages – most often opened with balloon angioplasty and/or coronary artery bypass surgery; 1 million heart angiograms performed annually at cost > $10bn, but money may be wasted; study results: in large fraction of medically stable patients with coronary disease urged to undergo coronary angiography, the procedure can be safely deferred; non-invasive testing to determine functional state of heart (exercise stress test, echocardiogram, Holter monitor) far more revealing of type of therapy needed than dangerous, invasive search for blocked arteries; if heart not functioning well, then angiogram is needed to see if surgery is required; blockages found by angiogram are usually not relevant to patient's risk of MI.

- **Coronary Artery Surgery Study** (CASS): heart patients with healthy hearts, but with one, two, or all three major heart vessels blocked, did surprisingly well without surgery – regardless of number or severity of blockages, each group had same very low annual death rate of 1%; same year, average death rate from bypass surgery was 10.1% (1 death per 10 operations) – operation recommended to save lives 5–10 times more deadly than disease; bypass surgery and balloon angioplasty are irrelevant to course of disease in all but most serious cases; patients electing not to have surgery live just as long, or longer, than those having surgery.

- **Severity of blockage does not estimate reduction in blood flow in artery:** there is no correlation between blood flow and severity of heart artery blockage; angiogram does not provide clinically relevant information (coronary artery with 96% blockage can have one of the most brisk blood flows, while a similar artery, with only 40% blockage, can have severe flow restriction); relevant "information cannot be determined accurately by conventional angiographic approaches".

- **Critical factor whether patient needs bypass surgery or angioplasty** is how well left ventricular pump is working, not degree of blockage or number of arteries affected; bypass is only helpful when ejection fraction < 40% (90% of bypasses done when ejection fraction is > 50% – adequate for circulatory needs, therefore surgery unnecessary); bypass surgery and/or angioplasty necessary based on stronger criteria increase long-term survival and symptomatic relief for 85%; complications: 61% of bypass patients subsequently suffer nervous system disorders; 2–5% of bypass patients die during or soon after operation and 10% have MI.

- **Dietary/lifestyle changes:** significantly reduce risk of MI and other causes of death due to atherosclerosis (*Textbook*, Ch. 133); nutritional supplements and botanical medicines improve heart function in even the most severe angina cases; i.v. EDTA chelation – controversial, but clinical research has proven its efficacy.

- **When an angiogram is unavoidable:** goal = prevent damaging effects; high-potency multiple vitamin-mineral, additional vitamin C (500 mg t.i.d.+) and CoQ_{10} (300 mg q.d. 2 weeks prior to surgery and for 3 months after); garlic and high dosages vitamin E (> 200 IU) to be avoided prior to surgery due to inhibition of platelet aggregation; vitamin C plummets by 70% 24 h after bypass surgery and persists for 2 weeks; after surgery, vitamin E and carotene levels do not change significantly – fat-soluble and retained longer; vitamin C depletion may deteriorate wound repair and defenses against free radicals and infection; CoQ_{10} can prevent oxidative damage during reperfusion – return of blood after bypass surgery induces oxidative damage to vascular endothelium and myocardium; increased risk for subsequent coronary artery disease; CoQ_{10} (150 mg q.d.) prevents reperfusion injury and lowers incidence of ventricular arrhythmias during recovery period; mixture of purified bovine aortic glycosaminoglycans (dermatan sulfate, heparin sulfate, hyaluronic acid, chondroitin sulfate) (100 mg q.d.) helps prevent reperfusion injury and restore structural integrity of endothelium.

Nutritional supplements

- **Carnitine (Crn):** vitamin-like compound that transports fatty acids across mitochondrial membrane and stimulates metabolism of long-chain fatty acids by mitochondria; Crn deficiency decreases mitochondrial fatty acid levels and energy production; normal heart function depends on adequate Crn; the normal heart stores more Crn than it needs; heart ischemia induces decreased Crn and energy production in heart and increased risk for angina and heart disease; Crn (900 mg q.d.) improves angina and heart disease, allows heart muscle to utilize limited oxygen more efficiently,

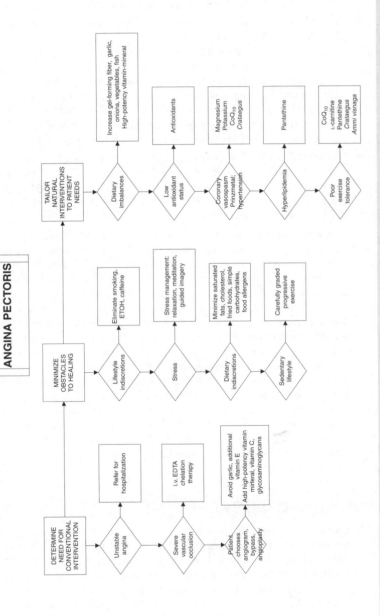

improves exercise tolerance and heart function – Crn is an effective alternative to drugs (beta-blockers, calcium-channel antagonists, and nitrates), especially in patients with chronic stable angina pectoris; Crn (40 mg/kg per day) may prevent production of toxic fatty acid metabolites that activate phospholipases, disrupt cell membranes, impair heart contractility and compliance, increase susceptibility to irregular beats, and eventual death of heart tissue.

- **Pantethine:** stable form of pantethine = active form of pantothenic acid = fundamental component of coenzyme A (CoA); CoA transports fatty acids within cell cytoplasm and mitochondria; pantethine reduces hyperlipidemia (pantothenic acid does not); 900 mg pantethine q.d. reduces serum triglyceride and cholesterol while increasing HDL with no toxicity; inhibits cholesterol synthesis and accelerates fatty acid breakdown in mitochondria; heart pantethine decreases during ischemia.

- **Coenzyme Q_{10} (ubiquinone):** essential component of mitochondrial energy production; synthesized within body synthesis impaired by nutritional deficiencies, genetic or acquired defect, or increased tissue need; angina, hypertension, mitral valve prolapse, and congestive heart failure require increased tissue levels of CoQ_{10}; elderly have increased CoQ_{10} needs: CoQ_{10} decline with age contributes to age-related decline in immunity; CoQ_{10} deficiency is common in heart disease patients; high metabolic activity of heart tissue causes unusual susceptibility to CoQ_{10} deficiency; reduces frequency of anginal attacks by 53% in stable patients and increases treadmill exercise tolerance.

- **Magnesium (Mg):** deficiency may play a major role in angina, including Prinzmetal's; deficiency produces coronary vasospasms; may be cause of non-occlusive MI; sudden MI in death of men is linked to much lower heart Mg^{2+} and K^+ than matched controls; researchers recommend Mg as treatment of choice for angina due to coronary vasospasm; helps manage arrhythmias and angina due to atherosclerosis; i.v. Mg during first hour after acute MI reduces immediate and long-term complications and death rates; beneficial effects of Mg in acute MI: improves heart energy production within the heart, dilates coronary arteries improving heart oxygenation, reduces peripheral vascular resistance (decreasing demand on heart), inhibits platelet aggregation, reduces size of infarct, and improves heart rate and arrhythmias.

Botanical medicines

- ***Crataegus* species (hawthorn):** berry and flowering tops extracts reduce angina attacks, lower blood pressure and serum cholesterol levels; improve blood and oxygen supply of heart via dilation of coronary vessels; improve metabolic processes in heart; improve cardiac energy metabolism, enhancing myocardial function with more efficient use of oxygen; interact with key enzymes to enhance myocardial contractility (*Textbook*, Ch. 79).

● *Ammi visnaga* **(khella):** ancient Mediterranean medicinal plant used historically to treat angina and other heart ailments; constituents dilate coronary arteries; mechanism of action similar to calcium-channel blocking drugs; constituent khellin is extremely effective in relieving angina symptoms, improving exercise tolerance, and normalizing EKGs; higher doses (120–150 mg q.d.) pure khellin linked to mild side-effects (anorexia, nausea, dizziness); most clinical studies used high doses; several studies: only 30 mg khellin q.d. offers good results with fewer side-effects; khella extracts standardized for khellin content (12%) preferred at dose = 250–300 mg q.d.; works synergistically with hawthorn.

Intravenous EDTA (ethylenediaminetetra-acetic acid) chelation therapy

Alternative to bypass surgery/angioplasty; may be more effective and is definitely safer and less expensive; EDTA = amino acid-like molecule that binds with minerals (e.g. Ca, Fe, Cu, and Pb) and carries them to kidneys for excretion; commonly used for Pb poisoning, but found to help atherosclerosis in late 1950s – Dr Norman Clarke treated patients with angina, cerebral vascular insufficiency, and occlusive peripheral vascular disease, and 87% showed symptomatic improvement; patients with blocked leg arteries, particularly diabetics, avoided amputation; EDTA chelates out excess Fe and Cu that stimulate free radicals in presence of O_2; free radicals damage endothelium causing atherosclerosis; giving too much EDTA or giving it too fast is dangerous – kidney failure; no deaths or significant adverse reactions in > 500,000 patients treated under controlled protocols; improves blood flow throughout body: recommended for angina, peripheral vascular disease, and cerebral vascular disease; substantiated by numerous FDA approved studies. (Contact American College of Advancement in Medicine [ACAM], 23121 Verdugo Drive, Suite 204, Laguna Hills, CA 92653; 1-800-532-3688 [outside California] or 1-800-435-6199 [inside California].)

THERAPEUTIC APPROACH

Primary therapy = prevention, since angina is usually secondary to atherosclerosis; once developed, restore proper blood supply to heart and enhance energy production within heart; unstable angina (progressive increase in frequency and severity of pain over several days, increased sensitivity to precipitating factors, and prolonged coronary pain) mandates hospitalization.

● **Diet:** increase fiber, especially gel-forming/mucilaginous fibers (flaxseed, oat bran, pectin); increase onions, garlic, vegetables, fish; decrease saturated fats, cholesterol, sugar, other animal proteins; avoid fried foods and food allergens; patients with reactive hypoglycemia – eat regular meals and avoid simple carbohydrates (sugar, honey, dried fruit, fruit juice, etc.).

- **Lifestyle:** stop smoking, ETOH, coffee; decrease stress via progressive relaxation, meditation or guided imagery; carefully graded, progressive, aerobic exercise (30 min 3 times weekly): start with walking.
- **Nutritional supplements:**
  — coenzyme Q_{10}: 150–300 mg q.d. (Note: C_o Q_{10} blood levels must reach greater than 2.5 mcg\ml for efficacy)
  — L-carnitine: 500 mg t.i.d.
  — pantethine: 300 mg t.i.d.
  — magnesium (aspartate, citrate, or other Krebs cycle intermediate): 200–400 mg t.i.d.
- **Botanical medicines:**
  — *Crataegus oxyacantha* (t.i.d.):
     berries or flowers (dried): 3–5 g or as a tea
     tincture (1:5): 4–6 ml (1–1.5 tsp)
     fluid extract (1:1): 1–2 ml (0.25–0.5 tsp)
     solid extract (10% procyanidins or 1.8% vitexin-4'-rhamnoside): 100–250 mg
  — *Ammi visnaga* (t.i.d.):
     dried powdered extract (12% khellin content): 100 mg.

Aphthous stomatitis (aphthous ulcer/canker sore/ulcerative stomatitis)

DIAGNOSTIC SUMMARY

Single or clustered, shallow, painful ulcers anywhere in oral cavity; lesions 1–15 mm in diameter, fairly even borders, surrounded by erythematous border, often covered by pseudomembrane; lesions usually resolve in 7–21 days, but are often recurrent.

GENERAL CONSIDERATIONS

Common condition (20% of population); lesions histologically similar to those of Behçet's syndrome – lymphomononuclear infiltrate and hemagglutination antibodies against oral mucosa – suggest autoimmune mechanism; etiology = food sensitivities (especially gluten), stress, and/or nutrient deficiency.

THERAPEUTIC CONSIDERATIONS

- **Food and environmental allergens:** association of recurrent aphthous stomatitis (RAS) with increased serum antibodies to food antigens and atopy strongly suggests allergic reaction involved; IgE-bearing lymphocytes significantly increased in aphthous lesions; mast cells increased in tissue from prodromal stages of recurrent ulcers; mast cell degranulation is important in producing lesion; elimination diet gives good results; allergen doesn't have to be food; frequent allergens inducing RAS are benzoic acid, cinnamaldehyde, nickel, parabens, dichromate, sorbic acid; allergen elimination usually brings complete resolution or significant improvement.

- **Gluten sensitivity:** gluten sensitivity is the primary cause of RAS in many cases; incidence of RAS is increased in patients with celiac disease; jejunal biopsy of RAS patients reveals villous atrophy typical of celiac disease plus signs of immunological reactions to food antigens; gluten may

APHTHOUS STOMATITIS

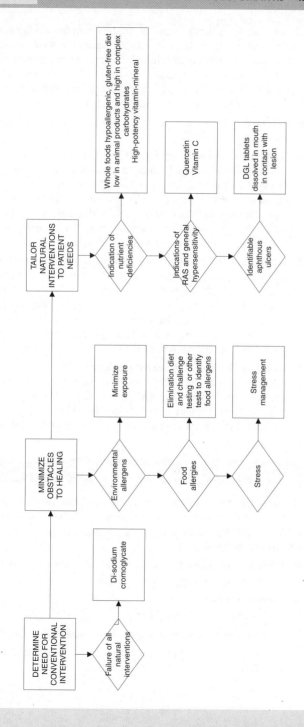

act directly on oral mucosa or produce functional changes in small intestine distinct from those of celiac disease; gluten-sensitive enteropathy induces nutritional deficiencies; withdrawing gluten causes complete remission of RAS in celiac patients and some improvement in other patients; even without villous atrophy, gluten sensitivity can produce RAS; measure alpha-gliadin antibodies in any patient presenting with RAS.

● **Stress:** precipitating factor in RAS, suggesting breakdown in host protective factors.

● **Nutrient deficiency:** oral cavity is often the first place where nutritional deficiency is visible – high turnover of mucosal epithelium; thiamin (B_1) deficiency is the most significant; low levels of transketolase (thiamin-dependent enzyme) in RAS compared with controls; nutrient deficiencies are much more common in RAS sufferers: 14.2% deficient in Fe, folate, B_{12}, or combination of these nutrients; 28.2% deficient in B_1, B_2, or B_6; when deficiencies are corrected, majority are completely remitted.

● **Quercetin:** inhibits mast cell degranulation, basophil histamine release, and formation of other mediators of inflammation; anti-allergy drug disodium cromoglycate has a very similar structure and function – effective in treating RAS; increased number of ulcer-free days with mild symptomatic relief; other flavonoids (acacetin, apigenin, chrysin and phloretin, but not catechin, flavone, morin, rutin or taxifolin) have anti-allergy effects similar to di-sodium cromoglycate.

● **Deglycyrrhizinated licorice (DGL):** may be effective in promoting healing of RAS: solution of DGL used as mouthwash (200 mg powdered DGL dissolved in 200 ml warm water) q.i.d. – 75% of patients experienced 50–75% improvement within 1 day, followed by complete healing of ulcers by third day; DGL tablets may be more convenient and effective.

THERAPEUTIC APPROACH

No single factor is solely responsible for initiating aphthous lesion, but underlying tendency to ulceration may be facilitated by these factors; underlying problem may be gluten sensitivity plus nutrient deficiencies; use anti-inflammatory nutrients.

● **Diet:** low in animal products, high in complex carbohydrates, free of known allergens and all gluten sources (i.e. grains).

● **Supplements:**

— vitamin C 1,000 mg q.d.

— high-potency multiple vitamin-mineral (*Textbook*, Ch. 44)

— DGL: one to two 380 mg chewable tablets held in direct contact with the lesion.

Ascariasis

DIAGNOSTIC SUMMARY

- **Intestinal phase:** vague upper abdominal discomfort, occasional vomiting, abdominal distension, and, rarely, intestinal obstruction. *Diagnosis* of intestinal infection is usually confirmed by finding *Ascaris* ova in stool; some patients discover worms when passed through mouth, nose or rectum.

- **Pulmonary phase:** transient cough, dyspnea, wheezing, urticaria, and transient pulmonary infiltrates. *Diagnosis* of *Ascaris* pneumonia may be confirmed by finding larvae and eosinophils in sputum or gastric aspirate.

- **Eosinophilic leukocytosis** (up to 50%) may be present, particularly during larval migration, but infrequently during chronic intestinal infection.

GENERAL CONSIDERATIONS

Ascariasis is parasitic infection by *Ascaris lumbricoides*, the largest and most common intestinal roundworm (class Nematoda, including *Ancylostoma duodenale*, *Ascaris lumbricoides*, *Enterobius vermicularis*, and *Strongyloides stercoralis*) 6–16 in long, found in warm, moist climates where soil pollution is common; 25% of the world's population (4 million Americans, especially in south-east) is infected; developing nations with poor sanitation – infection in children almost universal; parasites found in 20.1% of diagnostic stools samples (*Textbook*, Table 131.1).

- **Etiology:** Infection with *Ascaris* is found only in humans – contamination of food and fingers by human fecal matter containing mature eggs – where human feces used as fertilizer; motile larvae hatch in stomach and small intestine, from swallowed eggs, penetrate mucosa, journey through mesenteric venules and lymphatics to heart and then via blood vessels to lungs; they burrow through alveoli and migrate to trachea and throat; they are swallowed and return to jejunum to develop into mature nematode worms; within 2–3 months, female matures, producing huge numbers of eggs excreted in feces; eggs infective after 2–3 weeks in soil – can survive up to 7 years; adult worm lives 1+ years.

- **Pathophysiology and symptomatology:** worms cause capillary and alveolar damage passing through lungs – bronchopneumonia with fever, cough, dyspnea, wheezing and eosinophilic leukocytosis; chronic intestinal infestation is asymptomatic if infection is light; heavy infection – abdominal discomfort, with pain or distension and fullness, vomiting, weight loss, weakness, constipation, and diarrhea; *symptoms in children:* convulsions, fits or spasms, nervousness, irritability, twitching in various parts of body, itching of nose or anus, anal irritation, oral pallor, anorexia, ravenous appetite, restlessness at night, bruxism, frequent micturition, dry cough, malabsorption of fat, protein, carbohydrates, and vitamins common – anemia and growth retardation; worm may become entangled, blocking intestinal tract, gall bladder or appendix; pulmonary infiltrates (Löffler's syndrome) can develop in previously sensitized hosts; pulmonary phase – eosinophilia at 30–50% and may persist for 1 month.

- **Malnutrition:** *Ascaris* may interfere with host's food utilization, but studies yielded conflicting results; associated with growth retardation in marginally (protein) or malnourished children; deworming improves nitrogen and fat absorption and growth; *Ascaris*-infested children have decreased D-xylose absorption, lactose tolerance and mucosal lactase activity, and impaired absorption of vitamin A – contributes to xerophthalmia if diet poor in vitamin A; mechanism of malnutrition unclear; hypothetical mechanisms: functional alteration of mucosa (inflammation, direct mucosal surface blockage) leading to malabsorption, nutritional demands of worms depriving host of nutrients during child's growth cycle, anorexia and vomiting adversely affecting host's food intake; ascarids produce ascarase, which has an antitryptic effect, to protect parasite from proteolytic enzymes – may induce poor host protein digestion.

- **Asthma:** *Ascaris* is linked to asthma in children; *Ascaris* polysaccharide antigen strongly stimulates IgE production; repeated seasonal larvae proliferation can trigger allergic respiratory disease; allergic reactions to larvae penetrating lungs or increased sensitivity to inhaled allergens caused by exposure to *Ascaris* antigen may explain enhanced tendency to bronchoconstriction in susceptible individuals with ascariasis.

- **Environmental toxicity:** heavy metal toxicity may increase susceptibility to parasite infestation, inhibit body's attempts to limit infection, and allow increased migration of worms throughout body; industrial heavy metal emissions (Hg, Cu, Pb, Zn) decrease, in exposed lab animals, T- and B-cell population and macrophage phagocytic ability during migration phase of *Ascaris suum* compared with infected but untreated animals; exposed animals also manifested eightfold increase in density of migrating *Ascaris* larvae into lungs.

THERAPEUTIC CONSIDERATIONS

- **Diet:** helps prevent reinfection following therapy; diet with high unrefined carbohydrates and raw green vegetables, moderate protein, and no meat, dairy, or sugar – high resistance to worm infections; roundworms prefer acidic, sweet, and constipated environment – suggests alkaline diet with low sugar and high fiber; healthy diet prevents worm infection by improving immunity and preventing exposure – proper preparation, cooking, storage.

- **Fasting:** no human research; fasting pigs (water ad libitum) infested with *Ascaris suum* and *Oesophagostomum* spp. For 10 days decreases numbers and reproductivity of parasites at slaughter vs. controls, and worms are found in more distal locations in GI tract.

Botanical medicines

- **Traditional botanicals:** extracts of garlic, onion, pomegranate rind, turmeric (*Curcuma longa*), and various citrus rinds – anthelmintic properties against *Ascaris*; bromelain, papain, and other proteolytic enzyme complexes – dissolve outer layer of worms that shields them from proteases; fig powder – laxative effect; *Lactobacillus* – lactic acid inhibits growth of pathogens, decreases constipation tendency, promotes healthy bowel activity, preventing reinfection; some traditional anthelmintic botanicals – *Spigelia marilandica* (pinkroot), *Chenopodium ambrosoides* (wormseed), *Tanacetum vulgaris* (tansy), santonin (from flowers of *Artemesia maritima* and *Artemesia cina*) – either too toxic or ineffective in dosage considered safe; *Artemesia absinthium* (wormwood), *Inula helenium* (elecampane), and *Picraena excelpa* (quassia) – less toxic vermifuges specific for *Ascaris*; elecampane – safest for children, contains vermifuge helenin (also called alantolactone), which is similar to santonin but better, less toxic, and paralyzing to worm's CNS; wormwood and elecampane – bitter properties, having a tonic effect on GI tract that may enhance anthelmintic activity (*Textbook*, Table 131.2).

- **Papaya (*Carica papaya*) latex:** study with pigs with natural infection of *Ascaris suum* treated per os at doses of 2, 4, and 8 g papaya latex/kg body weight × 7 days; worm count reductions were 39.5, 80.1 and 100%, respectively; some pigs at highest dose showed mild diarrhea on the day following treatment; otherwise, no clinical or pathological changes observed in treated animals.

THERAPEUTIC APPROACH

- **Vermifuges** = toxic agents, which can be dangerous in material doses; fundamental precept of naturopathic medicine: avoid doing harm with

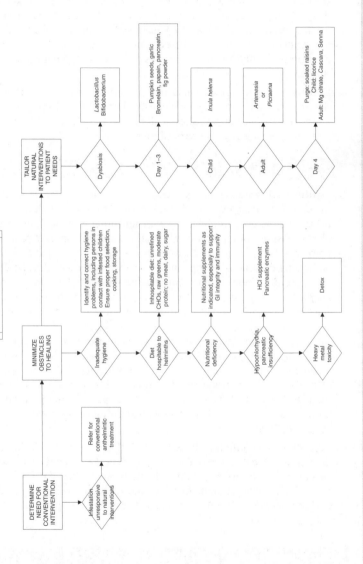

ASCARIASIS

DETERMINE NEED FOR CONVENTIONAL INTERVENTION

Infestation unresponsive to natural interventions

Refer for conventional anthelmintic treatment

MINIMIZE OBSTACLES TO HEALING

Inadequate hygiene → Identify and correct hygiene problems, including persons in contact with infested children Ensure proper food selection, cooking, storage

Diet hospitable to helminths → Inhospitable diet: unrefined CHOs, raw greens, moderate protein; no meat, dairy, sugar

Nutritional deficiency → Nutritional supplements as indicated, especially to support GI integrity and immunity

Hypochlorhydria, pancreatic insufficiency → HCl supplement Pancreatic enzymes

Heavy metal toxicity → Detox

TAILOR NATURAL INTERVENTIONS TO PATIENT NEEDS

Dysbiosis → *Lactobacillus* Bifidobacterium

Day 1–3 → Pumpkin seeds, garlic Bromelain, papain, pancreatin, fig powder

Child → *Inula helena*

Adult → *Artemesia* or *Picraena*

Day 4 → Purge: soaked raisins Child: licorice Adult: Mg citrate, *Cascara*, Senna

extreme measures; effective, simple, less toxic therapies should be used first; light *Ascaris* infestation common in childhood, frequently asymptomatic, and not necessarily serious in otherwise healthy children; drugs typically used – highly toxic and may, in heavily infected person, induce adult worm to migrate out of intestines into other body tissues with serious results; continuing infection implies improper hygiene.

- **Heavy infection** suggests underlying cause in host susceptibility and/or repeated exposure; simple de-worming alone will not cure or prevent rein-fection; consider living conditions, hygiene, diet, nutritional status, general state of health, heavy metal or other toxin exposure, GI function (e.g. con-stipation) and integrity (mucous membranes); examine all of child's close associates (home, school, recreation); re-examine feces 2 weeks and several months after completion of apparently effective treatment; other intestinal parasites are frequently associated with *Ascaris* and heavy *Ascaris* infection may mask other ova and parasites – false-negative lab reports; repeat stool exam after 3 months; use anthelmintic drugs for unresponsive situations.

- **Basic concept:** hygiene, inhospitable diet, botanical medicines to stun or poison worms, and purgative to expel helminths; most botanical anthelmintics do not affect eggs – repeat treatments to ensure clearing newly hatching larvae from existing eggs.

Days 1–3:   eat nothing but 3–5 oz pumpkin seeds, plus three to eight cloves raw garlic q.d.

- Empty stomach t.i.d.:
    — bromelain (1,200 MCU): 500 mg
    — papain: 500–1,000 mg
    — pancreatin (8× USP): 500 mg
    — fig powder: 1 tsp

- One botanical therapy t.i.d.:
    Children
    — *Inula helenium* (elecampane):
        powdered root: 1–2 g
        fluid extract (1:1): 1–2 ml

    Adults
    — *Artemesia absinthium* (wormwood):
        oil: 1–5 drops
        infusion: 0.5–1 tsp/cup
        powdered root: 1–2 g
        fluid extract (1:1): 2–4 ml
    — *Picraena excelsor* (quassia):
        powdered wood: 1–2 g.

Day 4: purging dose of licorice root (children), magnesium citrate, Senna, or *Cascara sagrada*; licorice root or coriander may be added to strong laxatives – more palatable and/or milder action; soaked raisins on day 4 prior to purge – sweetness lures remaining worms out of hiding and enhances expulsion.

Two weeks later: repeat entire 4-day program two more times – 2 weeks later and once more an additional week later; interim – preventive diet, continuing pumpkin seeds and garlic.

Asthma

DIAGNOSTIC SUMMARY

Recurrent attacks of dyspnea, cough, and expectoration of tenacious mucoid sputum; prolonged expiration phase with generalized wheezing and musical rales; eosinophilia, increased serum IgE, positive food and/or inhalant allergy tests.

GENERAL CONSIDERATIONS

Bronchial asthma is a hypersensitivity disorder characterized by bronchospasm, mucosal edema, and excessive excretion of a viscous mucus that can lead to ventilatory insufficiency; its prevalence is approximately 3% of the US population, and although it occurs at all ages, it is most common in children under 10; there is a 2:1 male:female ratio in children, which equalizes by the age of 30.

- **Major factors:** hypersensitivity of airways; beta-adrenergic blockade; cyclic nucleotide imbalance in airway smooth muscle; release of inflammatory mediators from mast cells.
- **Rate** in US is rising rapidly, especially in children; reasons for this: increased stress on immune system (greater chemical pollution in air, water, and food; earlier weaning and introduction of solid foods to infants; food additives; genetic manipulation of plants – food components with greater allergenic tendencies).
- **Pertussis vaccine:** children breast-fed from first day of life, fed exclusively breast milk for first 6 months and weaned after 1 year – relative risk of developing asthma = 1% in children receiving no immunizations, 3% in those receiving vaccinations other than pertussis, and 11% for those receiving pertussis; in group of 203 not immunized to pertussis, 16 developed whooping cough vs. only 1 of 243 in the immunized group.
- **Major categories:**
  — *extrinsic or atopic:* immunologically mediated with increased serum IgE
  — *intrinsic:* bronchial reaction due, not to antigen–antibody stimulation, but rather to such factors as chemicals, cold air, exercise, infection, agents that activate alternative complement pathway, and emotional upset.
- **Mediators:** mast cell-derived chemical mediators responsible for signs and symptoms; *preformed:* histamine (H), chemotactic peptides (eosinophilotactic

factor [ECF] and high-molecular-weight neutrophil chemotactic factor [NCF]), proteases, glycosidases and heparin proteoglycan; *membrane-derived:* lipoxygenase products (leukotrienes [LTs] and so-called slow-reacting substance of anaphylaxis [SRS-A]), prostaglandins (PGs), thromboxanes (TXs) and platelet-activating factor (PAF); actions = bronchoconstriction (H, LTC_4, LTD_4, LTE_4, $PGF_{2\alpha}$, PGD_2, PAF), mucosal edema from increased permeability (H, LTC_4, LTD_4, PAF), vasodilation (PGD_2, PGE_2), mucous plugging (H, HETEs, LTC_4), inflammatory cell infiltrate (NCF, ECF-A, HETEs, LTB_4, PAF), and desquamation of epithelium (proteases, glycosidases, lysosomal enzymes, basic proteins from neutrophils and eosinophils).

- **Mild episodic asthma vs. moderate to severe sustained asthma:** latter has subacute/chronic bronchial inflammation with infiltration of eosinophils, neutrophils and mononuclear cells; episodic – due to bronchial smooth muscle contraction.

- **Lipoxygenase products:** leukotrienes = most potent chemical mediators in asthma; SRS-A (LTC_4, LTD_4, LTE_4) 1,000 times more potent bronchoconstrictor than H; asthmatics have imbalance in arachidonic acid metabolism – relative increase in lipoxygenase products; platelets from asthmatics – 40% decrease in cyclooxygenase metabolites and 70% increase in lipoxygenase products; aggravated in "aspirin-induced asthma" – aspirin and NSAIDs inhibit cyclooxygenase while promoting lipoxygenase – shunt arachidonic acid to lipoxygenase pathway and excessive leukotrienes; tartrazine (ubiquitous yellow dye #5) = cyclooxygenase inhibitor and induces asthma, especially in children; tartrazine = anti-metabolite of vitamin B_6.

- **Autonomic nervous system:** parasympathetic vs. sympathetic innervation; beta-2-adrenergic receptors (localized in lung tissue and react to catecholamines); parasympathetic vagus nerve stimulation releases acetylcholine (Ach) which binds to receptors on smooth muscle, forming cGMP; increased cGMP and/or relative deficiency in cAMP causes bronchoconstriction and degranulation of mast cells and basophils; decreased sympathetic activity or diminished beta-2 receptor numbers or sensitivity also promote the cyclic nucleotide imbalance; some mediators block beta-2 receptors and elevate cGMP.

- **Adrenal gland:** cortisol = activator of beta receptors; epinephrine (Epi) = the prime stimulator of beta receptors; asthmatic attacks may be induced by relative deficiency of cortisol and Epi (which stimulates beta-2 receptors to catalyze formation of cAMP from AMP) leading to decreased cAMP:cGMP ratio and bronchial constriction.

THERAPEUTIC CONSIDERATIONS

General

Hypochlorhydria: 80% of tested asthmatic children had inadequate gastric acid secretion – hypochlorhydria and food allergies are predisposing factors.

- **Increased intestinal permeability:** "leaky gut" – increased antigen load on immune system; overwhelms immune system, increasing risk of additional allergies and bronchoconstrictive compound.

- ***Candida albicans*:** GI overgrowth implicated as causative factor in allergic conditions including asthma; acid protease produced by *C. albicans* is the responsible allergen.

- **Food additives:** must be eliminated; coloring agents, azo dyes – tartrazine (orange), sunset yellow, amaranth and new coccine (both red) – and non-azo dye pate blue; most common preservatives are sodium benzoate, 4-hydroxybenzoate esters, and sulfur dioxide; sulfites used in prepared foods; molybdenum deficiency may cause sulfite sensitivity – sulfite oxidase is the enzyme that neutralizes sulfites, and is molybdenum-dependent.

- **Salt:** increased intake worsens bronchial reactivity and mortality from asthma; bronchial reactivity to H is positively correlated with 24-h urinary Na and rises with increased dietary Na.

- **DHEA:** decreased levels common in postmenopausal women with asthma compared with matched controls; therapeutic benefit in asthma undemonstrated; important to immune function – positive effects possible.

Diet

- **Food allergy** (*Textbook*, Ch. 51): immediate onset sensitivities – due to (decreasing order of frequency) egg, fish, shellfish, nuts, peanuts; delayed onset – (decreasing order of frequency) milk, chocolate, wheat, citrus, food colorings; elimination diets identify allergens and treat asthma, especially in infants; elimination of common allergens during infancy (first 2 years) reduces allergic tendencies in high-risk children (strong familial history).

- **Vegan diet:** long-term trial (elimination of all animal products) significantly improved 92% of 25 patients who completed the study (nine dropped out) based on vital capacity, forced expiratory volume at 1 s (FEV_1), physical working capacity, haptoglobin, IgM, IgE, cholesterol, and triglycerides; also reduces tendency to infectious disease; 71% of patients responded in 4 months, 1 year required for 92%; diet excludes all meat, fish, eggs, dairy products, chlorinated tap water (drink spring water only), coffee, ordinary tea, chocolate, sugar, and salt; herbal spices allowed; water and herbal teas allowed up to 1.5 L q.d.; vegetables used freely = lettuce, carrots, beets, onions, celery, cabbage, cauliflower, broccoli, nettles, cucumber, radishes, Jerusalem artichokes, all beans except soya and green peas; potatoes allowed in restricted amounts; fruits used freely: blueberries, cloudberries, raspberries, strawberries, blackcurrants, gooseberries, plums, pears; apples and citrus fruits not allowed; grains restricted or eliminated; beneficial effects of vegan diet = elimination of food allergens, altered prostaglandin metabolism, increased intake of antioxidants and Mg.

Nutrition

- **Omega-3 essential fatty acids (ω-3 EFAs):** children who eat fish > once a week have 1/3 asthma risk of those who do not; fish oil supplements with EPA and DHA improve airway responsiveness to allergens and respiratory function; benefits due to increasing ratio of ω-3 to ω-6 EFAs in cell membranes, reducing arachidonic acid; ω-3 EFAs shift leukotriene synthesis from inflammatory 4-series to less inflammatory 5-series, improving asthma symptoms; benefits may take as long as 1 year before apparent – time to turn over cellular membranes in toward omega-3 fatty acids.

- **Tryptophan (Try) metabolism and pyridoxine (vitamin B$_6$) supplementation:** asthmatic children have metabolic defect in Try metabolism and reduced platelet transport for serotonin; Try is converted to serotonin (bronchoconstrictor in asthmatics); serotonin high in blood and sputum of asthmatics – elevated urinary 5-hydroxyindole acetic acid (5-HIAI), breakdown product of serotonin; urinary 5-HIAI correlates well with symptom severity; patients benefit from Try-restricted diet or B$_6$ supplements; plasma and RBC pyridoxal phosphate (PLP) in asthmatics much lower than in controls; 50–100 mg oral B$_6$ b.i.d. greatly decreases frequency and severity of wheezing and attacks and dosages of bronchodilators and corticosteroids; B$_6$ fails to demonstrate significant improvement in patients dependent upon steroids to control symptoms; theophylline depresses P5P; B$_6$ supplements reduce side-effects of theophylline (HAs, nausea, irritability, sleep disorders, etc.); tryptophan load test (*Textbook*, Ch. 28) may determine appropriateness and level of B$_6$ supplementation needed; urinary excretion of kynurenic and xanthurenic acids increases in patients responding to B$_6$.

- **Antioxidants:** oxidizing agents can stimulate bronchoconstriction and increase hyperactivity to other agents.

- **Vitamin C:** the major antioxidant in extracellular fluid lining airway surfaces; children of smokers have a higher rate of asthma (smoke depletes respiratory vitamins C and E) and symptoms in adults appear increased by exposure to environmental pro-oxidants and decreased by C supplements; nitrogen oxides = oxidants from endogenous and exogenous sources – vitamin C protects against nitrogen oxide lung damage in lab animals; asthmatic patients have much lower levels of serum and WBC ascorbate; clinically asthmatics have higher need for C; seven of 11 studies showed significant improvements in respiratory measures and symptoms using 1–2 g vitamin C q.d.; high-dose C therapy may lower H – H initially amplifies immune response, by increasing capillary permeability and smooth muscle contraction, and then suppresses accumulated WBCs to contain inflammation; vitamin C prevents H secretion by WBCs and increases H detox; vitamin C will only lower blood H if taken over a period of time.

- **Flavonoids:** key antioxidants to treat asthma – inhibit H release from mast cells and basophils stimulated by antigens, phospholipase A$_2$ in neutrophils, lipoxygenase, anaphylactic contraction of smooth muscle, phosphodi-esterase in lung (increasing cAMP), biosynthesis of SRS-A, Ca influx; quercetin spares vitamin C and stabilizes mast cell membranes; sources = quercetin, grape seed, pine bark, green tea, or *Ginkgo biloba*; proanthocyani-dins from grape seed or pine bark have affinity for lungs (*Textbook*, Ch. 106).

- **Carotenes:** powerful antioxidants which increase integrity of respiratory epithelium; act as substrates for lipoxygenase, possibly competing with arachidonic acid, decreasing leukotriene formation.
- **Vitamin E:** antioxidant, inhibitor of lipoxygenase and phospholipase.
- **Selenium:** reduced Se levels found in asthmatics; glutathione peroxidase (Se-dependent metalloenzyme) reduces hydroperoxy-eicosatetraenoic acid (HPETE) to hydroxy-eicosatetraenoic acid (HETE), thereby reducing leukotriene formation; decreased glutathione peroxidase common in asth-matics.
- **Vitamin B_{12}:** Jonathan Wright MD mainstay in childhood asthma; weekly 1,000 μg i.m. injections improve symptoms – less SOB on exer-tion, improved appetite, sleep, and general condition; B_{12} is especially effective in sulfite-sensitive patients; offers best protection when given orally (1–4 μg) prior to challenge; forms sulfite–cobalamin complex, blocking sulfite effect.
- **Magnesium:** i.v. Mg (2 g of Mg sulfate infused every hour up to total of 24.6 g) well-proven/clinically accepted to halt acute asthma attack as well as acute exacerbations of chronic obstructive pulmonary disease (COPD); i.v. Mg only necessary in emergency – acute MI or asthma; oral Mg effective to optimize body Mg stores – 6 weeks needed to elevate tissue Mg; supple-mentation warranted – dietary Mg intake is independently related to lung function and asthma severity.

Botanical medicines

Historical herbals = *Ephedra sinica* (Ma huang) in combination with herbal expectorants, e.g. *Glycyrrhiza glabra* (licorice), *Grindelia camporum* (grindelia), *Euphorbia hirta* (euphorbia), *Drosera rotundifolia* (sundew), *Polygala senega* (senega); ephedra alkaloids are effective bronchodilators for mild to moderate asthma and hay fever; peak bronchodilation in 1 h and lasts 5 h after adminis-tration.

- **_Glycyrrhiza glabra_ (licorice root):** documented anti-inflammatory and anti-allergic (*Textbook*, Ch. 90); primary active constituent is gly-cyrrhetinic acid – inhibits phospholipase A_2 which cleaves arachidonic acid from membrane phospholipid, initiating eicosanoid synthesis; licorice is also expectorant.
- **_Lobelia inflata_ (Indian tobacco):** alkaloid lobeline is an efficient expec-torant; long history of use in asthma, but promotes bronchoconstriction and is respiratory stimulant in vitro; binds to nicotine Ach receptors in

ganglions, promoting release of Epi and NE = therapeutic effects; effective alone, but traditionally used in combination with other botanical agents (*Capsicum frutescens* and *Symphlocarpus factida*).

- **Capsicum frutescens:** capsaicin induces long-lasting desensitization of airway mucosa to mechanical and chemical irritants; capsaicin depletes substance P (that increases vascular permeability and flow) in respiratory nerves; substance P = undecapeptide linked to "neurogenic inflammation" via direct effect and synergy with H on peripheral nervous system; respiratory and GI tracts have many substance P-containing neurons – believed to contribute to atopy (asthma and atopic dermatitis).

- **Zizyphi fructus (jujube plum):** traditional Chinese herb for treatment of asthma and allergic rhinitis; contains 100–500 nmol cAMP/g of dry weight, a concentration 10 times > than that of any other plant or animal tissue reported; contains beta-adrenergic receptor stimulator that also raises cAMP.

- **Thea sinensis (green tea):** adjunctive in asthma – methylxanthine and antioxidant constituents (*Textbook*, Ch. 70).

- **Allium family:** onions and garlic inhibit lipoxygenase and cyclooxygenase which generate TxA_2, PGD_2 and PGE_2; onion contains quercetin plus benzyl and other isothiocyanates (mustard oils); may inhibit biosynthesis of arachidonic acid metabolites.

- **Tylophora asthmatica:** Ayurvedic medicine for asthma and other respiratory disorders; mode of action unknown, thought to be due to alkaloids (tylophorine) – anti-H, antispasmodic activity and inhibits mast cell degranulation; good results – 200 mg tylophora leaves b.i.d. × 6 days improves symptoms and respiratory function during treatment and for 2 weeks after treatment; incidence of side-effects (nausea, partial diminution of taste for salt, slight mouth soreness) – 16.3% in tylophora group and 6.6% in placebo group; benefits of tylophora short-lived.

- **Ginkgo biloba:** unique terpenes (ginkgolides) antagonize platelet-activating factor (PAF), key mediator in asthma, inflammation, and allergies; ginkgolides compete with PAF for binding sites and inhibit events induced by PAF; improves respiratory function and reduces bronchial reactivity; dosage = 120 mg pure ginkgolides q.d. – dosage very expensive using 24% ginkgo flavonglycoside and 6% terpenoid GB extract.

- **Aloe vera:** may be effective for patients not dependent upon corticosteroids; extract produced from supernatant of fresh leaves stored in dark at 4°C × 7 days to increase polysaccharide fraction; 1 g of this extract produces 400 mg neutral polysaccharides vs. 30 mg produced from leaves not subjected to cold or dark; 5 ml of 20% solution of *Aloe vera* extract in saline b.i.d. × 24 weeks; 40% of patients without steroid dependence felt very much better; mechanism of action via restoring protective mechanisms, with augmentation of immune system.

- **Coleus forskohlii:** forskolin increases intracellular cAMP, relaxing bronchial muscles and relieving respiratory symptoms (*Textbook*, Ch. 77);

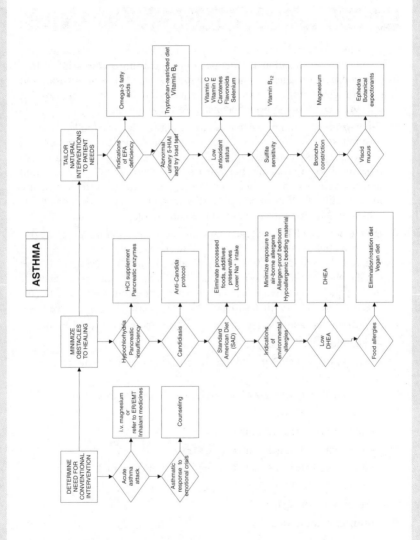

ASTHMA

DETERMINE NEED FOR CONVENTIONAL INTERVENTION

Acute asthma attack → I.v. magnesium or refer to ER/EMT Inhalent medicines

Asthmatic response to emotional crisis → Counseling

MINIMIZE OBSTACLES TO HEALING

Hypochlorhydria Pancreatic insufficiency → HCl supplement Pancreatic enzymes

Candidiasis → Anti-Candida protocol

Standard American Diet (SAD) → Eliminate processed foods, additives preservatives Lower Na⁺ intake

Indications of environmental allergies → Minimize exposure to air-borne allergens Allergen-proof bedroom Hypoallergenic bedding material

Low DHEA → DHEA

Food allergies → Elimination/rotation diet Vegan diet

TAILOR NATURAL INTERVENTIONS TO PATIENT NEEDS

Indications of EFA deficiency → Omega-3 fatty acids

Abnormal urinary 5-HIAl and try load test → Tryptophan-restricted diet Vitamin B₆

Low antioxidant status → Vitamin C Vitamin E Carotenes Flavonoids Selenium

Sulfite sensitivity → Vitamin B₁₂

Broncho-constriction → Magnesium

Viscid mucus → Ephedra Botanical expectorants

studies utilized inhaled doses of pure forskolin; efficacy of oral *C. forskohlii* extract yet to be determined; historical use and additional mechanisms of action recommend its use.

THERAPEUTIC APPROACH

Underlying defects and initiating factors must be determined and resolved: (1) defect allowing sensitization, (2) metabolic defect causing excessive inflammatory response, (3) triggering allergens with lifestyle, diet, and environment changes to avoid them, (4) modulating inflammatory process to limit severity, (5) effective treatment for bronchoconstriction of acute attack.

- **Environment:** minimize exposure to air-borne allergens (pollen, dander, dust mites); avoid dogs, cats, carpets, rugs, upholstered furniture, surfaces where allergens can collect; ensure bedroom is allergen-proof; encase mattress in allergen-proof plastic; wash sheets, blankets, pillow cases, and mattress pads weekly; consider Ventflex (hypoallergenic synthetic) bedding material; install air purifier, e.g. HEPA (high-efficiency particulate arresting) attachable to central heating/air-conditioning.

- **Diet:** eliminate all food allergens and additives and bananas if they aggravate condition; patient with many food allergies may need 4-day rotation diet; mild Try reduction (*Textbook*, Appendix 5) is helpful – essential if there is a metabolic defect in the Try metabolism; use garlic and onions liberally unless patient reacts to them; if patient willing, or asthma unresponsive, try vegan diet (for 4+ months), with possible exception of cold-water ocean fish.

- **Supplements** (adult doses; rule out potential allergens in supplements):
  — vitamin B_6: 25–50 mg b.i.d.
  — vitamin B_{12}: 1,000 μg q.d. (oral) or weekly i.m.; evaluate for efficacy after 6 weeks
  — vitamin C: 10–30 mg/kg body weight in divided doses
  — vitamin E: 200–400 IU q.d.
  — magnesium: 200–400 mg t.i.d.
  — quercetin: 400 mg 20 min before meals
  — grape seed extract (95% PCO content): 50–100 mg t.i.d.
  — carotenes: 25,000–50,000 IU q.d.
  — selenium: 200 μg q.d.

- **Botanical medicines:**
  — *Ephedra sinica* extract providing 12.5–25.0 mg ephedrine b.i.d.-t.i.d.; crude herb: 500–1,000 mg t.i.d.; can be combined with herbal expectorants indicated above
  — *Glycyrrhiza glabra*: powdered root (1–2 g); fluid extract (1:1): 2–4 ml; solid (dry powdered) extract (4:1): 250–500 mg

— *Camellia sinensis*: liberal use (green tea only)

— *Tylophora asthmatica*: 200 mg leaves or 40 mg dry ETOH extract b.i.d.

— *Coleus forskohlii* (standardized to 18% forskolin): 50 mg (9 mg forskolin) b.i.d. or t.i.d.

● **Counseling:** important for patients who respond to emotional crisis with asthmatic attacks and children with moderate to severe asthma, who may develop behavioral problems.

Acute attack: medical emergency; i.v. Mg or refer patient to ER/EMT immediately.

Atherosclerosis

DIAGNOSTIC SUMMARY

Associated with hypertension, weak pulse, and wide pulse pressure; symptoms and signs depend on arteries involved and degree of obstruction (angina, leg cramps [intermittent claudication], gradual mental deterioration, weakness or dizziness) or may also be asymptomatic; diagonal ear lobe crease.

GENERAL CONSIDERATIONS

The major causes of death in the US; "heart disease" refers to atherosclerosis of the coronary arteries; responsible for 43% of all deaths in US; largely a disease of diet and lifestyle.

- **Structure of an artery:** there are three major layers:
  - *intima* (internal lining) = layer of endothelial cells; glycosaminoglycans (GAGs) line exposed endothelial cells to protect from damage and promote repair; beneath surface cells – internal elastic membrane: layer of GAGs and ground substance compounds.
  - *media* = smooth muscle cells, interposed GAGs and other ground substance.
  - *adventitia* = external elastic membrane of connective tissue, including GAGs.
- **Process of atherosclerosis:** lesions initiated in response to injury to intima – weakening of GAG layer, leaving endothelial cell exposed to damage (free radicals, immune entities, physical, mechanical, viral, chemical, drug factors); sites of injury more permeable to plasma constituents (lipoproteins), binding lipoproteins to GAGs disintegrates ground substance matrix, increasing affinity for cholesterol; monocytes and platelets adhere to lesion, releasing factors stimulating smooth muscle cell migration from media into intima and replication; smooth muscle cells dump debris into intima, developing plaque; formation of fibrous cap (collagen, elastin, GAGs) over intimal surface; fat/cholesterol deposits accumulate; plaque grows until artery blocked; blockage 90% before symptomatic.
- **Causative risk factors:**
  - *major factors*: hypercholesterolemia, hypertension, smoking, diabetes, physical inactivity

— *other risk factors:* low antioxidant status, low essential fatty acids (EFAs), low Mg^+ and K^+, increased platelet aggregation, increased fibrinogen formation, elevated homocysteine (H), hypothyroidism, "type A" personality.

● **Clinical evaluation:** lab tests (total cholesterol, LDL, HDL, lipoprotein(a), fibrinogen, homocysteine, ferritin [iron-binding protein], lipid peroxides); exercise stress test, EKG, echocardiogram.

Risk factors

● **Smoking:** most important risk factor for coronary heart disease (3–5 × risk); smoker dies 7–8 years sooner than non-smoker; single major cause of cancer death in US (2 × risk); tobacco smoke contains > 4,000 chemicals, with > 50 carcinogens – damage intima directly or damage LDL, which damages arteries; toxins travel on plasma cholesterol; damages feedback mechanisms in liver that controls how much cholesterol is manufactured; promotes platelet aggregation and elevated fibrinogen; contributes to hypertension; environmental (secondary/passive) smoke increases heart disease mortality and morbidity; best results occur when people quit "cold turkey". Table 133.6 (*Textbook*) lists 10 tips to help patients stop smoking.

● **Hypercholesterolemia:** recommended levels – total cholesterol < 200 mg/dl, LDL < 130 mg/dl, HDL > 35 mg/dl, triglycerides < 150 mg/dl; VLDL and LDL transport fats from liver to body cells, while HDL returns fats to liver; ratio of total cholesterol to HDL and ratio of LDL to HDL = cardiac risk factor ratios – reflect whether cholesterol is being deposited into tissues or broken down and excreted; total cholesterol: HDL ratio should be < 4.2 and LDL:HDL ratio should be < 2.5; for every 1% drop in LDL, MI risk drops 2%; for every 1% increase in HDL, MI risk drops 3–4%; lipoprotein(a) (Lp(a)) is a plasma lipoprotein similar to LDL but with adhesive protein called apolipoprotein(a) (Apo(a)); elevated plasma Lp(a) is an independent risk factor for CHD, especially with elevated LDL; high Lp(a) has 10 times risk of elevated LDL (LDL lacks adhesive apo(a)); Lp(a) < 20 mg/dl is linked with low risk, 20–40 mg/dl moderate risk, and > 40 mg/dl extremely high risk.

● **Familial hypercholesterolemia (FH), familial combined hyperlipidemia (FCH), and familial hypertriglyceridemia (FT)** are common genetic inherited diseases (1 in every 500 people); FH involves defect in liver receptor protein that removes LDL from blood and helps decrease cholesterol synthesis; LDL receptors are damaged with aging and diseases (diabetes) and diet high in saturated fat/cholesterol decreases number of LDL receptors – reducing feedback telling liver cells no more cholesterol is needed; lifestyle/dietary changes increase function and/or number of LDL receptors; FCH defect = accelerated production of VLDL in liver; patients may have only hypertriglyceridemia, or only hypercholesterolemia, or both; FT has only hypertriglyceridemia with low HDL; FT defect = VLDL particles, made by liver, larger than normal and carrying more triglycerides; FT is worse in diabetes, gout, and obesity.

THERAPEUTIC CONSIDERATIONS

Lower cholesterol; reduce risk factors.

- **Diet:** decrease saturated fat and cholesterol by reducing or eliminating animal products; increase fiber-rich plant foods (fruits, vegetables, grains, legumes); weight reduction (if appropriate).

- **Lifestyle:** regular aerobic exercise, avoid smoking, reduce/eliminate coffee (caffeinated and decaf).

- **Saturated fat, cholesterol, and total fat:** with exception of nuts and seeds, plant foods are very low in fat; calories of nuts and seeds are derived from polyunsaturated EFAs.

- **Margarine, *trans* fatty acids and partially hydrogenated oils:** raise LDL, lower HDL, interfere with EFA metabolism, and suspected of carcinogenicity; restrict both butter and margarine; use natural polyunsaturated oils to meet EFA requirements – 1 tbsp high-quality flaxseed oil.

- **Cold-water fish and flaxseed oil:** cold-water ocean fish are sources of longer-chain omega-3 EFAs (eicosapentaenoic acid [EPA] and docosahexanoic acid [DHA]); lower cholesterol and triglycerides; prefer fish oils lab-certified against lipid peroxides, cold-water fish, and flaxseed oil.

- **Vegetables and fruits:** 2–3 servings fruit plus 3–5 servings vegetables daily; green leafy vegetables and yellow-orange fruits and vegetables are sources of carotenes (most widespread pigments in nature, including 30–50 the body can transform into vitamin A); red and purple vegetables and fruits are sources of flavonoids, powerful antioxidants; inverse correlation between flavonoid intake and death from MI.

- **Dietary fiber and complex carbohydrates:** "dietary fiber" = indigestible plant cell walls; soluble fiber found in legumes, fruit, and vegetables lowers cholesterol dose-dependently in patients with hypercholesterolemia; oat bran and oatmeal used in many studies; people with normal or low cholesterol – little change; for cholesterol > 220 mg/dl, 3 g soluble oat fiber (1 bowl oat bran cereal or oat meal) lowers total cholesterol by 8–23%; daily intake of 35 g fiber from fiber-rich foods is desirable.

- **Dietary animal protein:** body handles animal proteins differently from plant proteins; high intake of animal protein is linked to heart disease, cancer, hypertension, kidney disease, osteoporosis, and kidney stones; vegetarian diet linked to reduced risk; limit animal protein to < 4–6 oz/day, prefer fish, skinless poultry, and lean cuts.

- **Olive and canola oil:** best oils for cooking; composed of oleic acid, monounsaturated oil, resistant to heat and light damage; LDL largely composed of oleic acid is less susceptible to peroxidation.

- **Refined carbohydrates:** significant factor in atherosclerosis; high sugar intake elevates triglyceride, cholesterol, and insulin; elevated insulin is linked to elevated cholesterol, triglycerides, blood pressure, and CVD; limit sources of refined sugar; serum cholesterol is lowest among adults eating whole grain cereal for breakfast.

Nutritional supplements

- **Niacin:** lowers LDL, Lp(a), triglyceride, and fibrinogen, while raising HDL; the only lipid-lowering agent proven to reduce overall mortality; effects are long-lasting; better overall results despite the fact that some patients are unable to tolerate full dosage due to skin flushing; 33% increase in HDL; 35% reduction in Lp(a); side-effects of high doses are skin flushing 20–30 min post-ingestion, gastric irritation, nausea, and liver damage; "sustained release", "timed-release", or "slow-release" forms are more toxic to the liver; niacin can impair glucose tolerance – use with caution in diabetics; avoid with pre-existing liver disease or elevated liver enzymes – use gugulipid, garlic, or pantethine; safest form = inositol hexaniacinate, which is much better tolerated; check cholesterol and liver function every 3 months; niacin dosing = 100 mg t.i.d. – carefully increase dosage over 4–6 weeks to full therapeutic dose of 1.5–3 g q.d. in divided doses; inositol hexaniacinate dosing: 500 mg t.i.d. × 2 weeks, increase to 1,000 mg t.i.d.; take either form with meals; niacin should be considered premier lipid-lowering agent.

- **Pantethine:** stable form of pantetheine, the active form of vitamin B5 (pantothenic acid), the most important component of coenzyme A (CoA), involved in transport of fatty acids within cell cytoplasm and mitochondria; pantethine has significant lipid-lowering activity while pantothenic acid has very little; dose = 900 mg q.d.; reduces triglycerides by 32%, total cholesterol by 19%, LDL by 21%; increases HDL by 23%; especially useful for hyperlipidemia in diabetics; virtually no toxicity; mechanism of action – inhibits cholesterol synthesis and accelerates use of fat as energy source.

- **Vitamin C:** levels correspond to total cholesterol (TC) and HDL; the higher the ascorbate content of blood, the lower the TC and triglycerides and the higher the HDL; for each 0.5 mg/dl increase in blood ascorbate, HDL is increased 14.9 mg/dl in women and 2.1 mg/dl in men; most significant effects of high-dosage vitamin C may be reducing Lp(a) and antioxidant activity; reduces Lp(a) by 27%.

Botanical medicines

- ***Allium sativum* (garlic) and *Allium cepa* (onion):** garlic at daily dose of 10 mg alliin or total allicin potential of 4,000 μg lowers TC by 10–12%,

LDL and triglycerides by 15% each, and increases HDL by 10%; greatly improves LDL:HDL ratio; increase onion consumption; garlic dosage = 10 mg alliin or total allicin potential of 4,000 μg q.d. (German Commission E – 4,000 mg fresh garlic q.d. = 1–4 cloves; *Textbook*, Chs 62 and 63).

- **Gugulipid:** standardized extract of mukul myrrh tree (*Commiphora mukul*) of India; active components = Z-guggulsterone and E-guggulsterone; lowers TC by 14–27% in 4–12 weeks, LDL by 25–35%, and triglyceride by 22–30%; raises HDL by 16–20%; lipid reductions comparable to lipid-lowering drugs but without side-effects; mechanism of action – increases liver metabolism of LDL; guggulsterone increases liver uptake of LDL from blood; prevents formation of atherosclerosis and helps regress pre-existing plaques in animals; mildly inhibits platelet aggregation and promotes fibrinolysis – may prevent stroke or embolism; dosage based on guggulsterone content – gugulipid standardized to 25 mg guggulsterone per 500 mg tablet t.i.d.; no significant side-effects with purified gugulipid; crude guggul (e.g. gum guggul) is associated with side-effects (skin rashes, diarrhea, etc) (*Textbook*, Ch. 78).

Comparing natural cholesterol-lowering agents

- **Inositol hexaniacinate produces best overall effect:** along with dietary and lifestyle recommendations, niacin (1,000 mg t.i.d.) reduces TC by 50–75 mg/dl in patients with initial TC > 250 mg/dl within 2 months; initial TC > 300 mg/dl may take 4–6 months before reaching recommended levels; once TC < 200 mg/dl, reduce niacin dosage to 500 mg t.i.d. for 2 months; if cholesterol creeps above 200 mg/dl, restore dosage to 1,000 mg t.i.d.; if cholesterol remains < 200 mg/dl, then withdraw niacin completely; check cholesterol in 2 months; re-institute niacin if levels exceed 200 mg/dl.

- **Gugulipid** added to above protocol if after 4 months TC remains > 250 mg/dl; gugulipid also used for rare patient who cannot tolerate inositol hexaniacinate.

- **Pantethine:** for hypertriglyceridemia and cases of hyperlipidemia in diabetics (high-dose niacin adversely affects blood sugar control in some diabetics); normalizes platelet lipid composition and function, and blood viscosity.

- **Rule out hypothyroidism** in all cases of hyperlipidemia, especially Lp(a); overt hypothyroidism predisposes to CVD, due to increased LDL and decreased HDL; "subclinical" hypothyroidism (normal T_3 and FTI with raised TSH) is linked to significantly elevated LDL and Lp(a) (*Textbook*, Ch. 162).

GENERAL THERAPEUTIC CONSIDERATIONS

Antioxidant status: antioxidant nutrients (beta-carotene, Se, E, and C) protect against heart disease and slow down aging process; lipids are

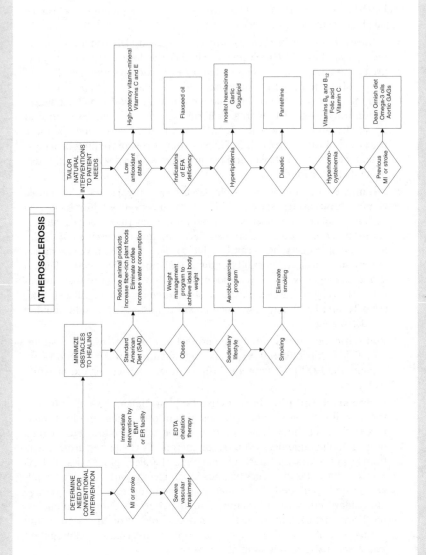

ATHEROSCLEROSIS

DETERMINE NEED FOR CONVENTIONAL INTERVENTION

MI or stroke → Immediate intervention by EMT or ER facility

Severe vascular impairment → EDTA chelation therapy

MINIMIZE OBSTACLES TO HEALING

Standard American Diet (SAD) → Reduce animal products / Increase fiber-rich plant foods / Eliminate coffee / Increase water consumption

Obese → Weight management program to achieve ideal body weight

Sedentary lifestyle → Aerobic exercise program

Smoking → Eliminate smoking

TAILOR NATURAL INTERVENTIONS TO PATIENT NEEDS

Low antioxidant status → High-potency vitamin-mineral / Vitamins C and E

Indications of EFA deficiency → Flaxseed oil

Hyperlipidemia → Inositol hexniacinate / Garlic / Gugulipid

Diabetic → Pantethine

Hyperhomocysteinemia → Vitamins B_6 and B_{12} / Folic acid / Vitamin C

Previous MI or stroke → Dean Ornish diet / Omega-3 oils / Aortic GAGs

particularly susceptible to free radical damage, forming lipid peroxides and oxidized cholesterol which damage artery walls and accelerate atherosclerosis; antioxidants block formation of damaging compounds; combination antioxidants provide greater protection than any single nutritional antioxidant; the two primary antioxidants are vitamins C ("aqueous phase") and E ("lipid phase") (*Textbook*, Ch. 99).

● **Vitamin E:** may offer greatest protection against LDL oxidation – easily incorporated into LDL molecule; the higher the dosage of vitamin E, the greater the degree of protection against LDL oxidative damage; doses of 400–800 IU required for significant effects; reduces LDL peroxidation and increases plasma LDL breakdown; inhibits excessive platelet aggregation; increases HDL; increases fibrinolytic activity; improves insulin sensitivity and plasma lipids in NIDDM; vitamin E levels may be more predictive of MI or stroke than TC; plays major role in treating heart disease, recovery from stroke, and peripheral vascular diseases (e.g. intermittent claudication).

● **Vitamin C:** first line of water-soluble antioxidant; partners = fat-soluble vitamin E and carotenes; works with antioxidant enzymes (glutathione peroxidase, catalase, and superoxide dismutase); regenerates oxidized vitamin E, thus potentiating antioxidant benefits of vitamin E; prevents LDL oxidation, even in smokers; significantly reduces risk of death from MI and stroke; lowers standardized mortality ratio (SMR) up to 48%, equivalent to increased longevity of 5–7 years for men and 1–3 years for women; lowers risk for CVD by acting as antioxidant, strengthening arterial collagen, lowering TC and Lp(a), lowering blood pressure, raising HDL, and inhibiting platelet aggregation.

● **Red wine:** flavonoids in red wine protect against LDL oxidation; serum antioxidant capacity (SAOX) effects – significantly better protection from consuming 1,000 mg vitamin C than one glass of either red or white wine.

● **Grape seed and pine bark extracts:** plant flavonoids called proanthocyanidins (or procyanidins); most potent proanthocyanidins = mixtures of proanthocyanidin dimers, trimers, tetramers, etc., called procyanidolic oligomers (PCOs); commercial PCO sources are extracts from grape seeds and bark of maritime (Landes) pine; uses of PCO extracts: vascular disorders (venous insufficiency, varicose veins, capillary fragility, diabetic retinopathy, macular degeneration); greater antioxidant effect than vitamins C and E; prevents damage to cholesterol and arterial lining; lowers blood cholesterol in animals and shrinks size of arterial cholesterol deposits; inhibits platelet aggregation and vasoconstriction in animals.

Platelet aggregation: excessive platelet aggregation is an independent risk factor for MI and strokes; aggregated platelets release compounds that promote atherosclerotic plaque or they can form obstructing clot; adhesiveness of platelets is determined by type of fats in diet and level of antioxidants; saturated fats and cholesterol increase platelet aggregation, while omega-3 oils have the opposite effect.

● **Essential fatty acids:** people who consume diets rich in omega-3 oils from fish or vegetable sources have reduced risk of heart disease; highest degree of coronary artery disease found in individuals with lowest concentration of omega-3 oils in their fat tissues; individuals with lowest degree of coronary artery disease have highest concentration of omega-3 oils; omega-3 fatty acids lower LDL and triglycerides, inhibit excessive platelet aggregation, lower fibrinogen levels, and lower systolic and diastolic BP in hypertensives; lowest rate of MI among people with high intake of alpha-linolenic acid (omega-3); oleic acid-containing oils (canola and olive oil) generate LDL that is less susceptible to peroxidation.

● **Vitamin B$_6$:** antioxidant nutrients, flavonoids, and B$_6$ inhibit platelet aggregation, lower BP and homocysteine; pyridoxine inhibits platelet aggregation by 41–48%, prolongs bleeding and coagulation time, but not over physiological limits, and has no effect on platelet count; pyridoxine lowers total plasma lipids and cholesterol.

● **Garlic:** inhibits platelet aggregation, increases microcirculation of the skin, and decreases plasma viscosity.

Fibrinogen formation: elevated fibrinogen is a major primary risk factor for CVD; stronger link to CVD deaths than cholesterol; natural therapies (e.g. exercise, omega-3 oils, niacin, and garlic) promoting fibrinolysis can prevent MI and strokes.

Hyperhomocysteinemia: homocysteine is an intermediate in conversion of methionine to cysteine; functional deficiency in folate, B$_6$, or B$_{12}$ induces increase in homocysteine – promoting atherosclerosis by directly damaging artery, reducing vessel integrity and interfering with formation of proper collagen; independent risk factor for MI, stroke, and peripheral vascular disease; found in 20–40% of patients with heart disease; folic acid (400 µg q.d.) alone could reduce number of MIs by 10%; folate, B$_{12}$, and B$_6$ work synergistically for proper homocysteine metabolism.

"Type A" personality: extreme sense of time urgency, competitiveness, impatience, and aggressiveness; twofold increase in coronary heart disease; regular expression of anger damaging to cardiovascular system; positive correlation between serum cholesterol level and aggression – the higher the aggression, the higher the cholesterol level; negative correlation between LDL/HDL ratio and controlled affect – the greater the ability to control anger, the lower the LDL/HDL ratio; those who learn to control anger experience reduction in the risk for heart disease; unfavorable lipid profile is linked to aggressive (hostile) anger coping style.

Other nutritional factors

● **Magnesium (Mg) and potassium (K):** absolutely essential to cardiovascular functioning; prevent heart disease and strokes; Mg and/or K supplementation is effective for angina, arrhythmias, CHF and hypertension; (K – *Textbook*, Ch. 159); average US Mg intake = 143–266 mg q.d.; Mg RDA = 350 mg for men and 300 mg for women; Mg sources are whole foods – tofu, legumes, seeds, nuts, whole grains, and green leafy vegetables; people dying of MI have low heart Mg; i.v. Mg is a treatment measure in acute MI – during first hour after hospital admission it reduces immediate and long-term complications and death rates; benefits of Mg for MI: improves heart energy production, dilates coronary arteries, reduces peripheral vascular resistance, inhibits platelet aggregation and blood clotting, reduces size of infarct, and improves heart rate and arrhythmias.

Preventing recurrent heart attack

Primary prevention of subsequent cardiovascular events is by controlling major risk factors – hyperlipidemia, hypertension, smoking, diabetes, and physical inactivity.

● **Aspirin (ASA):** statistically significant reduction in mortality; reduces mortality rate from all causes and cardiovascular deaths; mortality rate for all causes reduced by 30% with ASA at doses of 326–1500 mg q.d.; ASA linked with risk of GI bleeding due to peptic ulcer at all dosage levels; for preventing stroke, dosage necessary = 900 mg.

● **Natural alternatives to aspirin:** dietary modifications are not only more effective in preventing MI recurrence than ASA, but can reverse blockage of clogged arteries; Dean Ornish diet – low-fat vegetarian × 1 year (fruits, vegetables, grains, legumes, and soybean products with no animal products except egg white and 1 cup non-fat milk or yogurt q.d.) – 10% fat, 15–20% protein, and 70–75% complex carbohydrate; stress reduction techniques – breathing exercises, stretching, meditation, imagery, etc. for 1 h q.d. plus exercise at least 3 h/week; regimen induces regression in atherosclerosis of coronary vessels; American Heart Association's dietary recommendations are ineffective; people consuming a diet rich in omega-3 oils have significantly reduced risk of heart disease; the highest degree of CAD is in individuals with the lowest omega-3 oils in fat tissues; individuals with lowest degree of CAD have highest omega-3 oils; omega-3 fatty acids from plant sources (alpha-linolenic acid) offer the same protection as increased fish intake; Lyon Heart Study (Mediterranean/Cretan diet): whole-grain bread, root vegetables, green vegetables, fish, less meat (beef, lamb, pork replaced with poultry), fruit, butter and cream replaced with canola and olive oil.

● **Glycosaminoglycans (GAGs):** mixture of purified bovine GAGs native to aorta tissue (dermatan sulfate, heparin sulfate, hyaluronic acid, chondroitin sulfate, and related hexosaminoglycans) inhibit platelet aggregation; protect and promote normal artery and vein function; effective in treating cerebral and peripheral arterial insufficiency, venous insufficiency and varicose veins, hemorrhoids, vascular retinopathies including macular degeneration, and post-surgical edema; value primarily for patients recovering from MI or stroke, angiograms, coronary artery bypass surgery, or angioplasty; dosage = 100 mg q.d.; less impressive results in treating atherosclerosis with chondroitin sulfate at 3 g q.d. (1 g with meals t.i.d.).

- **Preventing a subsequent stroke:** *Ginkgo biloba* extract standardized to 24% ginkgo flavonglycosides and 6% terpenoids improves cerebral vascular insufficiency, short-term memory loss, depression, dizziness, ringing in ears, and HA; ginkgo enhances stroke recovery.

Other considerations

- **Angiography, coronary artery bypass surgery or angioplasty:** procedures used far more frequently than justified by appropriateness and efficacy (*Textbook*, Ch.129).
- **Intravenous EDTA chelation therapy:** *Textbook*, Chapter 129.
- **Ear lobe crease:** presence of diagonal ear lobe crease has been considered a sign of cardiovascular disease since 1973; ear lobe richly vascularized, and decreased blood flow over extended period collapses vascular bed, causing diagonal crease; 82% accuracy in predicting heart disease, with false-positive rate of 12% and false-negative rate of 18%; highly correlated with demonstrable heart disease and, less strongly, with previous MI; seen more commonly with advancing age, until age 80, when incidence drops dramatically; link to heart disease is age-independent; better predictor of heart disease than any other known risk factor, including age, smoking, sedentary lifestyle, hyperlipidemia, etc; presence does not prove heart disease, but strongly suggests it; correlation does not hold true with Asians, Native Americans, and children with Beckwith's syndrome.

THERAPEUTIC APPROACH

Tailor interventions to individual patient needs.

- **Dietary and lifestyle recommendations:** reduce or eliminate animal products; increase fiber-rich plant foods (fruits, vegetables, grains, legumes, and raw nuts and seeds); achieve ideal body weight; regular aerobic exercise; avoid smoking; eliminate coffee (caffeine and decaf); 1.4+ L water q.d.
- **Supplements** (high-potency multiple vitamin-mineral):
  — vitamin C: 500–1,000 mg t.i.d.

— vitamin E: 400–800 IU q.d.

— flaxseed oil: 1 tbsp q.d.

— inositol hexaniacinate: 500 mg t.i.d. with meals × 2 weeks, then increase to 1,000 mg t.i.d. with meals

— garlic: providing 4,000 µg allicin q.d. (or equal to 4000 µg of fresh garlic)

— *diabetics* – pantethine: 300 mg t.i.d.

Atopic dermatitis (eczema)

DIAGNOSTIC SUMMARY

Chronic, pruritic, inflammatory skin condition; skin is dry and hyperkeratotic; lesions include excoriations, papules, eczema (patches of erythema, exudation, and scaling with small vesicles formed within epidermis), and lichenification (hyperpigmented plaques of thickened skin with accentuated furrows); scratching and rubbing lead to lichenification, most commonly in antecubital and popliteal flexures; personal or family history of atopy.

GENERAL CONSIDERATIONS

Common condition (2.4–7% of population).

- **Immediate hypersensitivity disease:** serum IgE elevated in 80% of patients; all patients have positive skin, RAST, and other allergy tests; positive family history in two-thirds of eczema patients; many develop allergic rhinitis and/or asthma; most improve with elimination diet.

- **Physiological and anatomical abnormalities of skin:** type of abnormality determines manner in which atopic dermatitis (AD) is manifested in each patient – lowered threshold to itch stimuli (substance P excess?); hypersensitivity to alpha-adrenergic agonists and cholinergic agents via partial beta-adrenergic blockade (receptor site insensitivity); dry, hyperkeratotic skin with decreased water-holding capacity (dry – zinc or thyroid deficiency; hyperkeratotic – vitamin A deficiency?); tendency to lichenify in response to rubbing and scratching (membrane fragility?); skin heavily colonized by bacteria (coagulase-positive *Staphylococcus aureus*) (immune dysfunction).

- **Dennie's sign** (accentuated double pleat below margin of lower eyelid) and tendency towards vasoconstriction provoked by physical pressure ("white dermatographism").

- **Immunological abnormalities:** leukocytes have decreased cAMP due to increased cyclic AMP-phosphodiesterase activity and decreased prostaglandin precursors; decreased intracellular cAMP increases histamine release and decreases bactericidal activity.

- **Defect in serum bactericidal activity** (alternate complement pathway, ACP): inulin-containing herbs (burdock root [*Arctium lappa*] and dandelion root [*Taraxacum officinale*]) may restore bactericidal activity and increase cAMP – inulin activates ACP.

● **Predominance of pathogenic *Staphylococcus aureus*** in skin flora in 90% of patients – increased susceptibility to *Staphylococcus* infections.

● **Cell-mediated immunity defects:** increased susceptibility to cutaneous herpes simplex, vaccinia, molluscum contagiosum, and verruca vulgaris infections; reduced delayed-type hypersensitivity, cutaneous anergy, and decreased in vitro lymphocyte reactivity to mitogens and antigens; cell-mediated defects normalize during remission and abnormalize again during recurrences.

THERAPEUTIC CONSIDERATIONS

● **Food allergy:** major role in atopic dermatitis (*Textbook*, Ch. 51); breast-feeding acts as prophylaxis against atopic dermatitis (and allergies in general); breast-fed infants develop atopic dermatitis due to transfer of antigens in breast milk – mothers should avoid common food allergens (milk, eggs, peanuts, fish, soy, wheat, citrus, and chocolate); in older or formula-fed infants, milk, eggs, and peanuts are the most common foods inducing atopic dermatitis; virtually any food can be offending agent; diagnosis of food allergy – best via elimination diet and challenge; lab methods to identify food allergens in eczema: ELISA IgE and IgG_4 (*Textbook*, Ch. 15); food allergies linked to "leaky gut", i.e. increased gut permeability with increased antigen load on immune system and developing additional allergies; eliminating allergenic foods can stop development of new allergies; avoiding offending foods for 1 year may eradicate allergy – loss rate after 1 year is 26% for five major allergens (egg, milk, wheat, soy, peanut) and 66% for other foods.

● ***Candida albicans:*** GI overgrowth is the causative factor in allergies including atopic dermatitis; elevated anti-*Candida* antibodies are common in atopy; severity of lesions correlates with level of IgE antibodies to *Candida*; anti-*Candida* therapy (*Textbook*, Ch. 48) may significantly improve atopic dermatitis.

● **Essential fatty acids and prostaglandin metabolism:** AD patients have altered EFA and prostaglandin metabolism – increased linoleic acid levels to be increased with decreased longer-chain PUFAs (gamma-linolenic acid and arachidonic acid) and omega-3 oils (eicosapentaenoic acid [EPA] and docosahexanoic acid [DHA]); proportions of linoleic acid in total plasma lipids and phospholipids are greater, and those of oleic acid lower, than normal in AD patients; ratio of omega-3 to omega-6 fatty acids is lower in AD patients; no significant decreases in proportions of dihomo-gamma-linolenic acid and arachidonic acid observed in plasma lipids of atopic patients, suggesting delta-6-desaturase is not impaired; "fish oil", providing EPA and DHA or simply eating more fatty fish (mackerel, herring, salmon), increases omega-3 fatty acids in membrane phospholipids; degree of clinical improvement correlates with increased DHA in serum phospholipids; fish oils are more effective in raising DHA than flaxseed oil – EPA/DHA supplements or increasing consumption of cold-water fish may produce better results than flaxseed oil.

● **Inhibiting excess histamine release:** agents which stimulate cAMP production and/or inhibit cAMP phosphodiesterase reduce inflammatory process in AD by reducing shunting to histamine; *Coleus forskohlii* strongly enhances cAMP; many botanicals inhibit diesterase – licorice (*Glycyrrhiza glabra*) shows marked activity; flavonoids also inhibit cAMP phosphodiesterase – quercetin and hyperoside, the flavones orientin and vitexin, and the flavanone naringen; the common flavanol, rutin, has < 1/10 activity of quercetin; flavonoid extracts from *Vaccinium myrtillus*, *Rosa damascena*, *Ruta graveolens*, *Prunus spinosa* and *Crataegus pentagyna* are the most potent inhibitors of cAMP phosphodiesterase and also inhibit mast cell degranulation; flavonoid-rich extracts (grape seed, pine bark, green tea, *Ginkgo biloba*) may prove helpful; *Ginkgo* terpenes (ginkgolides) antagonize platelet-activating factor (PAF), the key mediator in AD; PAF plays central role in neutrophil activation, increasing vascular permeability, smooth muscle contraction (bronchoconstriction) and reduced coronary blood flow; ginkgolides compete with PAF for binding sites; mixtures of ginkgolides and *Ginkgo biloba* extract (standardized to 24% ginkgo flavonglycosides and 6% terpenoids) demonstrate significant anti-allergy effects.

● **Zinc:** low Zn is common in AD; EFA metabolism is essential in AD (Zn required for delta-6-desaturase).

Botanical medicines

Two categories: internal and external.

● **Licorice (*Glycyrrhiza glabra*):** useful in either application; internally, licorice has anti-inflammatory and anti-allergic effects (*Textbook*, Ch. 90).

● **Chinese herbal formula:** used in double-blind crossover trials; contains licorice, plus *Ledebourieella seseloides*, *Potentilla chinensis*, *Clematis chenisis*, *Clematis armandi*, *Rehmania glutinosa*, *Paeonia lactiflora*, *Lophatherum gracile*, *Dictamnus dasycarpus*, *Tribulus terrestris*, *Schizonepeta tenuiflora* – significant objective and subjective improvement in adults and children but many patients complained about unpalatability of decoction; base dosage upon level of delivered licorice; topical licorice: commercial preparations featuring pure glycyrrhetinic acid – effect similar to topical hydrocortisone for eczema, contact and allergic dermatitis, and psoriasis.

Miscellaneous factors

● **Hypothyroid** patients with eczema respond well to thyroid.

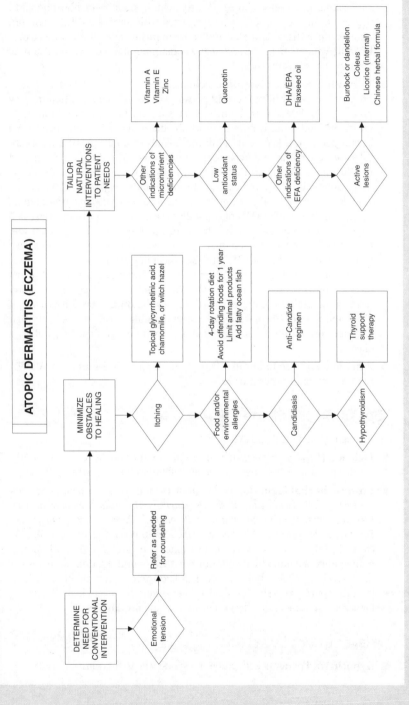

ATOPIC DERMATITIS (ECZEMA)

DETERMINE NEED FOR CONVENTIONAL INTERVENTION

- Emotional tension → Refer as needed for counseling

MINIMIZE OBSTACLES TO HEALING

- Itching → Topical glycyrrhetinic acid, chamomile, or witch hazel
- Food and/or environmental allergies → 4-day rotation diet / Avoid offending foods for 1 year / Limit animal products / Add fatty ocean fish
- Candidiasis → Anti-*Candida* regimen
- Hypothyroidism → Thyroid support therapy

TAILOR NATURAL INTERVENTIONS TO PATIENT NEEDS

- Other indications of micronutrient deficiencies → Vitamin A / Vitamin E / Zinc
- Low antioxidant status → Quercetin
- Other indications of EFA deficiency → DHA/EPA / Flaxseed oil
- Active lesions → Burdock or dandelion / Coleus / Licorice (internal) / Chinese herbal formula

- **Scratching:** extremely detrimental in AD – breaks skin, aiding bacterial ingress, and promotes lichenification; factors which limit itching promote healing and prevent recurrence.

- **Emotional tension:** aggravates itching in AD; AD patients show higher anxiety, hostility, and neurosis than matched controls.

THERAPEUTIC APPROACH

Relieve and prevent itching while treating underlying metabolic abnormalities; detect and control food and environmental allergens; normalize prostaglandin metabolism; balance immune system.

- **Diet:** 4-day rotation diet, eliminating all major allergens (milk, eggs, peanuts in 81% of cases); as patient improves, slowly reintroduce allergens and reduce stringency of rotation diet; limit animal products; add fatty fish (salmon, mackerel, herring, halibut).

- **Supplements:**
  — vitamin A: 50,000 IU q.d.
  — vitamin E: 400 IU q.d. mixed tocopherols
  — zinc: 50 mg q.d. – decrease as condition clears
  — quercetin: 200–400 mg t.i.d. 5–10 min before meals
  — EPA and DHA: 540 and 360 mg q.d. (or flaxseed oil 10 g q.d.)
  — evening primrose oil: 3,000 mg q.d.

- **Botanicals** (t.i.d.):
  — *Arctium lappa* or *Taraxacum officinale*:
      dried root: 2–8 g by infusion or decoction
      fluid extract (1:1): 4–8 ml (1–2 tsp)
      tincture: alcohol-based tinctures of dandelion are not recommended because of the extremely high dosage required
      juice of fresh root: 4–8 ml (1–2 tsp)
      powdered solid extract (4:1): 250–500 mg
  — *Coleus forskohlii* extract standardized to 18% forskolin: 50 mg (9 mg of forskolin)
  — *Glycyrrhiza glabra*:
      powdered root: 1–2 g
      fluid extract (1:1): 2–4 ml
      solid (dry powdered) extract (4:1): 250–500 mg.

- **Topical treatment:** glycyrrhetinic acid-containing commercial preparations; chamomile preparations (*Textbook*, Ch. 184); witch hazel preparations.
- **Helpful tips:** avoid sweating and rough-textured clothing; wash clothing with mild soaps only and rinse thoroughly; avoid exposure to chemical irritants; local application of soothing lotions ameliorates itching (zinc oxide); but minimize greasy preparations that block the sweat ducts.
- **Psychological:** determine if patient has significant anxiety, hostility, or neurosis; refer to counselor for therapy as needed.

Attention deficit disorders (hyperactivity and childhood learning disorders)

DIAGNOSTIC SUMMARY

● **Hyperactivity (attention deficit disorder with hyperactivity):** inattention, impulsiveness, and hyperactivity inappropriate for mental and chronological age.
● **Learning disability (attention deficit disorder without hyperactivity):** developmentally inappropriate brief attention span and poor concentration for mental and chronological age.

GENERAL CONSIDERATIONS

The term "ADD" encompasses a wide variety of terms used historically to describe similar disorders – hyperkinetic reaction of childhood, hyperkinetic syndrome, hyperactive child syndrome, minimal brain damage, minimal brain dysfunction, minimal cerebral dysfunction, and minor cerebral dysfunction; three separate ADD disorders exist – (1) ADD without hyperactivity, (2) ADD with hyperactivity, and (3) ADD, residual type; hyperactivity discussion is here concerned largely with food additives, food allergies, and sucrose; discussion of ADD without hyperactivity focuses on heavy metals; residual ADD (patient 18 years or older) is the continuation of the process; factors discussed under one disorder may be relevant to the other; recurrent otitis media (*Textbook*, Ch. 178) and antibiotic use are linked with greater likelihood of developing ADD.

HYPERACTIVITY (ATTENTION DEFICIT DISORDER WITH HYPERACTIVITY)

● **Incidence:** 3% of school-age children – over 2 million American children (mostly boys) take methylphenidate (Ritalin); much greater incidence in boys than in girls (10:1); onset by age 3; diagnosis not made until later when child enters school.

● **Characteristics:** hyperactivity, perceptual motor impairment, emotional lability, general coordination deficit, disorders of attention (short attention span, distractibility, lack of perseverance, failure to finish things off, not listening, poor concentration), impulsiveness (action before thought, abrupt shifts in activity, poor organizing, jumping up in class), disorders of memory and thinking, specific learning disabilities, disorders of speech and hearing, equivocal neurological signs and EEG irregularities.

● **Difficulties in school:** learning and behavior.

● **Food additives, food sensitivities, and sucrose consumption:** responsible for the majority of hyperactivity in the US:

● **Food additives:** 5,000 chemical additives used in USA; 1985 per capita daily consumption = 13–15 g; total annual consumption of food colors alone being 100 million lb; hypothesis of Benjamin Feingold MD: 40–50% of hyperactive children are sensitive to food additives and naturally occurring salicylates and phenolic compounds; research focused on only 10 food dyes vs. 3,000 additives of concern to Feingold; 50% of those who tried Feingold diet displayed decreased hyperactivity.

● **Sucrose:** interrelationship between sucrose consumption and artificial food dyes – destructive-aggressive and restless behavior well linked with amount of sucrose consumed; Langseth and Dowd findings: 75% of hyperactive children displayed abnormal glucose tolerance curves, with predominant abnormality being a low, flat curve; hypoglycemia promotes hyperkinesis via increased catecholamine secretion; refined carbohydrate is the major factor in promoting reactive hypoglycemia.

● **Food allergies (sensitivities):** artificial colorings and preservatives are the most common provoking substances, but few children are sensitive to these alone; food sensitivities provoke psychological symptoms; Eggers oligoantigenic diet (lamb, chicken, potatoes, rice, banana, apple, brassica family vegetable, calcium gluconate 3 g q.d., and multiple vitamin) for 4 weeks improved 82% of hyperactive children, with normal behavior achieved in one-third of these; HAs, abdominal pains, and fits also improved; reintroduction of allergenic foods caused return of symptoms and hyperactivity (*Textbook*, Ch. 51); 86% of hyperactive children have elevated eosinophils; more recent Eggers oligoantigenic diet consists of two meats (lamb and chicken), two carbohydrates (potatoes and rice), two fruits (banana and pears), vegetables (cabbage, sprouts, cauliflower, broccoli, cucumber, celery, and carrots), and water, supplemented with Ca, Mg, Zn and some basic vitamins – behavior improved in 63% of hyperactive children; provoking foods identified by sequential reintroduction; on a statistical basis, every study, both supportive and critical of the hypothesis, is marred by significant experimental design defects; critics of the hypothesis misuse apparently inconsistent statistical group results to ignore significance of clear (reproducible under double-blind conditions) individual results.

THERAPEUTIC APPROACH

Some hyperactive children consistently react with behavioral problems when challenged by specific food additives; eliminating all food additives is practically difficult; best results depend on accurate identification of offending agents (including food allergens), preferably with behavioral, rather than laboratory measurements; oligoantigenic diet (individualized to patient) × 4 weeks, followed by reintroduction/challenge of suspected foods (full servings at least once q.d., one food introduced per week); if symptoms recur or worsen upon reintroduction, the food should be withdrawn; if no improvement on oligoantigenic diet, child may be reacting to something in the diet or environment – further testing indicated; eliminate all refined sugars; add hypoallergenic multiple vitamin-mineral; factors discussed under "Learning disability" (below) should be considered – hyperactive children may have increased lead levels.

LEARNING DISABILITY (ATTENTION DEFICIT DISORDER WITHOUT HYPERACTIVITY)

Three major factors particularly relevant – (1) otitis media, (2) nutrient deficiency, and (3) heavy metals.

- **Otitis media (OM):** children with moderate to severe hearing loss can have impaired speech and language development, lowered IQ scores, and learning difficulties; early incidence of OM twice as common in learning-disabled children as in non-learning-disabled – must deal with otitis media preventively (see Otitis media chapter), since factors linked to hyperactivity are also linked to OM.

- **Nutrient deficiency:** any nutrient deficiency can impair CNS function; Fe is the most commonly deficient nutrient in American children; Fe deficiency effects = decreased attentiveness, less purposeful and narrower attention span, decreased persistence, and decreased voluntary activity responsive to supplementation; correcting even subtle nutritional variables has substantial influence on learning and behavior; "megavitamins" are of limited value.

- **Heavy metals:** strong relationship between childhood learning disabilities (and other disorders including criminal behavior) and body stores of heavy metals, especially lead (Pb); learning disabilities linked to high hair levels of mercury, cadmium, lead, copper, and manganese; poor nutrition is often linked to elevation of heavy metals – decreased consumption of food fac-

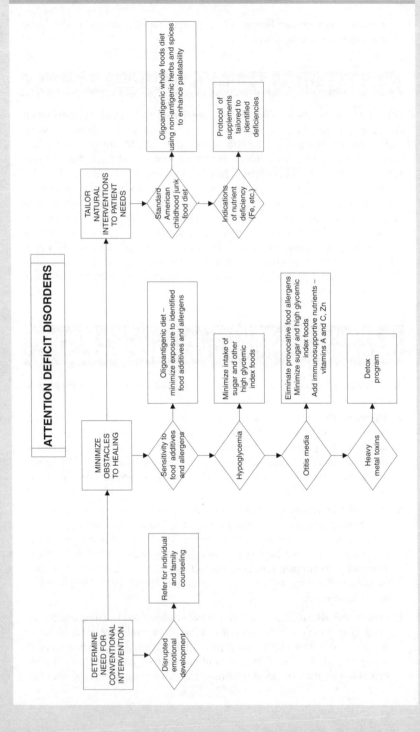

ATTENTION DEFICIT DISORDERS

DETERMINE NEED FOR CONVENTIONAL INTERVENTION

Disrupted emotional development → Refer for individual and family counseling

MINIMIZE OBSTACLES TO HEALING

Sensitivity to food additives and allergens → Oligoantigenic diet – minimize exposure to identified food additives and allergens

Hypoglycemia → Minimize intake of sugar and other high glycemic index foods

Otitis media → Eliminate provocative food allergens / Minimize sugar and high glycemic index foods / Add immunosupportive nutrients – vitamins A and C, Zn

Heavy metal toxins → Detox program

TAILOR NATURAL INTERVENTIONS TO PATIENT NEEDS

Standard American childhood junk food diet → Oligoantigenic whole foods diet using non-antigenic herbs and spices to enhance palatability

Indications of nutrient deficiency (Fe, etc.) → Protocol of supplements tailored to identified deficiencies

tors that chelate heavy metals or decrease their absorption (*Textbook*, Ch.18); screening for Pb toxicity is an essential part of evaluating a child with ADD symptoms or developmental delay (DD); hair mineral analysis or EDTA challenge more accurately reflects brain Pb toxicity than blood tests.

THERAPEUTIC APPROACH

Eliminate underlying otitis media (See Otitis media chapter); detect and eliminate any heavy metal toxicity (*Textbook*, Ch. 18); establish optimal nutrition for these children; counseling is indicated in most cases, ideally involving whole family.

Autism

DIAGNOSTIC SUMMARY

Syndrome of early childhood (first diagnosed no later than age 30 months) characterized by: profound failure to develop social relationships; language disorder with impaired understanding, echolalia, and pronominal reversal; rituals and compulsive phenomena; general retardation in intellectual development (most cases); male:female ratio = 4:1.

GENERAL CONSIDERATIONS

Originally thought to be primarily a psychiatric condition; recent hypothesis: organic defect in brain development – abnormal serotonin metabolism in brain; prognosis quite poor: only 1 in 20 improve by adulthood; prognosis related to IQ test results by experienced examiner; half of autistic children with IQ > 50 do moderately well or even attain normal adjustment, with appropriate behavioral therapy, psychotherapy, and special schooling; IQ < 50 – temporal lobe epilepsy eventually manifests; no specific medical treatment – phenothiazines only control severe aggressive and self-destructive behavior; vitamin B_6 and magnesium (Mg) (although not effective for all autistic children), used in combination, can greatly help significant portion.

THERAPEUTIC CONSIDERATIONS

● **Serotonin:** documented abnormalities = defect in serotonin metabolism; abnormal release and uptake of serotonin by platelets; abnormal kynurenine metabolism; increased serum serotonin and free tryptophan; abnormal urinary 5-hydroxyindolacetic acid (5-HIAA) levels; abnormal urinary serotonin metabolites; basic defect = decreased CNS serotonin activity despite elevated free tryptophan in serum; possible mechanisms to explain brain serotonin hypoactivity: (1) reduced tryptophan hydroxylase or l-aromatic amino acid decarboxylase activity causing impaired serotonin synthesis and, via feedback control, increased serum free tryptophan; (2) increased tryptophan oxygenase activity causing elevated kynurenine, reducing available tryptophan for serotonin synthesis and inhibiting tryptophan transport across blood–brain barrier; increased free tryptophan increasing tryptophan oxygenase activity, setting up positive feedback cycle; (3) increased degradation of serotonin by MAO or other enzymes; (4) abnormal blood levels of albumin and non-esterified fatty acids are directly involved in variation of serum free tryptophan; (5) lowered sensitivity of neuronal serotonin receptors, increasing serotonin synthesis through a feedback cycle; postulates (1) and (2) most plausible and most supported by scientific literature.

- **Folic acid, vitamin B_{12}, and vitamin C:** if defect due to decreased tryptophan hydroxylase activity (tetrahydrobiopterin [BH_4] dependent enzyme), then folate, ascorbate and B_{12} may increase enzyme activity by increasing BH_4; no studies with autistic children; increasing CNS BH_4 levels benefits patients with affective disorders and Parkinson's.

- **Pyridoxine:** if defect in decarboxylation or abnormal kynurenine metabolism, B_6 indicated; subgroup of autistic children improves with B_6 with reduced urinary homovanillic acid (HVA); only 20% show moderate improvement in symptom scores; 10% show dramatic clinical improvement; B_6 has greater effect used in combination with Mg; B_6 plus Mg improves behavior in fashion closely associated with decreases in HVA excretion and normalized evoked potential recordings (EP) amplitude and morphology; Mg or B_6 not very effective used alone; tryptophan load test indicated to screen for B_6-responsive patients and to monitor B_6 dosage (*Textbook*, Ch. 28); according to researcher Rimland 25–50% of children significantly helped, with 20% dramatically improving.

- **Serotonin metabolites:** may contribute to mental dysfunction; LSD, psilocybin, ergot, and other hallucinogens are serotonin analogs; some serotonin metabolites are hallucinogens; serotonin and its metabolites are produced in, and absorbed from, intestines.

- **Food allergies and intestinal permeability:** food allergies contribute to behavioral disorders; gluten and milk may be food allergens in these patients; diets with reduced/eliminated milk and gluten for 1 year increase social contact, decrease stereotypy, end self-mutilation (head banging) and decrease "dreamy state" periods with accompanying decrease in urinary peptide excretion; possible mechanism: autistics suffer from peptidase defects that fail to break down "exorphins" (exogenous opioids) in milk and wheat; exorphin peptides enter brain and disrupt brain chemistry; identify other food allergies that can increase intestinal permeability noted in autistics; increased gut permeability suggested as possible causative factor for autism.

THERAPEUTIC APPROACH

Information for developing effective therapy incomplete; electroconvulsive therapy should be discouraged.

AUTISM

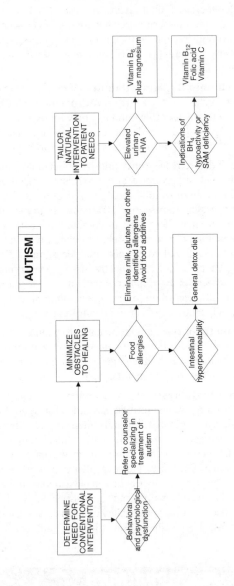

work-up for environmental and food allergies; eliminate dust mites – warm water washing at temperature of at least 58°C, air-filtering vacuum cleaners, air cleaner with HEPA filter, and humidity < 50%; remove all pets, carpeting and feather bedding, if necessary.

● **Sick building syndrome:** environmental chemicals within buildings can induce lethargy, HA, and blocked or runny nose – symptoms of chronic sinusitis.

● *Helicobacter pylori:* in atopic patients with symptoms of peptic ulcer, urticaria, sinusitis and exercise-induced anaphylaxis increased when patients were positive for *H. pylori; H. pylori*-specific IgE and IgG reactivity identified with endoscopy confirming *H. pylori* in stomachs or sinuses of those with *H. pylori* antibodies; antibiotic therapy for *H. pylori*-induced ulcers resolves allergy symptoms in a significant number of such patients.

THERAPEUTIC APPROACH

● **Therapeutic goals:** re-establish drainage and clear acute infection.

● **Methods:** local heat application, local use of volatile oils, antibacterial botanicals, and immune system support (*Textbook*, Ch. 53):

— isolate and eliminate food or air-borne allergens and correct underlying problem allowing allergy to develop (*Textbook*, Ch. 51).

— acute phase: eliminate common food allergens (milk, wheat, eggs, citrus, corn, and peanut butter) until more definitive diagnosis made.

— local applications of heat may alleviate short- and long-term symptoms of allergic rhinitis.

● **Supplements:**

— vitamin C: 500 mg every 2 h

— bioflavonoids: 1,000 mg q.d.

— vitamin A: 5,000 IU q.d. (or beta-carotene 25,000 IU q.d.)

— zinc: 30 mg q.d.

— thymus extract: 120 mg pure polypeptides with molecular weights < 10,000 or 500 mg crude polypeptide fraction q.d.

● **Botanicals:**

— *Echinacea* species (t.i.d.):

dried root (or as tea): 0.5–1 g

freeze-dried plant: 325–650 mg

juice of aerial portion of *E. purpurea* stabilized in 22% ethanol: 2–3 ml

tincture (1:5): 2–4 ml

fluid extract (1:1): 2–4 ml

solid (dry powdered) extract (6.5:1 or 3.5% echinacoside): 150–300 mg

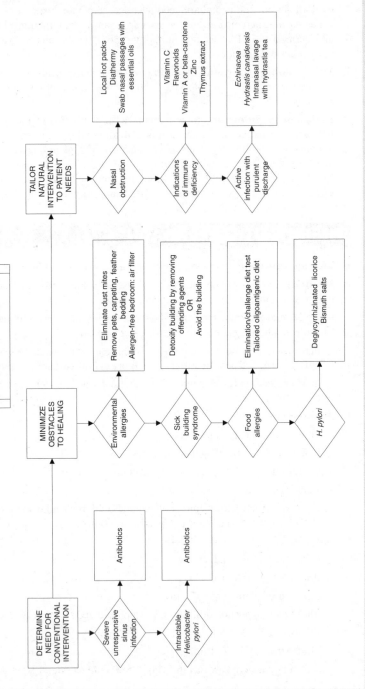

BACTERIAL SINUSITIS

DETERMINE NEED FOR CONVENTIONAL INTERVENTION

Severe unresponsive sinus infection → Antibiotics

Intractable *Helicobacter pylori* → Antibiotics

MINIMIZE OBSTACLES TO HEALING

Environmental allergies → Eliminate dust mites
Remove pets, carpeting, feather bedding
Allergen-free bedroom: air filter

Sick building syndrome → Detoxify building by removing offending agents OR Avoid the building

Food allergies → Elimination/challenge diet test
Tailored oligoantigenic diet

H. pylori → Deglycyrrhizinated licorice
Bismuth salts

TAILOR NATURAL INTERVENTION TO PATIENT NEEDS

Nasal obstruction → Local hot packs
Diathermy
Swab nasal passages with essential oils

Indications of immune deficiency → Vitamin C
Flavonoids
Vitamin A or beta-carotene
Zinc
Thymus extract

Active infection with purulent discharge → *Echinacea*
Hydrastis canadensis
Intranasal lavage with hydrastis tea

— *Hydrastis canadensis*: dosage based on berberine content – prefer standardized extracts:

dried root or as infusion (tea): 2–4 g

tincture (1:5): 6–12 ml (1.5–3 tsp)

fluid extract (1:1): 2–4 ml (0.5–1 tsp)

solid (powdered dry) extract (4:1 or 8–12% alkaloid content): 250–500 mg.

● **Local treatment:**

— intranasal douche with hydrastis tea

— swab passages with oil of bitter orange, Menthol or eucalyptus packs over sinuses (care should be taken to avoid irritation)

— hot packs

— diathermy: 30 min (discontinue if pain increases without drainage).

Benign prostatic hyperplasia

DIAGNOSTIC SUMMARY

- Symptoms of bladder outlet obstruction: progressive urinary frequency, urgency and nocturia, hesitancy and intermittency with reduced force and caliber of urine.
- Enlarged, non-tender prostate.
- Uremia if prolonged obstruction.

GENERAL CONSIDERATIONS

- **Affects over 50% of men in their lifetime:** incidence increases with advancing age: 5–10% at age 30, over 90% over age 85.
- **Androgen-dependent disorder of metabolism:** free testosterone (T) levels decrease with age; prolactin, estradiol, sex hormone-binding ligand, luteinizing hormone (LH), and follicle-stimulating hormone (FSH) levels increase; increased synthesis of potent androgen dihydrotestosterone (DHT) from T by 5-alpha-reductase and decreased hydroxylation metabolism of T and DHT due to inhibition by elevated estrogens.
- **Ultimate effect:** increased intraprostatic DHT; prostatic androgen receptors have a fivefold greater affinity for DHT than T; BPH tissue has three- to fourfold greater net ability to increase tissue levels of DHT.

DIAGNOSTIC CONSIDERATIONS

- Originates in periurethral and transition zones of prostate as early as the third decade of life.
- Develops from microscopic to palpable enlargement with age and androgen influence.
- Symptomatic in only 50–60% of men with macroscopic enlargement; many men symptomatic without macroscopic enlargement: hyperplasia constricts urethral lumen.

● Digital palpation for diagnosis is unreliable: half of men with palpable enlargement are symptomatic, and half without palpable enlargement are symptomatic.

● Rule out prostate cancer using prostate-specific antigen (PSA): normal < 4 ng/ml; elevation > 10 highly indicative of prostate cancer (90% of cases); there may be cancer without PSA elevation; mid-range elevations can occur with BPH, prostatitis, urinary retention, ejaculation, and exercise.

THERAPEUTIC CONSIDERATIONS

● **Natural course of untreated disease process:** bladder outlet obstruction, urinary retention, kidney damage.

● **TURP (transurethral resection of the prostate):** high rate of morbidity.

Nutritional factors

● Avoid pesticides; increase zinc and essential fatty acids; keep cholesterol levels < 200 mg/dl.

● **Diet:** high-protein diet (total calories: 44% protein, 35% carbohydrate, 21% fat) inhibits 5-alpha-reductase; low-protein diet (10% protein, 70% carbohydrate, 20% fat) stimulates the enzyme; speculative because never clinically tested on men with BPH.

● **Zinc:** reduces size of prostate and symptomatology in most patients; intestinal uptake is impaired by estrogens (increased in men with BPH), enhanced by androgens; inhibits 5-alpha-reductase; inhibits specific binding of androgens to the cytosol and nuclear receptors; inhibits prolactin secretion, reducing prostatic androgen uptake.

● **Alcohol:** beer raises prolactin levels; higher alcohol intake is definitely associated with BPH, especially beer, wine and sake.

● **Essential fatty acids:** can significantly improve symptoms in many patients; may correct underlying EFA deficiency since prostatic and seminal lipid levels and ratios are often abnormal.

● **Amino acids:** combination of glycine, alanine, and glutamic acid (two six-grain capsules t.i.d. for 2 weeks, one capsule t.i.d. thereafter) relieves many symptoms; mechanism of action unknown; amino acids may act as inhibitory neurotransmitters, reducing feelings of full bladder.

● **Cholesterol:** metabolites are cytotoxic, carcinogenic, accumulate in hyperplastic or cancerous prostate tissue; epoxycholesterols degenerate epithelial cells, triggering increased hyperplastic regeneration.

● **Soy:** rich in phytosterols (e.g. beta-sitosterol) that decrease cholesterol; improve BPH (20 mg beta-sitosterol t.i.d.); 3.5 oz serving of soybeans, tofu, or other soyfood provides 90 mg beta-sitosterol; associated with decreased risk of prostate cancer due to isoflavonoids genistein and daidzein ("phyto-estrogens") acting on estrogen receptors and inhibiting 5-alpha-reductase.

- **Pesticides** and other contaminants increase 5-alpha reduction of steroids.
- **Diethylstilbestrol (DES)** produces changes in rat prostates histologically similar to BPH.
- **Cadmium:** antagonist of zinc; increases activity of 5-alpha-reductase; effects on BPH unclear.

Botanical medicines

- **Order of relative efficacy:** serenoa > Cernilton > pygeum > urtica; each plant has a slightly different mechanism of action.
- Therapy must be tailored to individual patient needs.
- **Chance of clinical success** determined by the degree of obstruction indicated by residual urine volume: levels < 50 ml excellent; 50–100 ml quite good; 100–150 ml tougher to improve within 4–6 weeks; > 150 ml botanicals not likely to improve symptoms significantly.
- ***Serenoa repens* (saw palmetto):** liposterolic extract of fruit of palm significantly improves signs and symptoms; inhibits DHT binding to receptors; inhibits 5-alpha-reductase; interferes with intraprostatic estrogen receptors; 90% of mild to moderate cases improve in all symptoms (especially nocturia) within 4–6 weeks.
- **Cernilton flower pollen extract:** 70% overall success rate in 35 years of European experience; 70% reduction in nocturia and diurnal frequency; significant reductions in residual urine volume; some anti-inflammatory action; contractile effect on bladder while relaxing urethra; inhibits growth of prostate cells.
- ***Pygeum africanum:*** African evergreen tree; bark used historically for urinary tract disorders; bark components: fat-soluble sterols and fatty acids; all research based on extract standardized to 14% triterpenes including beta-sitosterol and 0.5% n-docosanol; effective in reducing symptoms and signs, especially early cases; serenoa gives greater relief, better tolerated, higher urine flow rate, less residual urine; serenoa does not produce effects that *Pygeum* has on prostate secretion.
- ***Urtica dioica* (stinging nettles):** fewer studies; more effective than placebo; interacts with binding of DHT to cytosolic and nuclear receptors.

THERAPEUTIC APPROACH

- **Therapeutic goals:** normalize prostate nutrient levels; restore steroid hormones to normal levels; inhibit excessive conversion of T to DHT;

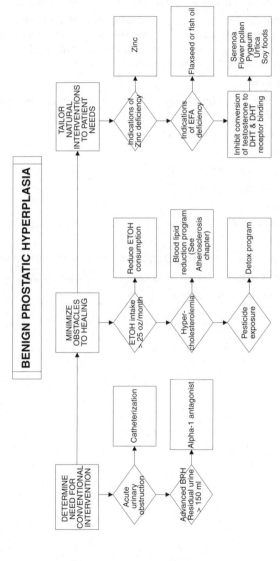

inhibit DHT receptor binding; limit promoters of the hyperplastic process, e.g. prolactin.

- **Severe BPH:** acute urinary retention may require catheterization; for relief, advanced case may not quickly respond to natural therapy, and may require short-term alpha-1 antagonist (e.g. Hytrin or Cordura) or surgery.

- **Diet:** initially high-protein, low-carbohydrate, low in animal fats, high in unsaturated oils; after patient responds, adopt a more normal diet; limit alcohol; avoid drug-, pesticide- and hormone-contaminated foods; limit cholesterol-rich foods; eat soy foods regularly.

- **Supplements:**
  - zinc: 50 mg/day (picolinate preferred, maximum of 6 months; monitor copper status)
  - flax oil: 1 tbsp two times/day
  - glycine: 200 mg/day
  - glutamic acid: 200 mg/day
  - alanine: 200 mg/day.

- **Botanicals:**
  - serenoa extract (standardized at 85–95% liposterols): 160 mg two times/day
  - flower pollen extract (e.g. Cernilton): 63 mg two to three times/day.
  - pygeum extract (standardized at 14% triterpenes): 100–200 µg q.d.
  - urtica extract: 120 µg b\d.

Carpal tunnel syndrome

DIAGNOSTIC SUMMARY

Numbness, tingling and/or burning pain on palmar surfaces of first three digits of hand; positive Tinel's sign (tingling or shock-like pain on volar wrist percussion); positive Phalen's sign (appearance of exacerbation of symptoms caused by flexion of wrist for 60 s and relieved by extension).

GENERAL CONSIDERATIONS

Carpal tunnel syndrome (CTS) is a uni- or bilateral paresthesia in palmar aspect of first three digits and lateral half of fourth digit of hand due to median nerve compression within carpal tunnel; pain may be felt in wrist, palm, and/or forearm proximal to the area of compression; possible loss of strength in abduction and opposition of thumb and atrophy of opponens pollicis muscle may develop.

- **Etiology:** any condition increasing volume of structures in carpal tunnel or causing tunnel narrowing can impinge median nerve; conditions decreasing tunnel volume: subluxation of carpals, separated distal radius and ulna, Colles' fracture, arthritic spurs, tumor, or thickening of flexor retinaculum; conditions increasing volume of contents of tunnel: fluid retention, fat deposition, carpal synovitis, or tenosynovitis; large percentage of cases are idiopathic – may involve vitamin B_6 deficiency or collagen dysplasia.

- **Risk factors and frequency of occurrence:** most obvious causes are traumatic injury and occupational injury through repetitive use; repetitive activities with flexed or extended wrist, hysterectomy without oophorectomy, and last menstrual period in menopausal women 6–12 months earlier; pregnant women, women taking oral contraceptives, menopausal women, and patients on hemodialysis; CTS is more prevalent among women and occurs frequently in age range 40–60 years.

DIAGNOSTIC CONSIDERATIONS

Pain and tingling or numbness in hand; symptoms worse at night and will awaken patient; relief from shaking or rubbing hand; can be bilateral; clumsiness due to inability to hold or feel an object.

- **Physical examination:** impaired sensation in distribution of median nerve; if prolonged condition, atrophy of thenar eminence and weakness of thumb abductor present; Tinel's and Phalen's tests accepted for diagnosing CTS in general practice; Tinel's sign = tingling in distribution of median nerve when tapping nerve in middle of palm over transverse carpal ligament; Phalen's test is positive when symptoms are reproduced by holding wrist in forced flexion for 60–90 s; Katz and Stirrat devised self-administered hand diagram that has 80% sensitivity and 90% specificity for classic or probable CTS; other tests include nerve conduction, CT scan, and MR imaging.

- **Differential diagnosis:** CTS paresthesia confused with paresthesia of brachial plexus in thoracic outlet syndrome or paresthesia of radial or ulnar nerves; hand pain may be presenting feature of reflex sympathetic dystrophy (shoulder–hand syndrome); impingement of median nerve below elbow where nerve passes under pronator teres muscle; specific dermatome pattern of CTS, without proximal dysfunction, should lead to history and tests establishing diagnosis of CTS; left-sided CTS may be confused with angina pectoris.

THERAPEUTIC CONSIDERATIONS

Majority of patients respond well to nutritional and conservative physical medicine; a few require surgical intervention; nutritional support needed to address underlying metabolic weakness.

Nutrition

- **Vitamin B supplementation:** Ellis and Folkers – 50 mg B_6 initially, increased to 200–300 mg as needed – significantly effective in treating CTS; vitamin B_2 useful, with even greater effect when B_6 and B_2 given together; B_2-containing enzymes convert B_6 to more active form, pyridoxal-5′-phosphate (P5P), the form of B_6 also used for CTS; therapeutic response may require 3 months; increased incidence of CTS parallels increased B_6 antimetabolites in environment – hydrazine dyes (FD&C yellow #5) and drugs (INH and hydralazine), dopamine, penicillamine, oral contraceptives, and excessive protein intake; researchers have found no correlation between blood levels of B_6 and presence of, or improvement in, CTS symptoms; given safety and positive clinical studies with B_6 in reasonable dosages (e.g. 25–50mg t.i.d.), trial of B_6 is warranted (especially before opting for surgery).

Physical medicine

- **Hydrotherapy:** inflammation and edema in CTS cause compression of local capillaries, decreasing nutrition to median nerve, making nerve fibers hyperexcitable; contrast hydrotherapy increases circulation and nutrition

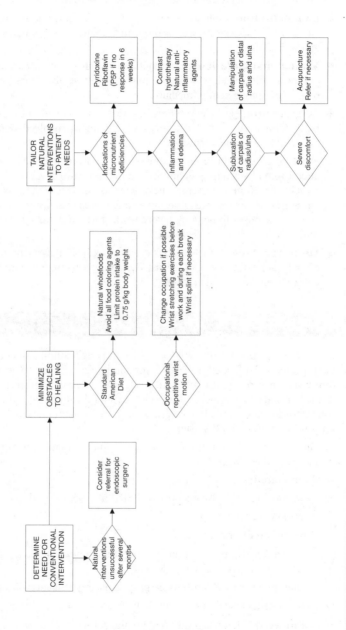

to the area and reduces pain; immersion in hot water for 3 min followed by immersion in cold water for 30 s, repeated three to five times.

- **Immobilization:** Cailliet – splinting wrist in a neutral position required day and night for several weeks; night-time splinting only when symptoms appear is ineffective.
- **Manual manipulation:** manipulation of subluxation of carpals or separation of distal radius and ulna may relieve pressure in carpal tunnel, relieving impingement of median nerve.
- **Acupuncture:** positive response in 35 of 36 patients (14 previously treated unsuccessfully with surgery); treatment involved puncture of PC-7 and PC-6 on affected side.
- **Stretching:** carpal tunnel pressure is twice normal in patients with CTS; after 1 min of stretching–loading exercises, pressure drops to normal and remains for 20 min; exercise = flexing wrists and fists with arms extended for 5 min; this slow, sustained movement prepares nerve for repetitive actions; exercises to be done before work starts and during every break; may reduce need for surgery by 50%.
- **Surgery:** last resort; incision has been through skin overlying transverse carpal ligament; Chow – less invasive endoscopic technique with high success rate and decreased morbidity.

THERAPEUTIC APPROACH

Prevention obviously best; avoid activities causing trauma to median nerve via repeated wrist flexion and extension, and direct trauma to wrist; maintain wrist posture; treatment instituted ASAP to avoid long-term damage to median nerve or associated muscles; avoid all sources of hydrazines; if treatment unsuccessful after several months, consider endoscopic surgery; anti-inflammatory agents useful.

- **Diet:** avoid foods containing yellow dyes and limit daily protein to maximum of 0.75 g/kg body weight.
- **Supplements:**
  — pyridoxine: 50–200 mg q.d. (use P5P if no response within 6 weeks)
  — riboflavin: 10 mg q.d.
- **Physical medicine:**
  — contrast hydrotherapy: immerse for 3 min in hot water followed by 30 s immersion in cold water, 3–5 × q.d.
  — manipulate carpals and ensure proper spacing of distal radius and ulna.
- **Acupuncture:** needle PC-7 and PC-6 on affected side.
- **Splint wrist** in neutral position night and day for unresponsive cases.
- **Regular wrist exercises.**

Celiac disease

DIAGNOSTIC SUMMARY

Chronic intestinal malabsorption disorder caused by intolerance to gluten; bulky, pale, frothy, foul-smelling, greasy stools with increased fecal fat; weight loss and signs of multiple vitamin and mineral deficiencies; increased levels of serum gliadin antibodies; diagnosis confirmed by jejunal biopsy.

GENERAL CONSIDERATIONS

Celiac disease (CD) is also known as non-tropical sprue, gluten-sensitive enteropathy, or celiac sprue; characterized by malabsorption and abnormal small intestine structure which reverts to normal on removal of dietary protein gluten; gluten and polypeptide derivative, gliadin, found in wheat, barley, and rye; symptoms appear in the first 3 years of life, after cereals are introduced to the diet; second peak = third decade; breast-feeding has prophylactic effect – breast-fed babies have decreased risk; early introduction of cow's milk is a major etiological factor; breast-feeding plus delay introducing cow's milk and cereals are preventive steps.

- **Epidemiology and genetics:** genetic etiology – increased frequency of serum histocompatibility antigens HLA-B$_8$ and DR$_{w3}$; HLA-B$_8$ found in 85–90% of celiac patients, but in 20–25% of normal subjects; HLA-B$_8$ gene locus linked to immunologic recognition of antigens and specific T-cell-regulated immune responses; low prevalence of HLA-B$_8$ in long-standing agrarian populations; frequency in northern and central Europe and NW Indian subcontinent much higher; wheat cultivation in high HLA-B$_8$ areas is a recent development (1000 BC); prevalence of celiac disease much higher in these areas than in other regions (e.g. 1:300 in SW Ireland and 1:2,500 in US).

- **Chemistry of grain proteins:** gluten = major component of wheat endosperm, composed of gliadins and glutenins; gliadin triggers CD; rye, barley, and oats – proteins triggering CD are secalins, hordeins, and avenins, respectively, and prolamines collectively; cereal grain family is *Gramineae* – close taxonomic relationship to wheat suggests ability to activate CD; rice and corn do not activate CD and are further removed taxonomically from wheat; gliadins = single polypeptide chains (mol. wt 30,000–75,000) with very high glutamine and proline; gliadins' four electrophoretic fractions: alpha-, beta-, gamma-, and omega-gliadin; alpha-gliadin may be fraction most capable of activating CD, but beta- and gamma-gliadin are also capable; omega-gliadin non-activating, but has highest glutamine and proline; hydrolyzed gliadin does not activate CD – suggesting deficient brush border peptidase or similar digestive defect.

● **Opioid activity:** pepsin hydrosylates of wheat gluten have opioid activity, the factor linking wheat ingestion to schizophrenia; hypothesis: gluten is a pathogenic factor in schizophrenia – substantiated by studies.

● **Pathogenesis:** abnormalities in immune response, not "toxic" property of gliadin; gliadin sensitization in humoral and cell-mediated immunity; T-cell dysfunction is the main factor in enteropathy; cell-mediated mechanisms can produce characteristic lesions: crypt hyperplasia, villous atrophy, and intraepithelial lymphocyte infiltration and mitosis; high titers of serum antibodies to gliadin and other food proteins are secondary to increased intestinal permeability induced by enteropathy produced by T-cell defect; immune complexes (antibody + gliadin) contribute to enteropathy via antibody-dependent cell-mediated cytotoxicity and activation of complement.

● **Clinical aspects:** CD lesions are often histologically indistinguishable from tropical sprue, food allergy, diffuse intestinal lymphoma, and viral gastroenteritis; CD can cause disaccharidase deficiency – lactose intolerance; increased intestinal permeability causes multiple food allergies; cow's milk intolerance may precede CD.

● **Associated conditions:** thyroid abnormalities, IDDM, psychiatric disturbances (including schizophrenia), dermatitis herpetiformis, and urticaria – linked to gluten intolerance; increased risk of malignant neoplasms in celiac patients: decreased micronutrient absorption – vitamin A and carotenoids (*Textbook*, Chs 67 and 121) and gliadin-activated suppressor cell activity; alpha-gliadin activates suppressor cells activation of celiac patients but not healthy controls or patients with Crohn's; casein and beta-lactoglobulin do not activate suppressor cells; depressed immune response increases susceptibility to infection and neoplasm.

DIAGNOSIS

Jejunal biopsy definitive; characteristic symptoms plus positive titer for antibodies to gliadin (anti-alpha-gliadin antibodies) avoid need for uncomfortable biopsy; ELISA test for alpha-gliadin antibodies – 100% sensitivity and 97% specificity; fluorescent immunosorbent test – 100% sensitivity and 84% specificity; both IgA and IgG gliadin antibody levels should be considered, not just one antibody assay; anti-endomysium antibodies are also reliable markers.

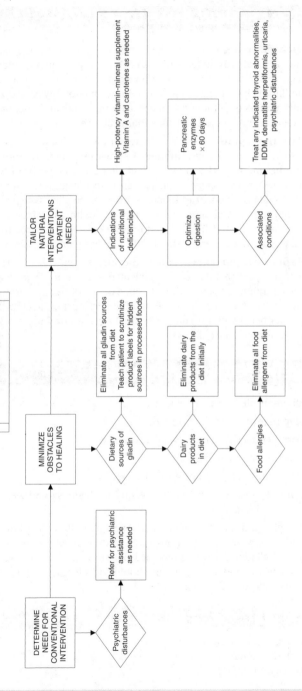

THERAPEUTIC CONSIDERATIONS

● **Diet:** gluten-free diet – no wheat, rye, barley, triticale, or oats; buckwheat and millet also excluded – buckwheat not in grass family and millet more related to rice and corn, but they contain prolamines with antigenicity similar to alpha-gliadin; modest amounts of oats may be tolerated without adverse effects; rotate other foods; eliminate milk and milk products until patient redevelops normal intestinal structure and function.

● **Patient response:** clinical improvement within a few days or weeks (30% respond within 3 days, another 50% within 1 month, and 10% within another month); 10% only respond after 24–36 months of gluten avoidance; failure to respond – consider: incorrect diagnosis, patient not adhering to diet or exposed to hidden sources of gliadin, associated disease or complication, such as zinc deficiency; multivitamin/mineral supplements treat underlying deficiency and provide cofactors for growth and repair; CD is refractive to dietary therapy if underlying zinc deficiency present.

● **Pancreatic enzymes:** pancreatic insufficiency in 8–30% of celiac patients; pancreatic enzyme supplements (2 capsules per meal with each cap containing: lipase 5,000 IU, amylase 2,900 IU, and protease 330 IU) enhance clinical benefit of gluten-free diet during first 30 days, but no greater benefit after 60 days; use of pancreatic enzymes first 30 days after diagnosis (*Textbook*, Ch. 101).

THERAPEUTIC APPROACH

● Eliminate all sources of gliadin.
● Eliminate dairy products initially.
● Correct underlying nutritional deficiencies.
● Treat associated conditions.
● Determine and eliminate all food allergens.
● If no response within 1 month, reconsider diagnosis and search for hidden sources of gliadin.

A strict gluten-free diet is difficult in the US – ubiquitous distribution of gliadin and other activators of CD in processed foods; read labels carefully for hidden sources of gliadin (soy sauce, modified food starch, ice cream, soup, beer, wine, vodka, whisky, malt, etc.); patients should consult resources for patient information on gluten-free recipes.

Patient resources

American Celiac Society
45 Gifford Avenue
Jersey City, NJ 07304

American Digestive Disease Society
7720 Wisconsin Avenue
Bethesda, MD 20014

Gluten Tolerance Group of North America
PO Box 23053
Seattle, WA 98102

National Digestive Disease Education and Information Clearing House
1555 Wilson Boulevard, Suite 600
Rosslyn, VA 22209

Cellulite

DIAGNOSTIC SUMMARY

"Mattress phenomenon" = pitting, bulging and deformation of skin; 90–98% of cases occur in women; feeling of tightness and heaviness in areas affected (particularly the legs); tenderness of skin when pinched, pressed upon, or vigorously massaged.

GENERAL CONSIDERATIONS

Cellulite is a cosmetic defect which is a cause for great distress among millions of European and American women; no inflammatory or infectious process involved (as in cellulitis); better termed "dermo-panniculois deformans" or "adiposis edematosa".

Histological features

● Subcutaneous tissue of thighs has three layers of fat, with two planes of connective tissue (CT) (ground substance) between them; construction of subcutaneous tissue of thigh differs between men and women; in women, uppermost subcutaneous layer consists of "standing fat-cell chambers", separated by radial and arching dividing walls of CT anchored to overlying CT of skin (corium); uppermost subcutaneous tissue in men is thinner, with network of criss-crossing CT walls and corium (CT structure between dermis and subcutaneous tissue) thicker than in women.

● "Pinch test" = pinching skin and subcutaneous tissue of woman's thighs exhibits "mattress phenomenon" – pitting, bulging, and deformation of skin; in most men, skin folds or furrows but will not bulge or pit.

● With aging, corium, already thinner in women than in men, becomes thinner and looser; fat cells migrate into this layer; CT walls between fat-cell chambers become thinner, allowing fat-cell chambers to hypertrophy; breakdown (thinning) of CT is a major contributor to cellulite and granular "buckshot" feel of cellulite.

● "Mattress phenomenon" = alternating depressions and protrusions in upper compartment of fat tissue; vertical orientation of women's fat-cell compartments and weakening of tissues allow protrusion of fat cells into lower corium.

- Distension of lymphatic vessels of upper corium and decrease in number of subepidermal elastic fibers.

Clinical features

Areas of body involved are the gluteal and thigh regions, lower abdomen, nape of neck, and upper arms – areas affected in gynecoid (female) obesity.

Four major stages:

- *Stage 0* – skin on thighs and buttocks has smooth surface when subject is standing or lying; pinch test – skin folds and furrows, but does not pit or bulge; "normal" stage of most men and slim women.

- *Stage 1* – skin surface smooth while standing or lying; pinch test clearly positive for mattress phenomenon (pitting, bulging, deformity of affected areas); normal for most females; in a male there may be a sign of deficiency of androgenic hormones; best classification most can expect, due to structural predisposition.

- *Stage 2* – skin surface smooth while lying, but when standing there is pitting, bulging, and deformity of affected skin; common in women who are obese or over 35–40 years of age.

- *Stage 3* – mattress phenomenon when lying or standing; very common after menopause and in obesity.

THERAPEUTIC CONSIDERATIONS

Best approach is prevention; number and size of fat cells largely determined by maternal prenatal nutritional status = significant predisposition; maintain slim subcutaneous fat layer via exercise and maintaining normal body weight throughout life (slim women and female athletes have little or no cellulite).

Lifestyle

- **Weight reduction and exercise:** primary mode of treatment; weight reduction should be gradual, especially in women over age 40 – rapid weight loss may exacerbate mattress phenomenon.

- **Massage:** very beneficial, particularly self-administered with hand or brush; improves circulation of blood and lymph; direction of massage – from periphery to heart.

Botanical medicines

Oral and topical herbs which enhance CT structures.

- *Centella asiatica:* extract containing 70% triterpenic acids (asiatic acid and asiatoside) is orally effective treating cellulite, venous insufficiency

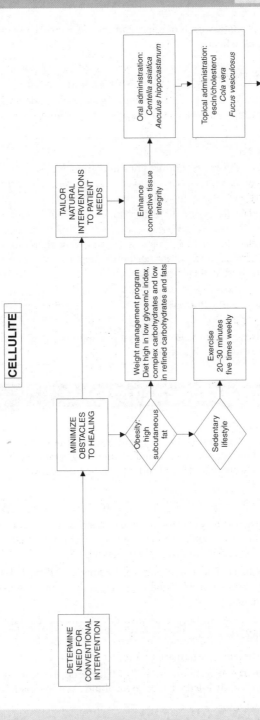

of lower limbs, and varicose veins; normalizes metabolism of CT – enhances tissue integrity by stimulating glycosaminoglycan (GAG) synthesis without promoting excess collagen synthesis or cell growth; GAGs are major components of amorphous intercellular matrix (ground substance) in which collagen fibers are embedded; net outcome = normal CT rich in GAGs; action in venous insufficiency and varicose veins = combination of CT effects and ability to improve blood flow through affected limbs.

- **Escin:** compound isolated from seeds of *Aesculus hippocastanum* (horse chestnut); anti-inflammatory and anti-edema properties; decreases capillary permeability by reducing number and size of small pores of capillary walls; venotonic – positive effect on varicose veins and thrombophlebitis; given orally, or escin/cholesterol complex applied topically; topical application of escin beneficial in treating bruises; decreases capillary fragility and swelling.

- ***Fucus vesiculosus* (bladderwrack):** seaweed used for obesity since 17th century; high iodine content may stimulate thyroid function; used in toiletries and cosmetics for soothing, softening, and toning effects; topical application used to treat cellulite – has not been confirmed by scientific investigation, but soothing, softening, and toning effects may be beneficial.

- ***Cola* species:** rich source of caffeine and related compounds that potentiate effect of catecholamine-induced lipolysis; topical caffeine is preferable to oral for cellulite, since effects will be primarily local.

THERAPEUTIC APPROACH

Cellulite is not a disease *per se*, but a cosmetic disorder due to tissue changes; excessive subcutaneous adipose or degeneration of subcutaneous CT leads to fat chamber enlargement and "mattress phenomenon"; reduce subcutaneous fat and enhance connective tissue integrity; varicose veins often coexist with cellulite – both conditions result largely from loss of integrity of supporting CT (*Textbook*, Ch. 193); "mattress phenomenon" in men is a sign of androgen deficiency – primary or secondary hypogonadism.

- **Diet:** high complex carbohydrates and low refined carbohydrates and fats; promote weight loss in obese patients.
- **Physical measures:**
  — exercise: 20–30 min aerobic exercise a minimum of 5 days/week
  — massage: regular self-massage of affected area.
- **Botanical medicines:**
  Oral administration
  — *Centella asiatica* extract (70% triterpenic acid): 30 mg t.i.d.
  — *Aesculus hippocastanum*

— bark of root: 500 mg t.i.d.

— escin: 10 mg t.i.d.

Topical application of salve, ointment, etc. (b.i.d.)

— cholesterol/escin complex: 0.5–1.5%

— *Cola vera* extract (14% caffeine): 0.5–1.5%

— *Fucus vesiculosus*: 0.25–75%.

Cervical dysplasia

DIAGNOSTIC SUMMARY

Abnormal Papanicolaou smear (stages II–IV); positive Schiller test.

Classification systems for Papanicolaou smears

Numerical	Dysplasia	CIN	Bethesda system
I	Benign	Benign	Normal
II	Benign with inflammation	Benign with inflammation	Normal
III	Mild dysplasia	CIN I	Low-grade SIL
III	Moderate dysplasia	CIN II	Low-grade SIL
III	Severe dysplasia	CIN III	High-grade SIL
IV	Carcinoma in situ	CIN III	High-grade SIL
V	Invasive cancer	Invasive cancer	Invasive cancer

CIN, cervical intraepithelial neoplasia; SIL, squamous epithelial lesion.

GENERAL CONSIDERATIONS

Cervical dysplasia (CD) is a precancerous lesion; risk factors similar to cervical cancer; lifestyle and nutritional factors in etiology of cervical carcinoma: early age of first intercourse, multiple sexual partners, herpes simplex type II and papilloma viruses, lower socioeconomic class, smoking, oral contraceptive use, and many nutritional factors; all risk factors are closely related.

- **Epidemiology:** 7,500 deaths per year; 16,000 cases of invasive cervical cancer and 45,000 cases of carcinoma in situ annually in the US; cervical cancer is the second most common malignancy in women aged 15–34 (can occur at any age); peak incidence of invasive lesions is age 45; in situ lesions peak age 30; invasive carcinoma rate is falling; incidence of carcinoma in situ increasing – increase in risk factors (early age at first intercourse, multiple sexual partners, oral contraceptive use, cigarette smoking).

- **Histology:** 95% of cervix cancers originate in squamocolumnar junction of cervical os; in adolescence, glandular epithelium covers much of exocervix; as adolescence progresses columnar epithelium replaced by squamous cells; actively growing area susceptible to multiple insults and carcinogenic substances – metaplastic nature of conversion process.

Risk factors

- **Sexual activity:** early age at first intercourse and/or multiple sexual partners – suggests sexually transmissible agent; arginine-rich histone or protamine released by sperm during degradation could be oncogenic agent.

- **Viruses:**
  - *herpes simplex type II (HSV-II):* 23% of women with herpes have CD or cancer, but 2.6% of those without infection; HSV-II antibody titers are much higher in women with CD or cancer than in controls; women with herpetic cervicitis have four to 16-fold increased risk of cervical cancer/dysplasia
  - *human papillomavirus (HPV):* agent in condyloma acuminata (venereal warts); detected in cervical tissue of the majority of patients with CD.

- **Smoking:** smokers have two to three times increased incidence compared with non-smokers (17 times in women aged 20–29) – depresses immunity, allowing sexually transmitted agent to promote abnormal cellular development; induces vitamin C deficiency; vaginal or endometrial cells may concentrate and secrete smoke carcinogens; unrecognized links between smoking and sexual behavior.

- **Oral contraceptives (OCs):** long-term use linked to increased risk of thromboembolism, gall bladder disease, MI, mental illness, hyperthyroidism, hypertension, and cervical cancer; OCs potentiate adverse effects of smoking and diminish numerous nutrient levels – vitamins C, B_6 and B_{12}, folate, riboflavin, and zinc.

THERAPEUTIC CONSIDERATIONS

Nutrition

Large proportion (67%) of patients with cervical cancer have abnormal anthropometric or biochemical parameters – height-to-weight ratios, triceps skin fold thickness, mid-arm muscle circumference, serum albumin levels, total iron-binding capacity, hemoglobin levels, creatinine height index, prothrombin time, and lymphocyte count; other patients marginal but "normal" nutritional status; multiple nutrient deficiencies are the typical situation; at least one abnormal vitamin level in 67% of patients, 38% have multiple abnormal parameters; nutrition plays major role in onset of CD/carcinoma; high-fat intake linked to increased risk; diet rich in fruits and vegetables protects against carcinogenesis – fiber, beta-carotenes, and vitamin C.

- **Vitamin A and beta-carotene:** minor association between dietary retinoids and CD risk; strong inverse correlation between beta-carotene intake and CD risk; only 6% of patients with untreated cervical cancer have < normal serum vitamin A; 38% have stage-related abnormal beta-carotene; low serum beta-carotene linked to three times increased risk for severe dysplasia; serum vitamin A and beta-carotene are much lower in CD patients than in controls; carotenes and retinols improve integrity and function of epithelial tissues, provide antioxidant properties, and enhance immune function (*Textbook*, Ch. 53); beta-carotene is more advantageous than retinoids – greater antioxidant properties, immune-enhancing effects and tendency to be concentrated in epithelial tissues.

- **Vitamin C:** diminished vitamin C intake and plasma levels in CD patients; inadequate vitamin C intake is an independent risk factor for premalignant cervical disease and carcinoma in situ; acts as an antioxidant, maintains normal epithelial integrity, improves wound healing, enhances immunity, and inhibits carcinogen formation.

- **Folic acid:** cervical cytological abnormalities related to folate deficiency precede hematological abnormalities; most common vitamin deficiency in the world, especially women who are pregnant or taking OCs; folate deficiency is the probable cause of many abnormal cytological smears rather than "true" dysplasia; OCs induce localized interference with folate metabolism – tissue levels at end-organ targets (cervix) are deficient; RBC folate decreased (especially with CD), while serum levels are normal or increased; OCs induce synthesis of macromolecule that inhibits folate uptake by cells; low RBC folate enhances effect of other CD risk factors – HPV infection: low RBC folate is a risk factor for cervical HPV infection; folate supplements (10 mg q.d.) improve/normalize cytological smears in CD patients; regression rates for untreated CD = 1.3% for mild and 0% for moderate; folate regression-to-normal rate reported 20%, 63.7%, and 100%; progression rate of untreated CD = 16% at 4 months; folate-supplemented rate = 0% (women remained on OCs); use vitamin B_{12} with folate to avoid folate masking underlying B_{12} deficiency.

- **Pyridoxine:** vitamin B_6 (RBC transaminase test) decreased in one-third of CD patients; decreased B_6 status affects metabolism of estrogens and tryptophan, and impairs immunity.

- **Selenium:** serum, dietary, and soil selenium inversely correlated with all epithelial cancers and much lower in CD patients; one anti-carcinogenic effect is increased glutathione peroxidase activity; toxic elements (lead, cadmium, mercury, gold) have selenium-antagonistic properties.

- **Copper:zinc ratio, zinc, retinol:** increased serum copper:zinc ratio is a non-specific reaction to inflammation or malignancy; serum copper:zinc ratio may be tool to establish extent of cancer; ratio > 1.95 indicated malignancy in 90% of patients studied; elevated ratios also seen in OC use, pregnancy, acute and chronic infections, chronic liver disease, and inflammatory conditions; serum Cu:Zn ratio should not be used to predict malignancy in these patients; decreased available zinc may cause retinol binding protein to be absent or undetectable in 80% of dysplastic tissue vs. 23.5% of normal tissue – inverse relationship between serum retinol/zinc and incidence of CD.

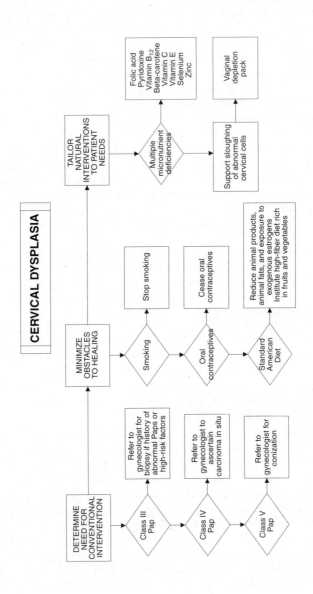

CERVICAL DYSPLASIA

Miscellaneous considerations

- **Vaginal depletion pack (vag pack):** long history of efficacy for CD; mechanism of action not yet elucidated; may promote sloughing superficial abnormal cervical cells; effective in most cases of CD (*Textbook*, App. 12).

THERAPEUTIC APPROACH

- **Pap class:** *class IV Pap* – ascertain carcinoma in situ by gynecologist; *class III Pap* – biopsy if patient has had recurrent abnormal Paps, has significant risk factors, or has been unresponsive to therapy; *carcinoma in situ or class V Pap* – conization.

- Eliminate all factors linked to CD (smoking and OCs); optimize patient's nutritional status – supplement folic acid, beta-carotenes, and vitamin C; vag pack will usually accelerate the rate of normalization of cervix; treat patients who undergo conization for underlying causes of CD; repeat Pap smears every 1–3 months, according to severity.

- **Diet:** decrease animal products – animal fats and exogenous estrogens increase high-fiber foods.

- **Supplements:**
  — folic acid: 10 mg q.d. for 3 months, then 2.5 mg q.d.
  — pyridoxine: 50 mg t.i.d.
  — vitamin B_{12}: 1 mg q.d.
  — beta-carotene: 200,000 IU q.d.
  — vitamin C: 1 g q.d.
  — vitamin E: 200 IU q.i.d.
  — selenium: 400 µg q.d.
  — zinc: 30 mg q.d.

- **Vaginal depletion pack:** weekly until Pap normalizes (unless patient has had conization; *Textbook*, App. 12 for formulation directions).

Chlamydial genital infections

DIAGNOSTIC SUMMARY

Mucopurulent discharge; dysuria; urinary frequency; negative cultures for *Neisseria gonorrhoeae* and *Ureaplasma urealyticum* (unless concomitant infection); positive direct immunofluorescent test in smears of urethral or cervical tissue; examination of Gram stain of discharge at 1,000 magnification in oil shows 4 WBC per field in urethritis and 10 WBC per field in cervicitis.

Pelvic inflammatory disease: dyspareunia; leukorrhea; moderate cramp-like, non-radiating lower abdominal pain; adenexal tenderness; slight elevation in temperature; slight elevation in WBC count and sedimentation rate; may be relatively asymptomatic.

GENERAL CONSIDERATIONS

Chlamydiae are a large group of obligate intracellular parasites related to Gram-negative bacteria; genus *Chlamydia* has two species: *psittaci* and *trachomatis*.

- *C. psittaci* infects birds and domestic/wild animals; humans can be infected – alveoli and reticuloendothelial cells – pneumonitis (psittacosis or ornithosis) has prolonged recovery period, and protracted infectious states (up to 8 years); infected animals very contagious (via inhalation); animal survivors become healthy carriers.

- *C. trachomatis* linked mainly to human disease; 15 immunotypes; genital serotypes are D–K; lymphogranuloma venereum (LGV) linked to chlamydia L_1–L_3; trachoma linked to serotypes A, B, Ba, C.

Epidemiology

- **Genital chlamydial infection:** 4 million cases annually in the US, 50 million worldwide; most common STD in developed countries; primary site of infection is the urethra in men and the cervix in women; incubation period 7–28 days.

  — LGV involves most invasive strains, and is important STD in tropics; rare in developed countries; symptoms in genitalia and inguinal lymph nodes – severe unilateral lymphadenopathy, nodes can rupture and, if scarring of nodes, elephantiasis of lower extremities can develop.

— serotypes of genital strain responsible for half of pneumonias in infants; baby afebrile with slow onset in second or third month; respiratory rate increased with rales and protracted staccato cough.

- **Trachoma:** *C. trachomatis* infection of ocular epithelial cells is not an STD; passed by direct eye–hand–eye contact or via infected vectors (flies); leading cause of blindness worldwide – 500 million people; infection deforms eyelids causing them to turn under; consequent abrasion of cornea leads to blindness; not to be confused with chlamydial conjunctivitis in neonates transmitted by genital infections of mothers ("paratrachoma"); incubation = 3–14 days; untreated – lasts for a month; course of conjunctivitis with serotypes D–K usually benign, but chronic cases cause permanent changes in conjunctiva or cornea; blindness does not occur, but effective treatment is important; neonate is infectious, requiring careful hygiene.

Microbiology

Organism size = 350 nm; considered to be a bacteria because contains both DNA and RNA, possesses a cell wall, susceptible to sulfonamides and broad spectrum antibiotics; inhabits columnar and pseudostratified columnar epithelium – called "parasite of mucosal surfaces" and "energy parasite" (unable to synthesize ATP and GTP); complex life cycle – multiplication only inside host cells, using cells' energy processes; life cycle has two phases – elementary bodies (EBs) and reticulate bodies (RBs) ("initial bodies"); EBs are extracellular travel forms that do not multiply but enter new host cells; RBs are non-infectious and multiply within cell; EBs enter cells and reorganize as RBs to reproduce by binary fission; RBs convert into EBs and are released from cell to begin cycle again; complete cycle takes 48–72 h; RBs reside in cytoplasmic vacuole with membrane composed of components of host cell's membrane – protects *Chlamydia* from host defenses and causes low levels of antibodies and chronicity of infection; membrane modification could trigger autoimmunity.

Non-infectious impacts of chlamydial infections

Chlamydial infections linked to intestinal overgrowth and several chronic diseases – rheumatoid arthritis in some patients, Reiter's syndrome, and coronary artery disease.

DIAGNOSIS

Clinical

Diagnosis difficult and obscure; infected women – 50% symptomatic and remaining have only increased vaginal secretions; mucopurulent cervical discharge is the most common sign ("mucopurulence" may be normal response to increased progesterone; increased PMN leukocytes in cervical mucus are common in women taking exogenous progesterone); other symptoms: urinary frequency and abdominal pain; thick cervical discharge more suspicious than thin; yellow/greenish discharge more suspicious than clear; other concomitant STDs or bacterial vaginosis common; *Chlamydia*-positive sexual contact gives valid grounds to expect infection; 60% of women with tubal infertility and serologic evidence of previous chlamydial infection have no history of acute salpingitis.

Laboratory

Expense, lab expertise, and collection techniques and transport are barriers to reliable reporting; 27 commercial tests available for *Chlamydia* in US; categories of tests: culture, DNA probes, direct fluorescent antibody (DFA), immunohistochemical detection of antigen (EIA, Chlamydiazyme, rapid tests), polymerase chain reaction (PCR or LCR); culture is gold standard and only test admissible for legal purposes; nucleic acid amplification technologies more sensitive, while cultures relatively insensitive (70–85%); cultures 100% specific:

- **CDC recommends** culture for female urethral specimens, asymptomatic men, nasopharyngeal specimens from infants, rectal specimens and vaginal sources of prepubertal girls; test selection parameters: age, gender, symptoms, legal issues, patient consent to consider; collection techniques vary with each test and gender.

- **Culture in women:** endocervix preferred; because blood interferes, brushes not advised; pooling of urethral swab with endocervix will increase culture sensitivity; swab types used for male urethra also used in females; for females, swab inserted 1 cm and rotated once; for males, anterior urethra is best; male should not urinate an hour prior to testing; dry swab inserted 3–4 cm and rotated; include host cells that harbor organism–secretions and exudate insufficient.

Procedure for the laboratory diagnosis of chlamydial infections of the genital tract

1.	Use a cotton-tipped swab with an aluminum or plastic stick
2.	Wipe the cervix and urethra clean of discharge
3.	Take the urethra sample by inserting the swab 3–5 cm and rotating it vigorously. Take the cervical sample from the endocervical canal, leaving the swab in for at least 30 s; carefully remove it without touching the vaginal wall
4.	Transport to the laboratory in plastic
5.	Order the fluorescein-labeled monoclonal antibody smear test (Microtrak)

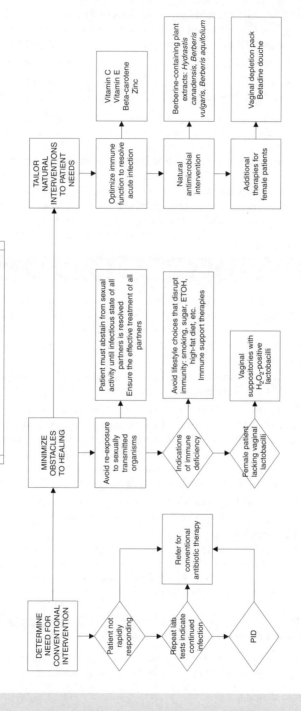

- EIAs and DNA probes are good screens but must be confirmed in low-prevalence populations if positive and person asymptomatic; endocervical PCR and LCR most sensitive and specific, but most expensive.
- Lab tests evolving rapidly – keep up-to-date with your laboratory.

The male

Chlamydia trachomatis is isolated from male urethra, epididymis, prostate, and rectum; rectal *Chlamydia* is asymptomatic and considered relatively innocuous; non-gonococcal urethritis (NGU) twice as common as GC urethritis, and half of all NGU has chlamydial etiology; > 800,000 cases of symptomatic chlamydial urethritis annually in men; other causes are *Ureaplasma urealyticum*, herpes simplex, and *Trichomonas vaginalis*; 45% of patients with GC urethritis have concomitant *Chlamydia* – urethral signs and symptoms of *Chlamydia* similar to GC (discharge and/or pyuria/dysuria); if symptoms present, will be 1–3 weeks after exposure; 25% asymptomatic; sexual partners should be identified and treated.

THERAPEUTIC CONSIDERATIONS

Alternative therapies for *C. trachomatis* are rarely found in scientific literature; recurrence of *Chlamydia* in men and women given antibiotics is a significant problem; question of reinfection vs. recurrence of previous infection; one study indicates recurrence, not reinfection – suggests use of non-drug or adjunctive therapies.

- **Immune support:** immune function essential (*Textbook*, Ch. 53); important nutrients are zinc and vitamin E.
- **Berberine:** local and oral applications of berberine-containing herbs; berberine is effective in treating ocular *C. trachomatis* (*Textbook*, Ch. 91); no studies on use of berberine in genital *Chlamydia*, but reasonable to expect efficacy; local application – berberine douches and vaginal depletion pack (*Textbook*, App. 12); oral treatment – tinctures, powdered dried root, and fluid and solid extracts of *Hydrastis canadensis*, *Berberis vulgaris*, and *Berberis aquifolium*.
- **Providone iodine:** Betadine, or other sources of providone iodine, is effective antichlamydial agent; used to clean cervix and in douche.
- **Lactobacilli:** Women without vaginal *Lactobacillus* more likely to have vaginal *C. trachomatis*; vaginal suppositories with H_2O_2-positive *Lactobacillus* may prevent recurrence and reinfection; most commercial products have *Lactobacillus* unable to produce H_2O_2 or dairy strains unable to bind to vaginal epithelium.

THERAPEUTIC APPROACH

Reinfection is a common complication – identification and treatment of sexual partners mandatory; abstinence recommended until mutual treatment complete; infection may become asymptomatic and recurrence post-therapy is common – lab monitor to ensure eradication; patient follow-up and education important.

- **Supplements:**
    - vitamin C: 1,000 mg q.i.d.
    - vitamin E: 400 IU q.d.
    - beta-carotene: 200,000 IU q.d.
    - zinc: 30 mg q.d. (picolinate).
- **Botanical medicine:**
    - *Hydrastis canadensis* dosages (t.i.d.):
      dried root: 2.0–3.0 g tincture (1:5): 6–12 ml
      fluid extract (1:1): 1.0–2.0 ml
      solid extract (4:1): 250 mg.
- **Additionally, for women:**
    - vaginal depletion pack: three times/week until negative cultures and then once/week as needed.
    - Betadine douche: 2 tbsp/quart of water alternating with vag packs.

> **Note:** *C. trachomatis* is responsible for 50% of all cases of acute salpingitis; ineffective treatment and undiagnosed infection can lead to tubal fibrosis and infertility. If patient not rapidly responding to treatment, if significant PID, or if repeat direct immunofluorescence shows continued infection, patient should be treated with antibiotics in addition to above therapies.

Chronic candidiasis

GENERAL CONSIDERATIONS

Candida is normal in GI tract and vagina; overgrowth, depleted immunity, damaged GI mucosa allow absorption of yeast cells, particles, toxins; result is "yeast syndrome" – "feel sick all over", fatigue, allergies, immune system malfunction, depression, chemical sensitivities, and digestive disturbances; women eight times more likely than men to have syndrome: estrogen, birth control pills, greater antibiotic use.

- **Causal factors:** multifactorial; correct factors predisposing overgrowth; requires more than killing yeast with antifungals, synthetic or natural; prolonged antibiotic use is the key factor in most cases – suppresses normal intestinal bacteria that control yeast, suppresses immunity, generates antibiotic-resistant microbes, may contribute to Crohn's disease.
- **Related syndromes:** small intestinal bacterial overgrowth and "leaky gut" associated with *Candida* overgrowth; may produce identical symptoms to the yeast syndrome.

DIAGNOSIS

- **Screening method:** comprehensive questionnaire (see *Textbook*, App. 2: *Candida* questionnaire).
- **Best method:** clinical evaluation – knowledge of yeast-related illness, detailed medical history, patient questionnaire.
- **Comprehensive stool and digestive analysis (CSDA):** more clinically useful; evaluates digestion, intestinal environment and absorption; indicates underlying digestive disturbance; may pinpoint other causes (e.g. small intestinal bacterial overgrowth, "leaky gut" syndrome).
- **Laboratory techniques (used only to confirm):** stool cultures for *Candida*, antibody to *Candida*, *Candida* antigens in the blood; rarely needed; confirm what history, physical exam, CDSA reveal; confirm *Candida* is factor, monitor therapy.

THERAPEUTIC APPROACH

- Comprehensive approach more effective than just killing yeast with drug or natural agent; address causes.

- Eradicate *Candida* with natural therapies; follow-up stool culture and analysis confirm *Candida* eliminated.
- If symptoms remain after yeast eliminated, condition unrelated to *Candida*; consider small intestinal bacterial overgrowth, pancreatic enzymes and berberine-containing plants.
- Address predisposing factors, recommend *Candida* control diet, support organ systems as needed.

Diet

- **Sugar:** chief nutrient of *Candida*; restrict sugar; avoid refined sugar; restrict honey, maple syrup, fruit juice.
- **Milk and dairy products:** high lactose content promotes *Candida*; contain food allergens; may contain trace levels of antibiotics disrupting GI bacteria, promoting *Candida*.
- **Mold and yeast-containing foods:** avoid foods with high yeast or mold – alcohol, cheese, dried fruits, peanuts.
- **Food allergies:** common in patients with yeast syndrome; ELISA tests for IgE- and IgG-mediated food allergies.

Hypochlorhydria

- Gastric HCl, pancreatic enzymes and bile inhibit *Candida*, prevent its penetration into intestinal mucosa; decreased secretion allows yeast overgrowth; anti-ulcer/antacid drugs induce *Candida* overgrowth in the stomach; pancreatic enzymes: proteases keep small intestine free from parasites.
- Supplement as needed HCl, pancreatic enzymes, substances promoting bile flow; use CDSA as guide.

Enhancing immunity

- **Immune function** essential; rule out other chronic infections due to depressed immunity.
- **Decreased thymus function:** major factor in depressed cell-mediated immunity; history of repeated viral infections (e.g. acute rhinitis, herpes, prostatic or vaginal infections).
- **Vicious cycle:** triggering event (e.g. antibiotic, nutrient deficiency) induces immune suppression, allowing yeast overgrowth, competition for nutrients, secretion of mycotoxins and antigens that tax immune system.
- **Restore immunity:** improve thymus function: prevent thymic involution with antioxidants (carotenes, vitamins C and E, zinc, selenium), nutrients for synthesis or action of thymic hormones, and concentrates of calf thymus tissue.

Promoting detoxification

- Liver damage is the underlying factor; non-viral liver damage reduces immunity, allowing *Candida* overgrowth; liver support: healthy lifestyle, avoid alcohol, regular exercise, vitamin-mineral, lipotropic formula, silymarin, 3-day fast at change of each season.

- **Lipotropic factors:** promote flow of fat and bile through liver – "decongesting" effect; increase intrahepatic levels of SAM (*S*-adenosylmethionine, major lipotropic compound) and glutathione (major detoxifying compound); daily dose: 1,000 mg choline and 1,000 mg of either methionine and/or cysteine.

- **Silymarin:** extract of milk thistle (*Silybum marianum*); protects liver from damage; enhances detoxification; dosage: 70–210 mg silymarin t.i.d.

- **Promote elimination:** high-fiber plant foods; fiber formulas as needed.

Probiotics

Colon microflora affect immunity, cholesterol metabolism, carcinogenesis, aging; species: *L. acidophilus, B. bifidum* (dosage of 1–10 billion viable organisms); application: promote proper intestinal environment, post-antibiotic therapy, vaginal yeast infections, urinary tract infections.

Natural anti-yeast agents

- **Herxheimer ("die-off") reaction:** worsening symptoms; due to rapid killing of *Candida* and absorption of yeast toxins, particles and antigens; to minimize – follow dietary recommendations for 2 weeks before anti-yeast agent; support liver; start anti-yeast medication at a low dose, and gradually increase over 1 month to full level.

- **Caprylic acid:** natural fatty acid antifungal; readily absorbed by intestines; use timed-release or enteric-coated for release throughout GI tract; dosage for delayed-release = 1,000–2,000 mg with meals.

- **Berberine-containing plants (*Hydrastis canadensis, Berberis vulgaris, Berberis aquifolium, Coptis chinensis*):** berberine alkaloids are broad-spectrum antibiotics against bacteria, protozoa, fungi, including *Candida*; dosage based on berberine content: solid extract (4:1 or 8–12% alkaloids), 250–500 mg t.i.d.

- **_Allium sativum_ (garlic):** significant antifungal activity and inhibition of *Candida*; dosage based on allicin content – at least 10 mg allicin or a total allicin potential of 4,000 µg or one clove (4 g) fresh garlic.

- **Enteric-coated essential oils (oregano, thyme, peppermint, rosemary):** antifungal agents; oregano oil is 100 times more potent than caprylic acid; enteric coating ensures delivery to small and large intestines; dosage – 0.2–0.4 ml b.i.d. between meals.

CHRONIC CANDIDIASIS

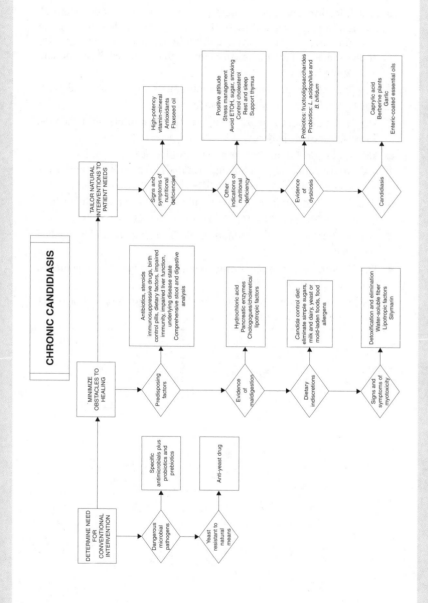

THERAPEUTIC SUMMARY

- *Step 1:* Identify and address predisposing factors: antibiotics, steroids, immune-suppressing drugs, birth control pills (unless there is an absolute medical necessity); comprehensive stool and digestive analysis; dietary factors, impaired immunity, impaired liver function, or an underlying disease state.

- *Step 2: Candida* control diet – eliminate simple sugars, milk and dairy, yeast or mold-laden foods, food allergens.

- *Step 3:* Nutritional support – high-potency multiple, antioxidants, 1 tbsp flaxseed oil daily.

- *Step 4:* Support immunity – promote positive attitude and stress coping; avoid alcohol, sugar, smoking, elevated cholesterol; rest and sleep; support thymus (750 mg crude polypeptide fractions daily).

- *Step 5:* Detoxification and elimination – 3–5 g water-soluble fiber (guar, psyllium, pectin) at night; lipotropic factors, silymarin.

- *Step 6:* Probiotics – 1–10 billion viable *L. acidophilus* and *B. bifidum* cells daily.

- *Step 7:* Anti-yeast therapy – nutritional and/or herbal supplements; anti-yeast drug if needed.

- Repeat stool cultures and antigen levels to monitor progress; stronger prescription antibiotics if needed.

Chronic fatigue syndrome

DIAGNOSTIC SUMMARY

Mild fever, recurrent sore throat, painful lymph nodes, muscle weakness, muscle pain, prolonged fatigue after exercise, recurrent headache, migratory joint pain, depression, sleep disturbance (hypersomnia or insomnia).

Definition: CDC criteria (*Textbook*, Table 49.1) ignore many common clinical symptoms (*Textbook*, Table 49.2); Australian definition = fatigue which disrupts daily activities in absence of other pathosis associated with fatigue.

ETIOLOGY

- **Epstein–Barr virus:** EBV-herpes viruses produce latent lifelong infections; host's immune system normally holds latent infection in check; immunocompromise allows recurrence; viral infection itself can disrupt immunity; elevated EBV antibody observed in diseases of immune dysfunction; elevated antibody titers to viruses observed in CFS patients; antibody testing useful as measure of immune function and host resistance, but not reliable for diagnosis of CFS.

- **Other infectious agents under investigation:** human herpes virus-6, Inoue–Melnich virus, *Brucella*, *Borrelia burgdorferi*, *Giardia lamblia*, cytomegalovirus, enterovirus, retrovirus.

- **Immune system abnormalities:** elevated antibodies to viral proteins; decreased natural killer (NK) cell activity; low or elevated antibody levels; increased or decreased levels of circulating immune complexes; increased cytokines (e.g. interleukin-2); increased or decreased interferon; altered helper/suppressor T-cell ratio.

- **CFS, fibromyalgia (FM), and multiple chemical sensitivities (MCS):** only difference in diagnostic criteria for FM and CFS is musculoskeletal pain in FM and fatigue in CFS; diagnosis of FM or CFS depends on type of physician consulted; 70% of patients with FM and 30% with MCS meet CDC criteria for CFS; 80% of both FM and MCS patients meet CFS criterion of fatigue for > 6 months with 50% reduction in activity; > 50% of CFS and FM patients have adverse reactions to various chemicals.

- **Other causes of CFS:** pre-existing pathosis, depression, stress/low adrenal function, impaired liver function and/or environmental illness, impaired immunity, food allergies, hypothyroidism, hypoglycemia, anemia and nutritional deficiencies, sleep disturbances, cause unknown.

DIAGNOSIS

- Identify as many factors as possible contributing to fatigue.
- **Complete physical exam:** swollen lymph nodes (chronic infection); diagonal crease in both ear lobes (impaired blood flow).
- **Lab:** avoid expensive tests unless absolutely necessary, CBC and chemistry panel (including serum ferritin for menstruating women); avoid tests to confirm diagnosis that will not affect treatment; assess liver detox function, bowel dysbiosis and GI permeability (*Textbook*, Chs 9, 16 and 21).

THERAPEUTIC CONSIDERATIONS

- Multifactorial conditions require tailored multiple therapies.
- Energy level and emotional state determined by internal focus and physiology: mental focus on fatigue; physiology – chemicals, hormones, posture, breathing (shallow), address mind and body.
- **Depression:** a major cause of chronic fatigue (CF); common in CFS; most common cause of CF in absence of pre-existing pathosis.
- **Stress:** underlying factor in patient with depression, low immune function, or other cause of CF (*Textbook*, Ch. 60); evaluate stress effects with "Social Readjustment Rating Scale" by Holmes and Rahe.
- **Impaired liver function and/or environmental illness:** exposure to toxins causes "congested liver"/"sluggish liver"/"impaired hepatic detoxification", leading to cholestasis and decreased phase I and/or phase II enzyme activity; use clinical judgment and lab tests (serum bilirubin, AST, ALT, LDH, GGTP, serum, bile acid assay, clearance tests) (*Textbook*, Ch. 16); patient complaints: depression, general malaise, headaches, digestive disturbances, allergies and chemical sensitivities, premenstrual syndrome, constipation; hair mineral analysis: heavy metals – if inconclusive, use 8-h lead mobilization test with chelating agent EDTA (edetate calcium disodium), which measures lead excreted in urine for 8 h after injection of EDTA.
- **Excessive GI permeability:** measured by lactulose/mannitol absorption test (*Textbook*, Ch. 21); common finding in CFS; utilize food allergy control, nutrients to stimulate GI regeneration, support hepatic phase I and II detox, and oligoantigenic rice protein food replacement formula.

- **Impaired immune function and/or chronic infection:** fatigue is body's response to infection: immune system works best when body rests; use questions in *Textbook*, Table 49.8, and lab tests in Chapter 20.

- **Chronic *Candida* infection:** impaired immunity allows GI *Candida* overgrowth; diagnosis difficult: no single specific test; stool cultures and elevated *Candida* antibody levels plus detailed history and patient questionnaire (see Chronic candidiasis chapter).

- **Food allergies:** CF is a key feature of food allergies = "allergic toxemia"; fatigue, muscle/joint aches, drowsiness, difficulty concentrating, nervousness, depression; 85% of people with CFS have allergies (*Textbook*, Ch.15).

- **Hypothyroidism:** common cause of CF often overlooked; failure to treat reduces efficacy of other interventions (see Hypothyroidism chapter).

- **Hypoglycemia:** must be ruled out as it contributes to depression: depressed people suffer from hypoglycemia and depression is most common cause of CF.

- **Hypoadrenalism:** disruption of hypothalamic–pituitary–adrenal axis (HPA) may be major feature of CFS; symptoms of glucocorticoid deficiency: debilitating fatigue, stressing event followed by feverishness, arthralgias, myalgias, adenopathy, post-exertional fatigue, exacerbation of allergic responses and disturbances of mood and sleep, pathophysiological antecedents (acute infection, stress, pre-existing/concurrent psychiatric illness) may converge into CFS; patients have reduced evening cortisol levels, low 24-h urinary free cortisol excretion, elevated basal ACTH, increased adrenal cortical sensitivity to ACTH, but reduced maximal response, and attenuated net integrated ACTH response to corticotropin-releasing hormone; may reflect secondary adrenal insufficiency: adrenal ACTH receptors hypersensitive from inadequate exposure to ACTH and overall adrenal atrophy.

- **Mind and attitude:** mental attitude influences immunity and energy level; many with CFS are either depressed or have lost sense of enthusiasm for life.

Diet

Energy level directly related to food quality; eliminate caffeine and refined sugar: degree of fatigue is related to quantity of caffeine; cessation of coffee may cause caffeine withdrawal symptoms: fatigue, headache, intense desire for coffee for a few days.

Nutritional supplements

- **High-potency vitamin-mineral:** deficiency of any nutrient can produce fatigue and susceptibility to infection.

- **Extra vitamin C:** 3,000 mg/day in divided doses.
- **Magnesium:** 500–1,200 mg/day in divided doses; even subclinical deficiency can cause CF, low RBC Mg^{2+} (more accurate measure than routine blood analysis), common with CF and CFS; benefit noted after 10 days; prefer bound to aspartate, citrate or Krebs intermediates.

Other therapies

- **Breathing, posture, and bodywork:** diaphragm breathing, good posture, bodywork (massage, spinal manipulation, etc.).
- **Exercise:** moderate level improves mood, ability to handle stress; increases (up to 100%) NK activity; stimulates immune system; intense exercise can have opposite effect.

Botanical medicines

- *Eleutherococcus senticosus* **(Siberian ginseng):** supports adrenals; non-specific adaptogen, increases T-helper cells and NK activity – valuable in treating CFS.
- *Glycyrrhiza glabra* **(licorice):** antiviral and glucocorticoid-potentiating properties (*Textbook*, Ch. 90); use whole root, as glucocorticoid-potentiating glycyrrhizic and glycyrrhetinic acids are removed from DGL.

THERAPEUTIC APPROACH

Comprehensive diagnostic and therapeutic approach: identify underlying factors; optimize hepatic detox, control food allergy, restore GI function; support immune function (*Textbook*, Ch. 53).

- **Diet:** Identify and control food allergies; increase water; eliminate caffeine and ETOH; whole organic foods; control hypoglycemia – eliminate sugar and refined foods, and take regular healthy small meals and snacks; use medical food replacement (e.g. UltraClear) for several weeks to speed detox.
- **Lifestyle:** diaphragmatic breathing; proper posture; regular low intensity exercise.
- **Supplements:**
  - high-potency vitamin-mineral (*Textbook*, Ch. 44)
  - vitamin C: 500–1,000 mg t.i.d.
  - vitamin E: 200–400 IU/day
  - thymus extract: 750 mg crude polypeptides q.d. or b.i.d.
  - magnesium bound to citrate or Krebs intermediates: 200–300 mg t.i.d.
  - pantothenic acid: 250 mg/day.

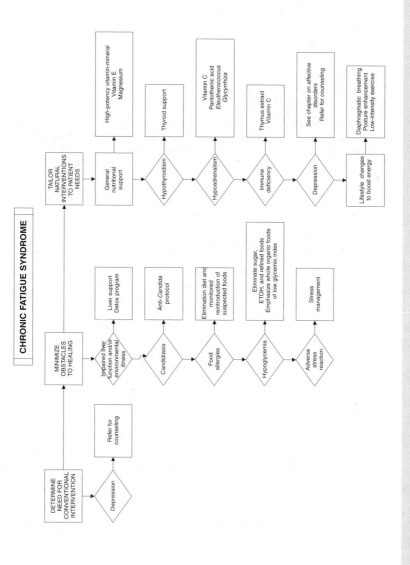

- **Botanicals:**
  - *Eleutherococcus senticosus*:
    dried root: 2–4 g
    tincture (1:5): 10–20 ml
    fluid extract (1:1): 2.0–4.0 ml
    solid (dry powdered) extract (20:1 or standardized to >1%
    eleutheroside E):
    100–200 mg
  - *Glycyrrhiza glabra*:
    powdered root: 1–2 g
    fluid extract (1:1): 2–4 ml
    solid (dry powdered) extract (4:1): 250–500 mg.

- **Counseling:** directly or referral to professional counselor to reinforce pattern of mental, emotional, and spiritual affirmations.

Congestive heart failure

DIAGNOSTIC SUMMARY

- Left ventricular failure – exertional dyspnea, cough, fatigue, orthropnea, cardiac enlargement, rales, gallop rhythm, and pulmonary venous congestion
- Right ventricular failure – elevated venous pressure, hepatomegaly, dependent edema
- Both left and right ventricular failure – combinations of above
- Diagnosis confirmed by echocardiograph.

Stages of congestive heart failure as defined by the New York Heart Association

Stage I	Symptom-free at rest and with treatment
Stage II	Impaired heart function with moderate physical effort; SOB with exertion common; no symptoms at rest
Stage III	Even minor physical exertion results in SOB and fatigue; no symptoms at rest
Stage IV	Symptoms (SOB) and signs (lower extremity edema) present when patient is at rest.

SOB, shortness of breath.

GENERAL CONSIDERATIONS

Congestive heart failure (CHF) is the inability of the heart to effectively pump enough blood; contractile function of heart is governed by five factors: (1) contractile state of myocardium; (2) pre-load of ventricle; (3) end-diastolic volume; (4) impedance to left ventricular ejection; (5) heart rate (HR).

- **Causes of CHF:** long-term hypertension; previous MI; disorder of heart valve; cardiomyopathy; and chronic lung disease.
- **Precipitating or exacerbating factors:** increased demand, anemia, fever, infection, fluid overload, increased Na^+ intake, high environmental temperature, renal failure, hepatic failure, thyrotoxicosis, arteriovenous shunt, respiratory insufficiency, emotional stress, pregnancy, obesity, arrhythmias, pulmonary embolism, ETOH ingestion, nutrient deficiency,

uncontrolled hypertension, beta-adrenergic blockers, anti-arrhythmic drugs, Na-retaining drugs (steroids, NSAIDs).

- **Consequences of reduced cardiac output (CO):** reduced renal blood flow and glomerular filtration, causing Na and fluid retention; activation of renin–angiotensin–aldosterone system increases peripheral vascular resistance, ventricular afterload, and levels of circulating vasopressin, a vasoconstrictor and antidiuretic.

- **Compensatory mechanisms** for the reduced CO are tachycardia, increased sympathetic NS activation, ventricular dilation, and hypertrophy; mixed blessing – increased sympathetic activity increases CO by increasing HR and force of contraction plus increased vascular resistance.

- **Signs and symptoms of CHF:** depend on which ventricle has failed; left – pulmonary congestion and edema; right – systemic venous congestion and peripheral edema; weakness, fatigue, and SOB common to both, as well as biventricular failure.

DIAGNOSTIC CONSIDERATIONS

CHF most effectively treated via natural measures in early stages; early diagnosis and prevention by addressing causative factors are imperative; first symptom = SOB; chronic non-productive cough also a first presenting symptom; extensive cardiovascular evaluation – complete physical exam, looking for characteristic signs (peripheral signs of heart failure, enlarged and sustained left ventricular impulse, diminished first heart sound, gallop rhythm, etc.), EKG, and echocardiogram.

THERAPEUTIC CONSIDERATIONS

Initial stages of CHF – natural measures for underlying causes (e.g. hypertension) or improving myocardial metabolic function (*Textbook*, Ch. 129) often quite effective; later stages, conventional treatment – diuretics, angiotensin-converting enzyme (ACE) inhibitors and/or digitalis glycosides – indicated in most cases; measures described here used as adjunct in more severe cases; excellent clinical results expected in NYHA Stages I and II using natural measures described below.

Nutritional supplements

Improve myocardial energy production – CHF always characterized by energy depletion, often from nutrient or coenzyme deficiency; dietary recommendations for hypertension appropriate for most CHF patients, especially if CHF due to hypertension; diet low in Na^+ and high in K^+; restrict Na^+ intake to < 1.8 g q.d.

- **Magnesium:** low WBC Mg common in CHF patients; Mg levels correlate directly with survival rates; Mg deficiency linked to cardiac arrhythmias, reduced cardiovascular prognosis, worsened ischemia, and increased mortality in acute MI; deficiency probably due to inadequate intake and increased wasting via overactivation of renin–angiotensin–aldosterone system, common in patients with heart failure; supplementation also prevents Mg depletion caused by conventional drug therapy for CHF – digitalis, diuretics, and vasodilators (beta-blockers, calcium-channel blockers, etc.); Mg supplements produce positive effects in CHF patients on conventional drugs, even if serum Mg normal; critical nutrient for producing ATP; dosage = 200–400 mg t.i.d. (citrate).

- **Thiamine:** thiamin (vitamin B_1) deficiency has cardiovascular effects – "wet beri-beri", Na^+ retention, peripheral vasodilation, and heart failure; furosemide (Lasix, most widely prescribed diuretic) causes B_1 deficiency in animals and patients with CHF; severe B_1 deficiency uncommon (except in alcoholics), but many do not get RDA (1.5 mg) especially elderly in hospitals/nursing homes; significant percentage of geriatric population are deficient in B vitamins; daily doses of 80–240 mg of B_1 q.d. improves clinical picture: 13–22% increase of left ventricular ejection fraction; increased ejection fraction linked to greater survival rate in CHF; benefit, lack of risk and low cost of 200–250 mg B_1 q.d. warrant its use in CHF.

- **Carnitine (Crn):** essential for transport of fatty acids into myocardial mitochondria for ATP production; normal heart stores more Crn and CoQ_{10} than it needs; heart ischemia quickly decreases Crn and CoQ_{10}; Crn supplements improve cardiac function in CHF patients; the longer Crn used, the more dramatic the improvement; 500 mg t.i.d. × 6 months increases max. exercise time by 16–25% and ventricular ejection fraction by 12–13%.

- **Coenzyme Q_{10}:** most studies used CoQ_{10} as adjunct to conventional drugs; most recent and largest study: 2,664 patients in NYHA classes II and III in open study in Italy; daily dosage = 50–150 mg orally × 90 days (majority of patients, 78%, took 100 mg q.d.); proportions of patients with improved clinical signs and symptoms = cyanosis – 78.1%, edema – 78.6%, pulmonary edema – 77.8%, hepatomegaly – 49.3%, venous congestion – 71.81%, SOB – 52.7%, heart palpitations – 75.4%, sweating – 79.8%, subjective arrhythmia – 63.4%, insomnia – 66.2%, vertigo – 73.1%, nocturia – 53.6%; improvement of at least three symptoms in 54% of patients – significantly improved quality of life with CoQ_{10}; low incidence of mild side-effects – only 1.5%.

- **Arginine:** amino acid of value in CHF; CHF patients less able to achieve peripheral vasodilation during exercise; body makes natural vasodilator nitric oxide from arginine; 5.6–12.6 g q.d. oral L-arginine increases peripheral blood flow by 29%; 6-min walking distance increases by 8% and arterial compliance increases 19%.

CONGESTIVE HEART FAILURE

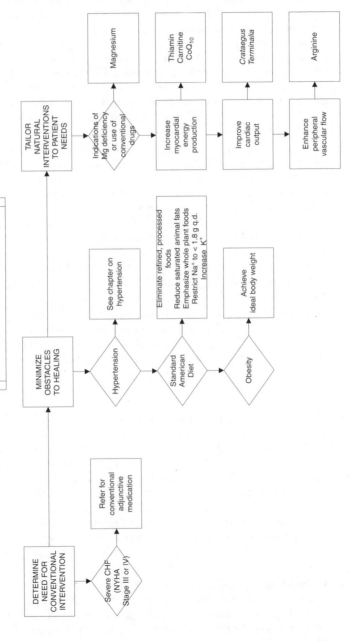

Botanical medicines

- *Crataegus oxyacantha* (hawthorn): quite useful in early stages as sole agent and later stages in combination with digitalis cardioglycosides; crataegus extract standardized to 15 mg procyanidin oligomers per 80 mg capsule b.i.d. × 8 weeks was better than placebo in improving heart function; mildly reduces systolic and diastolic BP; no adverse reactions at recommended dosage; patients with CHF (NYHA stage II) – 600 mg standardized crataegus extract q.d. × 56 days was better than placebo (25 vs. 5 watts), increasing patient working capacity on bicycle ergometer.

- *Terminalia arjuna:* traditional Ayurvedic botanical for cardiac failure; CHF patients (class IV NYHA) receiving extract (500 mg every 8 h) from bark for 2 weeks or placebo – extract group experienced (echocardiogram) statistically significant improvement in end-systolic volume and left ventricular ejection fractions; uncontrolled phase of study using combination of *T. arjuna* and conventional drugs for 2 years found nine patients showing remarkable improvement to NYHA class II and other three improving to class III.

THERAPEUTIC APPROACH

Diet and natural agents effective in early stages (NYHA stages I and II); in latter stages, adjunct drug therapy necessary; treatment designed to address underlying pathophysiology and improve myocardial function through improved energy production.

- **Diet:** achieve ideal body weight; restrict Na^+ intake (< 1.8 g q.d.); increase plant foods; reduce saturated fat; follow other guidelines for lowering BP.

- **Nutritional supplements:**
  - magnesium: 200–400 mg t.i.d.
  - thiamin: 200–250 mg q.d.
  - L-carnitine: 300–500 mg t.i.d.
  - coenzyme Q_{10}: 150–300 mg q.d.

- **Botanical medicines:**
  - hawthorn extract (1.8% vitexin-4′-rhamnoside or 10% procyanidin content): 100–200 mg t.i.d.

Cystitis

DIAGNOSTIC SUMMARY

Burning pain on urination; increased urinary frequency, nocturia; turbid, foul-smelling, or dark urine; lower abdominal pain; urinalysis shows significant pyuria and bacteriuria.

GENERAL CONSIDERATIONS

Bladder infections in women are common: 10–20% of all women have urinary tract discomfort at least once a year; 37.5% of women with no history of UTI will have one within 10 years; 2–4% of healthy women have elevated bacteria in urine – unrecognized UTI: women with history of recurrent UTI have episode once a year; recurrent bladder infections significant problem – 55% eventually involve kidneys; recurrent kidney infection causes progressive damage – scarring and, for some, kidney failure; UTIs much less common in males, except infants – indicate anatomical abnormality, prostate infection or rectal intercourse.

Causes

Urine secreted by kidneys is sterile until reaching urethra; bacteria can ascend urethra or, much less commonly, reach urinary system via bloodstream; bacteria introduced into urethra from fecal contamination or, in women, vaginal secretions; factors influencing ascending infection are anatomical or functional obstructions to flow (pooling of urine) and immune dysfunction; major defenses: free flow, large urine volume, complete bladder emptying, optimal immune function, urine flow washes away bacteria, inner surface of bladder has antimicrobial properties, urine pH inhibits growth of many bacteria, in men prostatic fluid has antimicrobial substances, and body quickly secretes WBCs to control bacteria.

● Risk factors: pregnancy (twice as frequent), sexual intercourse (nuns have 1/10 incidence), homosexual activity (males), mechanical trauma or irritation, and (most important) structural abnormalities of urinary tract blocking free urine flow.

● Reflux of infected urine from bladder upward infects kidney and establishes recurrence.

DIAGNOSIS

Bladder infection diagnosis imprecise – clinical symptoms and presence of significant amounts of bacteria in urine do not correlate; only 60% of women with UTI symptoms actually have abundant bacteria in urine; 20% have serious kidney involvement; diagnosis is according to signs, symptoms and urinary findings; microscopic exam of infected urine – high WBCs and bacteria; urine culture determines quantity and type of bacteria; *E. coli* (from colon) most common; fever, chills, and low back pain – kidneys; recurrent infections – i.v. urogram to rule out structural abnormality.

Collection of urine specimen for culture

Optimal = voided midstream specimen: clean urethral meatus and vaginal vestibule before collecting; spread labia and cleanse area with two gauze sponges moistened with cleansing solution and a dry gauze sponge; wash by making single front-to-back motion with each of two moist sponges and then dry sponge; while labia still held apart, small amount of urine allowed to pass into toilet (or bedpan); then midstream specimen collected in sterile container and immediately closed; collection via catheterization is more invasive and carries 1–2% chance of initiating UTI; suprapubic aspiration is the most accurate method but most invasive.

Examining collected urine

Several methods – dipsticks, microscope, and culture; most accurate is to examine urine within 1 h; if exam to be delayed, refrigerate at 5°C; culturing requires urine not be refrigerated for more than 8 h.

- **Dipsticks:** reagent strips dipped into urine and removed; parts of dipstick impregnated with chemicals that react with specific substances in urine to produce various colors; careful matching of dipstick color to color standard at appropriate time is essential; invaluable for qualitative and rough quantitative analysis – pH, protein, glucose, ketones, bilirubin, hemoglobin, nitrite, and urobilinogen; some dipsticks detect WBCs and bacteria (including semi-quantitative cultures); many organisms reduce urine nitrate to nitrite (*Citrobacter* spp., *Escherichia coli*, *Klebsiella pneumonia*, *Proteus* spp., *Pseudomonas* spp., *Serratia marcescens*, *Shigella*, *Staphylococcus* spp. – most); measuring nitrite is inexpensive and a rapid detector of bacteriuria – confirm by culture.

- **Microscopic exam:** perform within first hour; a drop of fresh urine or a drop of resuspended sediment from centrifuged fresh urine placed on slide, covered with cover glass, and examined with high-dry objective under reduced illumination: > 10 bacteria per field in unstained specimen suggests bacteria count > 100,000/ml; Gram stain under oil immersion objective: WBCs indicate infection; abundant protein and/or WBC casts indicate renal involvement – commonly pyelonephritis.

● **Urine culture:** only quantitative cultures used; diluted urine introduced to suitable medium and incubation; colonies counted and multiplied by dilution factor, giving bacterial count/ml; bacteriuria significant if > 100,000/ml; but 1,000 colonies/ml is clinically significant in presence of UTI symptoms; semi-quantitative tests using dipsticks or glass slides coated with culture media commonly used; colonies counted or appearance compared 12–24 h later; recurrent or chronic infection – sensitivity studies; 95% of UTIs – single bacterial species involved; mixed bacterial species grown – probable contamination; *Staphylococcus epidermidis*, diphtheroids and *Lactobacillus* common in distal urethra but rarely cause UTI; most common organisms are *Escherichia coli*, *Proteus miribili*, *Klebsiella pneumonia*, *Enterococcus*, *Enterobacter aerogenes*, *Pseudomonas aeruginosa*, *Proteus* sp., *Serratia marcescens*, *Staphylococcus epidermidis*, *S. aureus*.

THERAPEUTIC CONSIDERATIONS

Primary goal is to enhance normal host defenses – enhance urine flow via proper hydration, promote protective urine pH, prevent bacterial adherence to bladder endothelium, and enhance immune system; use antimicrobial botanical medicines as needed.

Chronic interstitial cystitis: persistent form of cystitis not due to infection; focus on enhancing integrity of interstitium and endothelium; eliminating food allergens is warranted – food allergies can produce cystitis in some patients; *Centella asiatica* extracts improve integrity of connective tissue that composes interstitium and heal bladder ulcerations (*Textbook*, Ch. 74).

General measures

● **Increase urine flow:** increase amount of liquids consumed – pure water, herbal teas, fresh fruit and vegetable juices diluted with equal amount of water; drink 2+ L – at least half as water; avoid soft drinks, concentrated fruit drinks, coffee, and ETOH.

● **Cranberry juice:** effective in several clinical studies; 0.5 L q.d. cranberry juice beneficial in 73% of male and female UTI subjects; withdrawal of cranberry juice from people who benefited resulted in recurrence in 61%; in order to acidify urine, 1+ L cranberry juice must be consumed at one sitting; concentration of hippuric acid in urine from drinking cranberry juice is insufficient to inhibit bacteria; constituents in cranberry juice reduce ability of *E. coli* to adhere to bladder and urethral endothelium; only cranberry and blueberry contain this inhibitor; blueberry juice is a suitable alternative to

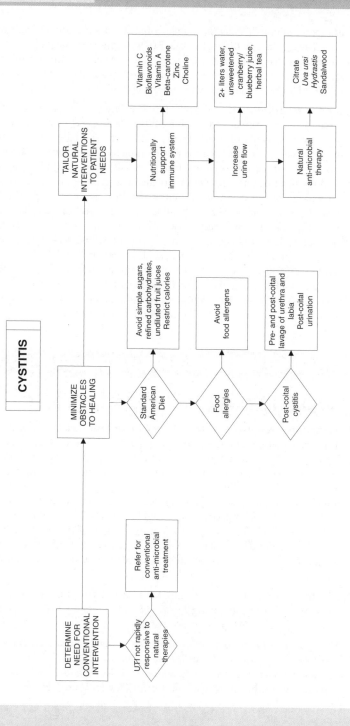

CYSTITIS

DETERMINE NEED FOR CONVENTIONAL INTERVENTION

UTI not rapidly responsive to natural therapies → Refer for conventional anti-microbial treatment

MINIMIZE OBSTACLES TO HEALING

Standard American Diet → Avoid simple sugars, refined carbohydrates, undiluted fruit juices Restrict calories

Food allergies → Avoid food allergens

Post-coital cystitis → Pre- and post-coital lavage of urethra and labia Post-coital urination

TAILOR NATURAL INTERVENTIONS TO PATIENT NEEDS

Nutritionally support immune system → Vitamin C Bioflavonoids Vitamin A Beta-carotene Zinc Choline

Increase urine flow → 2+ liters water, unsweetened cranberry/blueberry juice, herbal tea

Natural anti-microbial therapy → Citrate *Uva ursi* *Hydrastis* Sandalwood cranberry juice in bladder infections; 300 ml cranberry juice in 153 women (average age 78.5) with bacteriuria (10^5/ml urine) dramatically decreased bacteria and frequency of recurrence; avoid sweetened cranberry juice that suppresses immunity; prefer fresh cranberry (sweetened with apple or grape juice) or blueberry juice; cranberry extracts available.

- **Acidify or alkalinize? –** it is difficult to acidify urine – popular methods (ascorbic acid, cranberry juice) have little effect on pH at commonly prescribed doses; alkalinizing urine is more effective, especially in women without pathogenic bacteria in urine; best method for alkalinizing = citrate salts (potassium citrate and sodium citrate) – rapidly absorbed and metabolized without affecting gastric pH or producing laxative effect; excreted partly as carbonate, raising urine pH; K^+ citrate and/or Na^+ citrate used to treat lower UTIs and often used as "holding exercise" until urine culture complete; 4 g sodium citrate every 8 h for 48 h – 80% of 64 women had relief of symptoms, 12% had deterioration of symptoms, and 91.8% rated treatment acceptable; significant symptomatic relief in 80% of another 159 women studied who were abacteriuric; urine culture can be restricted to women who fail to respond to alkalinization; many herbs used to treat UTIs (*Hydrastis canadensis, Arctostaphylos uva ursi*) contain antibacterial components which work most effectively in alkaline environment.

ENHANCE IMMUNE FUNCTION (*Textbook*, Ch. 53)

Botanical medicines

- *Arctostaphylos uva ursi* **(bearberry or upland cranberry):** urinary antiseptic component is arbutin, composing 7–9% of leaves; arbutin hydrolyzed to hydroquinone and glucose in the body; hydroquinone most effective in alkaline urine; crude plant extracts are more effective medicinally than isolated arbutin; especially active against *E. coli*; has diuretic properties; prophylactic effect of standardized extract on recurrent cystitis – effective over 1-year period of study without side-effects; regular use may prevent bladder infections; avoid excessive dosages of *uva ursi* – as little as 15 g (0.5 oz) dried leaves can be toxic in susceptible individuals; toxic signs include tinnitus, N/V, sense of suffocation, SOB, convulsions, delirium, collapse.

- *Allium sativum* **(garlic):** antimicrobial activity against many disease-causing organisms, including *Escherichia coli, Proteus* sp., *Klebsiella pneumonia, Staphylococcus* sp., *Streptococcus* sp.

- *Hydrastis canadensis* **(goldenseal):** very effective antimicrobial agent; effective against *Escherichia coli, Proteus* sp., *Klebsiella* sp., *Staphylococcus* sp., *Enterobacter aerogenes* (requires large dosage), and *Pseudomonas* sp.; berberine works better in an alkaline urine (*Textbook*, Ch. 91).

THERAPEUTIC APPROACH

Most cases of cystitis are relatively benign, but must be properly diagnosed, treated, and monitored; patient must notify physician of any change in condition; if culture positive, follow up with another culture 7–14 days after treatment started; citrates can be used to ameliorate symptoms; occasional acute bladder infection is easily treated; chronic cystitis is a significant challenge – must find underlying cause: structural abnormalities, excessive sugar intake, food allergies, nutritional deficiencies, chronic vaginitis, local foci of infection (prostate, kidneys), current or childhood sexual abuse.

- **General measures:** large amounts of fluids (2+ L q.d.) including 0.5+ L unsweetened cranberry or 0.25+ L blueberry juice q.d.; recurrent postcoital cystitis – urinate after intercourse; wash labia and urethra with strong tea of *Hydrastis canadensis* (2 tsp/cup) before and after; if this is inadequate, use dilute solution of povidone-iodine.

- **Diet:** avoid all simple sugars, refined carbohydrates, full-strength fruit juice (diluted acceptable), and food allergens; restrict calories; eat liberal amounts of garlic and onions.

- **Nutritional supplements:**
    - vitamin C: 500 mg every 2 h
    - bioflavonoids: 1,000 mg q.d.
    - vitamin A: 25,000 IU q.d.
    - beta-carotene: 200,000 IU q.d.
    - zinc: 30 mg q.d.
    - choline: 1,000 mg q.d.

- **Botanical medicines (t.i.d.):**
    - *Uva ursi*:
        dried leaves or as a tea: 1.5–4.0 g (1–2 tsp)
        freeze-dried leaves: 500–1,000 mg
        tincture (1:5): 4–6 ml (1–1.5 tsp)
        fluid extract (1:1): 1.0 ml (0.25–0.5 tsp)
        powdered solid extract (10% arbutin): 250–500 mg
    - *Hydrastis canadensis*:
        dried root (or as tea): 1–2 g
        freeze-dried root: 500–1,000 mg
        tincture (1:5): 4–6 ml (1–1.5 tsp)
        fluid extract (1:1): 0.5–2.0 ml (0.25–0.5 tsp)
        powdered solid extract (8% alkaloid): 250–500 mg
    - sandalwood oil: 1–2 drops.

Bacteriologic susceptibility to nutrients and botanical medicines

Bacteria species	Agent
Abacterial	Citrates
Enterobacter aerogenes	
Enterococcus	
Escherichia coli	*Allium sativum*
	Hydrastis canadensis
	Uva ursi
Klebsiella pneumonia	*Allium sativum*
	Hydrastis canadensis
Proteus miribili	*Allium sativum*
	Hydrastis canadensis
Pseudomonas aeruginosa	*Hydrastis canadensis*
Staphylococcus saprophyticus	*Allium sativum*
	Hydrastis canadensis

Dermatitis herpetiformis

DIAGNOSTIC SUMMARY

- Pruritic, blistering rash usually on extensor surfaces.
- Most common in middle-aged Caucasian males, although may present in individuals of any age.
- IgA deposits in papillary skin; confirmed by immunofluorescence.
- Asymptomatic "celiac" disease (gluten-sensitive enteropathy) in 75–90% of patients.

GENERAL CONSIDERATIONS

Dermatitis herpetiformis (DH) is a dermatological condition due to GI immunological disorder; jejunal biopsy in DH patients – villous atrophy characteristic of celiac disease, but GI symptoms rare; absorption studies (*Textbook*, Ch. 21) used to assess degree of enteropathy; average age of onset of rash = 7.2 years; predilection for elbows, knees, and buttocks; skin biopsy – granular IgA deposits.

THERAPEUTIC CONSIDERATIONS

- **Gluten:** most important factor is to eliminate all sources of gluten; Frazer's criteria for diagnosing gluten-sensitive enteropathy (improvement on gluten-free diet and relapse after reintroduction) indicate rash and villous atrophy are largely gluten-dependent; gluten elimination improves virtually all patients, including disappearance of reticulin and gluten antibodies in DH; gliadin polypeptide of gluten = key antigen; indirect immunofluorescence shows antibodies to gliadin in sera of 45% of DH patients with DH; titer and correlation increase with increasing disease severity; 81% of patients with severe jejunal abnormalities show antibodies to gliadin; gluten connection never mentioned in medical textbooks; gluten-free diet superior to drugs like dapsone and its severe side-effects.

  — Effects of gluten-free diet = 65+% of patients experience complete resolution and remainder substantially improved; complete resolution of DH enteropathy; harsh medicines can be eliminated or substantially reduced; most patients experience improved sense of well-being.

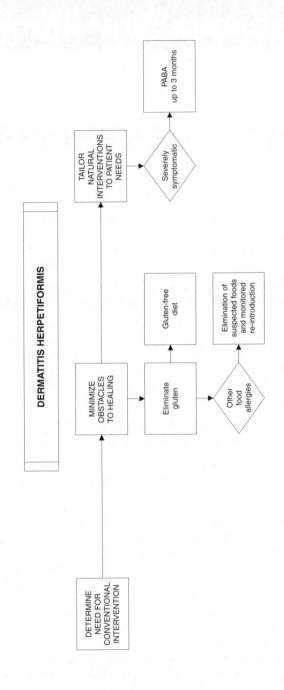

DERMATITIS HERPETIFORMIS

—Those using gluten-free diet rather than drugs are protected against developing lipomas.

- **Food allergy:** 35% of patients not adequately helped by gluten-free diet – only half of patients totally eliminate cutaneous IgA deposits and develop normal jejunal tissue; other food allergies develop via increased leakage of macromolecules across damaged GI mucosa; milk significant in some patients (ELISA); 75% of DH patients have serum antibodies to gliadin, bovine milk, or ovalbumin; elemental diet followed by careful food reintroduction gives better results than gluten-free diet.

- **PABA:** para-aminobenzoic acid used successfully to control DH, even in those not controlling dietary gluten; provides only symptom control and no repair of villous atrophy; not recommended treatment of choice – adjunct in unresponsive or severe cases.

THERAPEUTIC APPROACH

Eliminate all gluten and gliadin sources; identify and eliminate other food allergens (*Textbook*, Ch. 15); use therapeutic regimen similar to atopic dermatitis; patience is necessary since response may take several weeks to 6 months.

- **Diet:** normal, healthy, unprocessed diet free of all grains and allergic foods.
- **Supplements:**
   —PABA: 5 g q.d. until remission (maximum of 3 months).

Diabetes mellitus

DIAGNOSTIC SUMMARY

- Fasting (overnight): venous plasma glucose concentration $\geq$ 140 mg/dl on at least two separate occasions.
- Following ingestion of 75g glucose: venous plasma glucose concentration $\geq$ 200 mg/dl at 2 h post-ingestion and at least one other sample during 2-h test.
- Polyuria, polydipsia, and polyphagia.

GENERAL CONSIDERATIONS

Diabetes is a chronic disorder of carbohydrate, fat, and protein metabolism characterized by fasting elevations of blood glucose, greatly increased risk of heart disease, stroke, kidney disease, and loss of nerve function. Causes: pancreas does not secrete enough insulin, or cells of body resistant to insulin – sugar cannot enter cells, causing serious complications; > 10 million Americans have diabetes, but < half know this or ever consult physician.

Classification

Two major categories:

— type I (insulin-dependent diabetes mellitus, IDDM) – most often in children and adolescents

— type II (non-insulin-dependent diabetes mellitus, NIDDM) – onset after age 40.

Features	Type I	Type II
Age at onset	Usually under 40	Usually over 40
Percentage of all diabetics	Less than 10%	Greater than 90%
Seasonal trend	Fall and winter	None
Family history	Uncommon	Common
Appearance of symptoms	Rapid	Slow
Obesity at onset	Uncommon	Common
Insulin levels	Decreased	Variable
Insulin resistance	Occasional	Often
Treatment with insulin	Always	Not required
Beta-cells	Decreased	Variable

Features	Type I	Type II
Ketoacidosis	Frequent	Rare
Complications	Frequent	Frequent

- **IDDM (type I):** complete destruction of pancreas beta-cells, which manufacture insulin; patients require lifelong insulin, must manage blood sugar daily, modifying insulin types and dosage schedules according to results of regular blood sugar testing; 10% of diabetics are type I; current causal theory = injury to beta-cells plus defect in tissue regeneration; autoimmune component – antibodies to beta-cells present in 75% of cases, compared with 0.5–2.0% of normals; antibodies to beta-cells may develop in response to cell destruction due to other mechanisms (chemical, free radical, viral, food allergy).

- **NIDDM (type II):** 90% of diabetics; insulin elevated – loss of sensitivity to insulin by cells of body; obesity is the major contributor – 90% of type II diabetics are obese; achieving ideal body weight is linked to restoring normal blood sugar in most cases; diet of primary importance, implemented diligently before drug use; most type II diabetics can be controlled by diet alone.

- **Other types of diabetes:**
  - *secondary diabetes*: secondary to conditions/syndromes (pancreatic disease, hormone disturbances, drugs, malnutrition)
  - *gestational diabetes*: glucose intolerance during pregnancy
  - *impaired glucose tolerance*: includes prediabetic, chemical, latent, borderline, subclinical, and asymptomatic diabetes.

Individuals with impaired glucose tolerance have blood glucose and GTT intermediate between normal and clearly abnormal; reactive hypoglycemia may be prediabetic condition.

Incidence and epidemiology

Incidence is 4.5% in the US, of which 90% is NIDDM; prevalence rising – seventh leading cause of death in US; number of diabetics doubles every 15 years; linked to Western lifestyle – uncommon in cultures consuming "primitive" diet; in cultures switching to "foods of commerce", rate of DM increases.

Hypoglycemia–diabetes link

Western diet rich in refined sugar, fat, and animal products, and low in dietary fiber; refined carbohydrates are contributing factors to diabetes, reactive hypoglycemia, and obesity; refined sugars quickly absorbed, causing rapid rise in blood sugar; body response – greatly increase pancreas insulin secretion; excess insulin drives blood sugar down toward hypoglycemia; response is a rapid fall in blood glucose – adrenals secrete epinephrine (adrenaline), causing rapid increase in blood glucose; adrenals become "exhausted" by repeated stress; lack of response by exhausted adrenals leads to reactive hypoglycemia; further glucose stress induces insulin insensitivity and pancreas "exhaustion" – reactive hypoglycemia turns into diabetes.

DIAGNOSIS

● **Fasting blood glucose:** normal fasting blood glucose = 70–105 mg/dl; fasting blood glucose > 140 mg/dl on two separate occasions is diagnostic of diabetes; levels < 50 mg/dl indicate fasting hypoglycemia.

● **Glucose tolerance test (GTT):** very sensitive test for DM, but very stressful to patient and has relatively low specificity; 75 g glucose dose dissolved in 300 ml of water, for adults (1.75 g/kg ideal body weight for children), after overnight fast in subjects consuming 150+ g carbohydrate q.d. for 3 days prior to test; patient normal if 2-h plasma glucose < 140 mg/dl and no value > 200 mg/dl; confirmatory diagnosis of DM requires levels > 200 mg/dl at 2 h and at least once between zero time and 2 h; medications impairing glucose tolerance (diuretics, glucocorticoids, nicotinic acid, and phenytoin) may invalidate results.

● **Glucose-insulin tolerance test (G-ITT):** blood sugar levels alone are often not adequate for diagnosing blood sugar disorders; G-ITT is more sensitive in diagnosing hypoglycemia and diabetes than GTT; G-ITT uses 6-h glucose tolerance test plus measurements of insulin levels; two-thirds of subjects with suspected diabetes or hypoglycemia and normal GTT demonstrate abnormal ITT; down-side of G-ITT = cost.

● **Skin tags:** fibroepithelial papillomas common in diabetic men; multiple, large, hyperpigmented, lateral skin tags in male patient suggestive of diabetes – lab test to rule out.

CAUSES OF DIABETES

Genetic considerations

IDDM and NIDDM are genetically very different; IDDM has a positive association with $HLA-DR_3$, $HLA-DW_3$, $HLA-DR_4$, $HLA-B_8$ and $HLA-B_{15}$, and negative associations with $HLA-B_7$ and $HLA-DR_{21}$; 50% of juvenile diabetics are $HLA-B_8$; these correlations are not seen in NIDDM, but genetic factors play an even greater role; in twins under age 40, concordance rate of 20–50% in identical twins and 5% in fraternal twins with IDDM contrasted to concordance rate near 100% in identical and only 10% in fraternal twins with NIDDM; environmental factors are important in induction of DM – diet high in refined, fiber-depleted carbohydrate is diabetogenic in susceptible genotypes; high-fiber, complex carbohydrate-rich diet is protective; obesity is significant factor – 90%

of NIDDM types are obese; normal individuals – significant weight gain induces carbohydrate intolerance, higher insulin, and insulin insensitivity in fat and muscle tissue; progressive insulin insensitivity is an underlying factor in genesis of NIDDM; weight loss alone can correct abnormalities, improving metabolic disturbances of DM or converting overt diabetes into subclinical diabetes.

Etiological factors

IDDM due to insulin deficiency – hereditary beta-cell predisposition to injury plus defect in tissue regeneration; causes of injury: hydroxyl and other free radicals, viral infection, and autoimmune reactions; dietary intake of *N*-nitroso compounds in smoked/cured meats are diabetogenic in susceptible individuals, producing beta-cell damage; many chemicals, such as rodenticide vacor, are implicated.

- **Viral infection:** viral etiology initially suspected due to seasonal variation in onset of disease (October–March); during these months, viral diseases (mumps, hepatitis, infectious mononucleosis, congenital rubella, and Coxsackie virus infections) are more prevalent; viruses are capable of infecting beta-cells and inducing DM.

- **Autoimmunity:** possible especially in HLA-B$_8$ individuals; antibodies to pancreatic cells (all types) present in 75% of IDDM cases compared with 0.5–2.0% of normals; antibodies decline after first few weeks of disease, suggesting beta-cell destruction and depletion of antigenic stimulus; antibodies may arise from cell destruction due to other mechanisms when concealed cellular antigens exposed.

- **Early weaning and bovine milk exposure:** exposure to bovine albumin peptide in neonates may trigger autoimmunity and type I DM; animal/lab evidence suggestive, but human studies conflicting; early cow's milk exposure may be determinant of subsequent type I DM and may increase risk 1.5 times; patients with type I DM more likely to have been breast-fed < 3 months and exposed to cow's milk or solid foods before 4 months.

NIDDM: insulin insensitivity evidenced by high levels of circulating insulin and reversibility of hyperglycemia by dietary changes and/or weight loss sufficient to restore insulin sensitivity.

- **Obesity:** major role in etiology of NIDDM; linked to insulin insensitivity; adipose size and distribution may be important; types of obesity: hypertrophic obesity (enlarged fat cells) and hyperplastic obesity (increased number of fat cells); hypertrophic more closely linked to metabolic complications of obesity (diabetes, hyperinsulinemia, glucose intolerance, hypertension, hyperlipidemia); another system based on two categories of fat distribution – android type (deposition in upper body: abdomen – obese male) and gynecoid type (distribution in lower body: gluteal and femoral – obese female); activity of abdominal adipocyte affected by metabolic variables – plasma insulin and triglycerides; gluteal/femoral adipocytes sensitive to steroids (corticosteroids and estrogen); DM incidence higher in men and women with hypertrophic, android-type obesity; weight loss (decreased body fat percentage) is the prime objective in treating most NIDDM patients – improves all aspects of NIDDM and may cure.

● **Dietary fat:** percentage of calories from fat (saturated fat) linked to NIDDM and predicts conversion from impaired glucose tolerance to NIDDM; high-fat, low-carbohydrate diet increases risk of NIDDM.

● **Chromium (Cr) deficiency:** Cr level is a major determinant of insulin sensitivity; essential micronutrient, cofactor in all insulin-regulating activities; deficiency widespread in US; trivalent chromium (Cr^{3+}) is the only form exhibiting biological activity; integral component of "glucose tolerance factor" (GTF); GTF has two molecules of nicotinic acid plus cysteine, glutamine, and glycine; supplemental Cr improves glucose tolerance, decreases fasting glucose, cholesterol and triglycerides, and increases HDL by increasing insulin sensitivity in normal, elderly and NIDDM patients; but Cr is not a panacea for NIDDM.

● **Uremia:** potent inhibitor of insulin sensitivity – circulating small peptide unique to patients with kidney failure; assess and monitor renal function in all diabetics.

● **Prenatal factors:** prenatal malnutrition (hyperglycemia) may be promoter of types I and II DM later in life; adults during "hypocaloric war and post-war period (1941–48)" have much less DM than those born during hypercaloric years before and after: > 50% drop in incidence of DM; much lower incidence of childhood DM during periods in which maternal hyperglycemia is carefully controlled and fetus protected from hyperinsulinism: > 50% drop in incidence of childhood DM.

MONITORING THE DIABETIC PATIENT

Causal relationship between hyperglycemia and DM complications; monitoring and controlling hyperglycemia are critical to preventing complications; adequacy of control determined by simple lab tests.

● **Urinary glucose:** archaic and insufficient measure of diabetic control – diabetics have higher renal threshold for glucose than normal 180 mg/dl.

● **Home glucose monitoring:** reagent strips and capillary blood using simple spring-triggered device with disposable lancet; best sites are lateral sides of distal phalanges (avoid nail beds); sample placed on reagent strip and color change measured using reflectance meter; some reagent strips use visual inspection via dual-color scale.

● **Glycosylated hemoglobin:** proteins with glucose molecules attached (glycosylated peptides) elevated several-fold in DM; glycosylated hemoglobin (HgbA1c) used to monitor blood glucose over long period; normal

= 5–7% of hemoglobin; mild glucose elevations increase HgbA1c to 8–10%; severe elevations increase HgbA1c up to 20%; average RBC life span = 120 days, therefore HgbA1c assay is time-averaged value for glucose over preceding 2–4 months: simple, useful method for assessing treatment efficacy and patient compliance; also used to diagnose DM; oral GTT more sensitive than HgbA1c assay in DM diagnosis, but more stressful to patient; elevated HgbA1c almost always indicates DM: used by many physicians as alternative to GTT, especially for pregnant women.

COMPLICATIONS OF DIABETES

Risk of complications = reflection of glucose control; good glucose control greatly reduces risk; monitoring and controlling hyperglycemia are critical to preventing complications.

Acute complications

● **Hypoglycemia:** much more common in type I than type II – type I diabetic injects insulin; excess insulin, missing meals, and over-exercising induce hypoglycemia; insulin dosing must be gauged correctly; daytime hypoglycemic symptoms: sweating, nervousness, tremor, and hunger; nighttime hypoglycemia may be asymptoms or display night sweats, unpleasant dreams, or early morning HA; secretion of hormones which raise blood glucose levels (epinephrine, norepinephrine, growth hormone, cortisol) is increased – blood sugar rebounds, leading to hyperglycemia = Somogyi phenomenon; suspect Somogyi whenever there are wide swings in glucose over short periods of time during day; improved insulin therapy, insulin pump, and home monitoring afford better sugar control and decreased frequency of Somogyi phenomenon.

● **Diabetic ketoacidosis:** more likely in the type I; caused by lack of insulin and build-up of ketoacids; if progressive, ketoacidosis can cause metabolic problems and coma; potential medical emergency requiring prompt recognition; coma preceded by a day or more of polyuria, thirst, marked fatigue, N&V; home urine dipsticks measure ketones in urine.

● **Non-ketogenic hyperosmolar syndrome:** mortality rate > 50% makes non-ketogenic a true medical emergency; result of profound dehydration from deficient fluid intake or precipitating events (pneumonia, burns, stroke, recent surgery, certain drugs – phenytoin, diazoxide, glucocorticoids, and diuretics); onset insidious over period of days or weeks; symptoms: weakness, polyuria and thirst, and worsening signs of dehydration (weight loss, loss of skin elasticity, dry mucous membranes, tachycardia, hypotension).

Chronic complications

Atherosclerosis, retinopathy, neuropathy, nephropathy, and foot ulcers; two primary mechanisms: glycosylation of proteins and intracellular accumulation of sorbitol.

● **Glycosylation of proteins:** excessive non-enzymatic binding of glucose to proteins changes their structure and function; adverse effects = inactivation of enzymes, inhibition of regulatory molecule binding, cross-linking of glycosylated proteins, trapping of soluble proteins by glycosylated extracellular matrix, decreased susceptibility to proteolysis, abnormalities of nucleic acid function, altered macromolecular recognition, increased immunogenicity.

● **Sorbitol:** by-product of glucose metabolism formed within cell via aldose reductase; in non-diabetics, sorbitol is metabolized by polyol dehydrogenase to fructose, allowing sorbitol excretion from cell; in hyperglycemia, sorbitol accumulates and plays major role in chronic complications of DM; accumulation to high concentrations persists even if glucose levels return to normal; high concentration creates osmotic gradient drawing water into cells to maintain osmotic balance; cells release small molecules (amino acids, inositol, glutathione, niacin, vitamin C, Mg^{2+}, K^+) to maintain osmotic balance – these compounds protect cells from damage; their loss increases susceptibility to damage; intracellular accumulation of polyols is a major factor in the complications of DM – lens epithelium, Schwann cell of peripheral nerve, papilla in kidney, islets of Langerhans in pancreas, and mural cell of retinal blood vessels; measurement of RBC sorbitol is valuable indicator of diabetic control – RBC and nerve cell sorbitol correlate well.

● **Atherosclerosis:** 2–3 times higher risk of dying prematurely of atherosclerosis than non-diabetics; reduce risk factors linked to MI and stroke (LDL and triglycerides) and increase HDL – healthy diet and lifestyle.

● **Diabetic neuropathy:** loss of peripheral nerve function, tingling sensations, numbness, loss of function, pain, and muscle weakness; occasionally affects deeper nerves – impaired heart function, alternating bouts of diarrhea and constipation, inability to empty bladder, and impotence; earliest and best measured signs of neuropathy are decreased nerve conduction velocities; due to sorbitol accumulation, which leads to myoinositol loss; inositol supplements may improve nerve conduction velocity, but underlying sorbitol issue must be addressed.

● **Diabetic retinopathy:** can result in blindness – leading cause of blindness in US; 1 in 20 type I and 1 in 15 type II diabetics develop retinopathy; lesions divided into background or "simple" retinopathy (microaneurysms, hemorrhages, exudates, and retinal edema) and proliferative or "malignant" retinopathy (newly formed vessels, scarring, retinitis proliferens, vitreous hemorrhage, and retinal detachment); laser photocoagulation may reduce diabetes-induced blindness; patients with these signs should be referred to ophthalmologist – moderate or severe growth of new vessels on or within one disc diameter of optic disc, mild growth of new vessels on or within one disc diameter of optic disc if fresh hemorrhage present, moderate or severe growth of new vessels elsewhere if fresh hemorrhage present; laser photocoagulation probably not indicated in milder retinopathy since occasional side-effects (vitreous hemorrhage, vitreous contraction with retinal detachment, macular edema, and visual field loss) may outweigh benefits.

- **Diabetic neuropathy:** usually limited to peripheral nerves; most common is peripheral polyneuropathy; typically bilateral – paresthesias, severe hyperesthesias, and pain; dulled perception of vibration, pain and temperature, worse in lower extremities; bilateral atrophy of first interosseous muscle of hand is characteristic; nerve conduction delayed; delayed Achilles reflex similar to hypothyroidism; occasional autonomic neuropathy – postural hypotension, decreased cardiovascular response to Valsalva maneuver, resting tachycardia, alternating bouts of diarrhea and constipation, inability to empty bladder, and impotence.

- **Diabetic nephropathy:** common complication and a leading cause of death in DM; four types of possibly overlapping lesions: glomerulosclerosis, arteriosclerosis of efferent and afferent arterioles, arteriosclerosis of renal artery and its intrarenal branches, and peritubular deposits of glycogen, fat, and mucopolysaccharides; Kimmelsteil–Wilson syndrome = edema, hypertension, proteinuria, and renal failure as complications of DM; periodic monitoring of patient's kidney function (BUN, uric acid, creatinine, and creatinine clearance) important.

- **Diabetic foot ulcers:** ischemia and peripheral neuropathy are key factors; incidence of gangrene of feet is 20 times that of matched controls; foot ulcers largely preventable with proper foot care, avoidance of injury and tobacco, employing methods to improve local circulation, and keeping feet clean, dry, and warm; wear only well-fitted shoes; tobacco constricts peripheral blood vessels and can cause Buerger's disease; improve circulation by avoiding sitting with legs crossed or other positions compromising circulation; massage feet lightly upwards and carefully apply hydrotherapy (*Textbook*, Ch. 42); *Ginkgo biloba* extract may help improve vascular flow.

THERAPEUTIC CONSIDERATIONS

Effective treatment requires careful integration of wide range of therapies and patient's willingness to alter diet and lifestyle; monitor carefully, particularly if on insulin or relatively uncontrolled DM; attend to symptoms, home glucose monitoring, and other blood tests; drug dosing will need alteration as natural therapies are implemented.

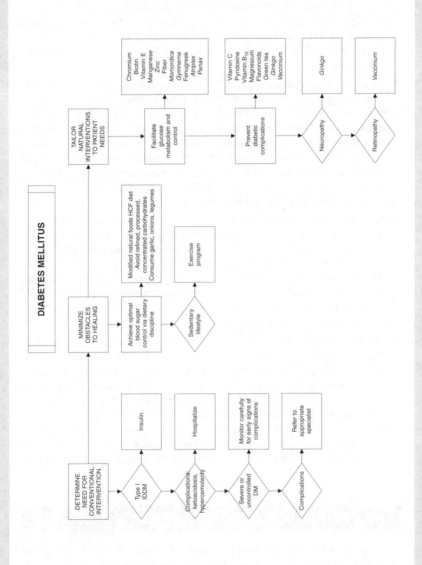

Diet

Fundamental to success in type I or II; DM highly correlated with low-fiber/high refined carbohydrate diet; diet high in plant cell-wall materials and complex carbohydrates and low in fat and animal products superior to oral hypoglycemic agents, insulin (when < 30 units/day), carbohydrate restriction, high protein, and ADA diet.

- **ADA diet:** inferior to HCF and MHCF; exchange system recognizes six food groups: milk, vegetables, fruit, bread, meat, and fat; Healthy Exchange System is a better version – emphasizes healthier food choices of unprocessed, whole foods; diet prescribed by allotting specific number of exchanges per list per day; restrict fat to < 35% of total calories; reduce saturated fats to 1/3 of fat intake, substituting poultry, veal, and fish for red meats; reduce cholesterol to < 300 mg q.d.; carbohydrate content = 40–50% of total calories; unrefined carbohydrates supplying 15–20 g q.d. of fiber; exclude refined/simple carbohydrates; weaknesses of ADA diet: not as effective as other diets, large percentage of calories derived from fat, low in fiber.

- **HCF diet:** high carbohydrate, high plant-fiber diet popularized by James Anderson MD; high in cereal grains, legumes, and root vegetables; restricts simple sugar and fat; 70–75% complex carbohydrates, 15–20% protein, and 10–25% fat, total fiber 100 g q.d.; positive metabolic effects are reduced postprandial hyperglycemia and delayed hypoglycemia, increased tissue sensitivity to insulin, reduced cholesterol and triglycerides with increased HDL, progressive weight reduction; Anderson promotes two HCF diets – (1) initial treatment of hospitalized patient (70% carbohydrate, 19% protein, 11% fat, 50 mg q.d. cholesterol and 35–49 g q.d. dietary fiber per 1,000 kcal); (2) home maintenance diet (55–60% carbohydrate, 20% protein, 20–25% fat, 75–200 mg q.d. cholesterol, 50 g q.d. dietary fiber); carbohydrate from grains (50%), fruits and vegetables (48%), and skimmed milk (2%); protein, fruits and vegetables (50%), grains (36%), and skim milk and lean meat (14%); fat from grains (60%), fruits and vegetables (20%), and skim milk and meat (12%); exchange system used; serum triglyceride is a sensitive indicator of dietary compliance – when patient deviates, serum triglycerides rise; type I patients also benefit from HCF diet – average insulin requirements drop by 38% plus much lower fasting, postprandial and urinary glucose than matched patients on control diets.

- **Modified high-fiber content diet (MHFC):** substitutes more natural (primitive/unprocessed) foods wherever possible in HCF diet; higher in legume fiber; limits processed grains; excludes fruit juices, low-fiber fruits, skimmed milk and margarine; legumes low in fat, high in complex carbohydrates and fiber, and effective in treating DM; fruit juices, low-fiber fruits, and processed grains (flour) rapidly elevate serum glucose and insulin; casein in skimmed milk raises cholesterol; *trans* fatty acids in margarine (and other synthetically saturated fats) also injurious.

- **Importance of dietary fiber:** DM related to inadequate dietary fiber intake; increase complex carbohydrates rich in fiber; "dietary fiber" = plant cell walls and indigestible residues from plant foods; types most beneficial to blood sugar control are water-soluble hemicelluloses, mucilages, gums, and pectins – slow down digestion and absorption of carbohydrates, preventing hyperglycemia, increasing sensitivity to insulin, preventing hyperinsulinemia, and improving glucose uptake by liver and other tissues; majority of fiber in most plant cell walls is water-soluble; good sources of water-soluble fiber = legumes, oat bran, nuts, seeds, psyllium seed husks, pears, apples, and most vegetables; daily intake – at least 50 g.

- **Fiber supplements vs. high-fiber diet:** fiber supplements (guar gum at 5 g/meal and pectin 10 g/meal) have positive impact on diabetic control; fiber-supplemented diets not as effective as HCF diet; reserved for type II patient unwilling to implement dietary changes and willing to settle for palliation; insulin dosage on fiber-supplemented diets reduced to 1/3 used on control (ADA) diets, but HCF diet helps discontinue insulin therapy in 60% of NIDDM patients, and greatly reduces doses in other 40% (*Textbook*, Ch. 57).

- **Glycemic index:** developed by David Jenkins in 1981 to measure rise of blood glucose after eating a particular food; standard value of 100 based on rise after ingestion of glucose; ranges from 20 for fructose and whole barley to 98 for baked potato; insulin response to carbohydrate foods similar to rise in blood sugar; guideline for diabetics and hypoglycemics; avoid foods with high values and choose instead carbohydrate foods with lower values; glycemic index should not be only dietary guideline – high-fat foods have low glycemic index but are not good choices for hypoglycemics or diabetics.

- **Fruits and fructose:** fructose does not cause rapid rise in blood sugar – fructose converted to glucose in liver to be used by body; most diabetics and hypoglycemics cannot tolerate sucrose, but most can tolerate moderate amounts of fruits and fructose; fructose and fruits better tolerated than white bread and other refined carbohydrates; produce less sharp elevations in blood sugar compared with starch; fructose enhances sensitivity to insulin by 34% when fed to NIDDM patients for 4 weeks.

Nutritional supplements

Patients have greatly increased need for many nutrients; improve blood sugar control; prevent or ameliorate many major complications of DM; diet is primary focus.

- **Chromium:** works closely with insulin, facilitating glucose uptake into cells; supplementing Cr decreases fasting glucose, improves glucose tolerance, lowers insulin, and decreases total cholesterol and triglycerides while increasing HDL; decreases HgbA1c, fasting glucose, 2-h postprandial glucose, fasting and 2-h postprandial insulin, and total cholesterol; reversing Cr deficiency by supplementing lowers body weight and increases lean body mass; effects are due to increased insulin sensitivity; Cr deficiency may be underlying factor in diabetes, hypoglycemia, and obesity; at least 200 µg q.d. necessary for optimal sugar regulation; depleted by refined carbohydrates, and lack of exercise; prefer Cr polynicotinate, Cr picolinate, and Cr-enriched yeast.

● **Vitamin C:** major function is manufacture of collagen, main protein substance of connective tissue; vital for wound repair, healthy gums, preventing excess bruising, immune function, manufacture of certain neurotransmitters and hormones, and absorption and utilization of other nutritional factors; transport of vitamin C into cells is facilitated by insulin – diabetics may have insufficient intracellular vitamin C = relative vitamin C deficiency despite adequate dietary consumption; chronic latent vitamin C deficiency causes increased bleeding tendency (increased capillary permeability), poor wound healing, microvascular disease, elevated cholesterol and depressed immune function; high doses (2,000 mg q.d.) reduce accumulation of sorbitol in RBCs of diabetics and inhibit glycosylation of proteins; corrects sorbitol accumulation independent of changes in diabetic control; encourage vitamin C-rich foods that also contain flavonoids and carotenes, which enhance effects of vitamin C; dietary sources of vitamin C: broccoli, peppers, potatoes, Brussels sprouts, citrus fruits.

● **Niacin and niacinamide (nicotinamide):** niacin (vitamin B_3)-containing enzymes important in energy production, metabolism of fat, cholesterol, and carbohydrate, and the synthesis of many body compounds (sex and adrenal hormones); essential component of GTF; niacinamide (Ncm) supplements may prevent type I diabetes and help restore beta-cells or at least slow down their destruction; Ncm prolongs non-insulin-requiring remission, lowers insulin, improves metabolic control, and increases beta-cell function; Ncm can induce complete resolution in some newly diagnosed type I diabetics; main difference between positive and negative studies in recent-onset IDDM is older age and higher baseline fasting C-peptide in positive studies; mechanism of action = inhibition of macrophage- and interleukin-1-mediated beta-cell damage, inhibition of nitric oxide production, and antioxidant activity; daily dose of nicotinamide = 25 mg/kg; children use 100–200 mg q.d.; inositol hexaniacinate (Inh) is useful in type I and type II DM to lower hyperlipidemia; niacin lowers cholesterol safely and extends life; Inh lowers cholesterol and improves blood flow in intermittent claudication; Inh improves sugar regulation and is much better tolerated than niacin; high-dose niacin can disrupt glucose control in diabetics; closely monitor glucose and discontinue if worsening of diabetic control.

● **Biotin:** functions in manufacture and utilization of carbohydrates, fats, and amino acids; synthesized in intestines by gut bacteria; vegetarian diet alters intestinal flora to enhance synthesis and promote absorption of biotin; supplements enhance insulin sensitivity and increase activity of glucokinase, the enzyme in first step of utilization of glucose by liver; glucokinase is low in diabetics; 16 mg q.d. biotin significantly lowers fasting glucose and improves glucose control in type I DM; in type II DM, similar effects at 9 mg q.d. biotin; insulin requirements must be adjusted.

- **Vitamin B$_6$:** supplements protect against diabetic neuropathy (such patients deficient in B$_6$); long-standing DM or signs of peripheral nerve abnormalities indicate B$_6$; dose = 150 mg q.d.; neuropathy of B$_6$ deficiency indistinguishable from DM neuropathy; B$_6$ inhibits glycosylation of proteins; safe treatment for gestational diabetes – 100 mg B$_6$ × 2 weeks.

- **Vitamin B$_{12}$:** deficiency characterized by numbness of feet, pins and needles sensations, or burning feeling – symptoms typical of DM neuropathy; B$_{12}$ supplements used with some success in DM neuropathy; absence of megaloblastic anemia not adequate criteria for ruling out deficiency; deficit within nerve cells precedes anemia by several years; measuring blood levels is more reliable; oral 1,000–3,000 µg q.d. may be sufficient, but i.m. vitamin B$_{12}$ may be necessary in many cases.

- **Vitamin E:** diabetics have an increased requirement for vitamin E; high-dose vitamin E (900 IU q.d.) improves insulin action and offers benefits that may prevent long-term DM complications; may be preventive of DM.

- **Magnesium:** involved in several areas of glucose metabolism; Mg deficiency is common in diabetics and Mg may prevent DM complications (retinopathy and heart disease); Mg levels lowest in those with severe retinopathy; RDA = 350 mg q.d. for adult males and 300 mg q.d. for adult females; diabetics may need twice this amount; sources: tofu, legumes, seeds, nuts, whole grains, green leafy vegetables; fish, meat, milk, refined foods, and most commonly eaten fruit – low in Mg; at least 50 mg q.d. B$_6$ needed – level of intracellular B$_6$ is intricately linked to Mg content of cell: without B$_6$, Mg will not enter cell.

- **Potassium (K):** supplements improve insulin sensitivity, responsiveness and secretion; insulin administration induces loss of K; high K intake reduces risk of heart disease, atherosclerosis, and cancer; estimated safe and adequate daily dietary intake = 1.9–5.6 g; K salts can cause N&V, diarrhea, and ulcers; side-effects not seen when K is increased via diet only – vegetable juices, foods, and food-based K supplements; most people can handle excess K, but patients with DM and kidney disease do not handle K normally and are more likely to experience heart disturbances and other consequences of K toxicity; patients with kidney disorders need to restrict K intake; most diabetics can consume high-K diet, but evaluate kidney function before prescribing K supplement.

- **Manganese:** a cofactor in many enzymes of glucose control, energy metabolism, and thyroid hormone function; Mn deficiency in lab animals results in DM and offspring with pancreatic abnormalities or no pancreas at all; diabetics have only half the Mn of normal persons; daily dose for diabetics = 30 mg.

- **Zinc:** involved in all aspects of insulin metabolism; protective against beta-cell destruction; antiviral effects; diabetics excrete excessive amounts of Zn in urine; supplements improve insulin levels in type I and type II DM; helps improve poor wound healing in diabetics; sources: whole grains, legumes, nuts, and seeds; supplemental dose for diabetics = 30 mg q.d. (min.).

● **Flavonoids:** normalize body's reaction to allergens, viruses, and carcinogens: anti-inflammatory, anti-allergic, antiviral, and anti-carcinogenic properties; quercetin promotes insulin secretion and potently inhibits sorbitol accumulation; increase intracellular vitamin C, decrease leakiness and breakage of small blood vessels, prevent easy bruising; support immune function; consume diet rich in flavonoids; supplemental dose = 1–2 g q.d. mixed flavonoids.

● **Essential fatty acids:** omega-6 and omega-3 fatty acids benefit diabetes; omega-6 gamma-linolenic acid (18:3n6) protects against diabetic neuropathy; omega-3 oils protect against atherosclerosis and augment insulin secretion in NIDDM; increase cold-water fish (salmon, herring, mackerel, halibut); supplement 480 mg gamma-linolenic acid (evening primrose, borage, blackcurrant oil); consume 1 tbsp (10 g) flaxseed oil q.d.

— *omega-6 fatty acids*: DM linked to substantial disturbance in essential fatty acid (EFA) metabolism, causing microvascular, hemorrheological, and other abnormalities that lead to reduced blood flow and neuronal hypoxia; endoneural hypoxia impairs axonal transport, produces demyelination, and reduces neural ATPase activity; EFA metabolic disturbance due to intracellular deficiencies of nutrients of EFA metabolism (C, Mg, B_6, Zn); key disturbance is impaired conversion of linoleic acid to gamma-linolenic (GLA), dihomo-gamma-linolenic (DHGLA), and arachidonic acids; as a result, providing GLA may bypass this disturbance.

— *omega-3 fatty acids*: lower total cholesterol, LDL, and triglyceride and raise HDL; decrease blood viscosity; increase tissue plasminogen activator; reduce endothelial permeability; improve insulin function; proper dosage and antioxidant support (vitamin E) critical to produce beneficial rather than deleterious effects; potential small deleterious effects – increased plasma glucose, total cholesterol, LDL, and serum apolipoprotein B – at larger doses (4–10 g q.d. EPA and DHA); at lower dosage of 2.5 g omega-3 fatty acids, fish oil inhibits platelet aggregation and thromboxane A_2 production, reduces elevated systolic BP, reduces triglycerides, and causes small but statistically significant increase in HBA1c and total cholesterol – benefits retained and deleterious effects reduced at lower dosage; there is threshold of benefit with EPA: dosages above 900 mg q.d. adversely affect glucose control and blood lipids; peroxide contaminants may be source of problem with fish oil supplements; fish consumption is more effective in improving several other factors involved in cardiovascular disease; inverse correlation between fish intake and impaired glucose tolerance and DM; fish consumption lowers mortality; low prevalence of IDDM and NIDDM in cultures consuming cold-water fish; flaxseed oil may offer similar benefits from alpha-linolenic acid (ALA) converted to EPA; linolenic acid has many of the same benefits as EPA plus several on its own; ALA is not as effective in increasing tissue EPA and lowering tissue arachidonic acid; daily intake of 30 g q.d. of fish = two 100 g servings/week; flaxseed oil daily dosage = 1 tbsp (roughly 10 g).

- **Carnitine:** supplementing diabetics significantly decreases total serum lipid and increases HDL; increases beta-oxidation of fatty acids, and may prevent ketoacidosis.

- **Inositol:** effective in experimental animal diabetic neuropathy, re-establishing normal myoinositol levels in deficient neurons; neuronal myoinositol deficiency may be due to glucose competition with myoinositol for active transport plus sorbitol accumulation, resulting in loss of intracellular myoinositol; oral supplements in human diabetics have not provided significant clinical improvement.

- **Lipoic acid (also known as alpha-lipoic acid and thioctic acid):** an approved drug in Germany for the treatment of diabetic neuropathy, several double-blind studies have shown lipoic acid supplementation (300–600 mg daily) to improve diabetic neuropathy. Lipoic acid's primary effect in improving diabetic neuropathy is thought to be the result of its antioxidant effects. However, it has also been shown to lead to an improvement in blood sugar metabolism, to improve blood flow to peripheral nerves, and actually to stimulate the regeneration of nerve fibers. Its ability to improve blood sugar metabolism is a result of its effects on glucose metabolism and an ability to increase insulin sensitivity.

Botanical medicines

Before the advent of insulin, DM was treated with plant medicines; effective natural treatment of diabetics requires careful integration of diet, nutritional supplements, lifestyle, and botanical medicine.

- ***Allium cepa* and *Allium sativum*:** onions and garlic have blood sugar-lowering action; active principles = sulfur-containing compounds, allyl propyl disulfide (APDS) and diallyl disulfide oxide (allicin), respectively; flavonoids may play a role; APDS lowers glucose by competing with insulin (also a disulfide) for insulin-inactivating sites in liver, increasing free insulin; ADPS in doses of 125 mg/kg to fasting humans drops blood glucose and increases serum insulin; allicin at doses of 100 mg/kg has similar effect; graded doses of onion extracts (1 ml of extract = 1 g whole onion) at levels found in diet (1–7 oz onion) reduce glucose in dose-dependent manner; effects similar in raw and boiled onion extracts; lower cholesterol and blood pressure (BP).

- ***Momordica charantia* (bitter melon, balsam pear):** green cucumber-shaped fruit covered with gourd-like bumps; native to Asia, Africa and South America; fresh juice and extract of unripe fruit lower blood sugar in human clinical trials; several compounds have confirmed anti-diabetic properties: charantin = hypoglycemic mixture of steroids more potent than oral hypoglycemic drug tolbutamide; insulin-like polypeptide-P lowers blood sugar when injected subcutaneously into type I diabetics with fewer side-effects than insulin – suggested as replacement for some patients; oral bitter melon preparations – good results in type II diabetics: glucose tolerance improved using 57 g of juice; 15 g of aqueous extract produces 54% decrease in postprandial blood sugar and 17% reduction in HbA1c; dose = 57 g shot of juice.

- **Gymnema sylvestre:** plant native to tropical forests of India; effective in type I and type II DM; applied to tongue, gymnemic acid blocks sensation of sweetness; subjects who had *Gymnema* extracts applied to tongue ate fewer calories at meals compared with controls; capsules or tablets do not produce same effect; enhances glucose control in diabetic animals; no effect in pancreasectomized animals – may enhance secretion of endogenous insulin; may regenerate beta-cells; reduces insulin requirements and fasting glucose, and improves glucose control in type I diabetics on insulin; in type I DM, *Gymnema* may enhance action of insulin; in type II DM, improves glucose control; reduces need for hypoglycemic drugs in some patients and eliminates need in others – sugar control with *Gymnema* extract alone; dosage for extract = 400 mg q.d. in type I and type II; does not have hypoglycemic effects in healthy volunteers; no side-effects reported.

- **Trigonella foenum-graecum:** fenugreek active principle is in defatted portion of seed, containing alkaloid trigonelline, nicotinic acid, and coumarin; defatted seed powder 50 g b.i.d. in IDDM reduces fasting glucose and improves glucose tolerance with 54% reduction in 24-h urinary glucose excretion and significant reductions in LDL, VLDL, and triglycerides; in non-insulin diabetics, 15 g powdered seed soaked in water significantly reduced postprandial glucose during meal tolerance test.

- **Atriplex halimus:** salt bush is branchy woody shrub native to Mediterranean, North Africa, and southern Europe; improves glucose regulation and glucose tolerance in type II diabetics; rich in fiber, protein, and trace minerals including chromium; dosage used in human studies = 3 g q.d.

- **Pterocarpus marsupium and epicatechin-containing plants:** *Pterocarpus* has long history of use in India for DM; flavonoid, (–)-epicatechin, from bark, prevents beta-cell damage in rats; epicatechin and extract of *Pterocarpus marsupium* actually regenerates functional pancreatic beta-cells in diabetic animals; catechin and epicatechin plus their glycosides and esters are flavan-3-ols that readily undergo epimerization (interconversion between chemically identical but sterically different forms); interconversion of (+) and (–) forms possible; these constituents are very strong antioxidants against hydroxyl radical-induced lipoperoxidation of alloxan-induced DM and many hepatotoxins; most flavan-3-ols may have anti-diabetic properties; dry weight percentage of epicatechin is high in *Camellia chinensis* (green tea) (1–3%) and *Acacia catechu* (burma cutch) (5%) – also good sources of catechins, gallo-catechins and epigallocatechins; commercial *Pterocarpus* is lacking in US – green tea suitable alternative; dosage = 2+ cups green tea q.d. = 240 mg green tea polyphenols.

● *Vaccinium myrtillus*: bilberry or European blueberry is shrubby perennial with blue-black berry; leaf tea orally administered reduces hyperglycemia in normal and diabetic dogs, even when glucose concurrently injected i.v.; berries may offer greater benefit; anthocyanoside myrtillin is the most active constituent: weaker than insulin when injected, but less toxic, even at 50×1 g q.d. therapeutic dose; single dose can produce benefits lasting several weeks; anthocyanosides increase intracellular vitamin C, decrease leakiness and breakage of capillaries, prevent easy bruising, and are potent antioxidants – support microvascular abnormalities of DM; improves night vision – anthocyanosides have affinity for blood vessels of retina, especially macula, and improve circulation to retina; beneficial in diabetic retinopathy; extract dose based on anthocyanosides, calculated by anthocyanidin percentage (typically 25%); dose = 80–160 mg t.i.d.

● *Ginkgo biloba*: improves blood flow to peripheral tissues; superior to placebo in intermittent claudication; prevents diabetic retinopathy in diabetic rats; dosage of extract standardized to 24% ginkgo flavoglycosides and 6% terpenoids = 40 mg t.i.d.

● **Ginseng:** in NIDDM, elevates mood, improves psychophysiological performance, and reduces fasting glucose and body weight; 200 mg dose improved HbA1c, serum amino-terminal propeptide concentrations, and physical activity.

Exercise

Improves many parameters and is indicated in IDDM and NIDDM; physically trained diabetics experience enhanced insulin sensitivity with consequent diminished need for exogenous insulin, improved glucose tolerance, reduced total cholesterol and triglycerides with increased HDL resulting in less atherogenesis, and improved weight loss (in obese diabetics); must be carefully adapted to fitness of patient; avoided during hypoglycemia; exercise increases tissue levels of Cr (in rats) and increases number of insulin receptors in IDDM patients.

THERAPEUTIC APPROACH

Careful integration of wide range of therapies; patient must be willing to improve lifestyle; type II DM is the end result of chronic metabolic insult; focus of protocol on NIDDM, but equally appropriate for IDDM with exception that, according to current information, type I diabetic will always require insulin; thorough diagnostic work-up essential – identify DM complications; study patient's diet, environment, and lifestyle; rule out agents inducing glucose intolerance; tailor diet, exercise, and supplement program to patient needs – current glucose tolerance; normalize patient's weight (*Textbook*, Ch. 175); severe or uncontrolled DM demands awareness of early indications of acute complications – acidosis and hyperosmolar non-ketogenic coma; hospitalize patient at first signs, monitor carefully if patient on insulin or DM relatively uncontrolled; Somogyi phenomenon can give misleading fasting and urinary glucose levels, causing inappropriate therapeutic actions and serious, life-threatening symptoms; home glucose monitoring, and HgbA1c are the best ways to monitor progress; as therapies take effect, drug dosages will have to be altered – good working relationship with prescribing doctor greatly aids healing; ultimate goal is to re-establish normal glycemia and prevent (or ameliorate) complications; do not suddenly take patient off diabetic drugs, especially insulin – according to current information, IDDM patient will never be able to stop insulin.

● **Diet:** HCF diet modified to incorporate more natural foods; avoid all simple, processed and concentrated carbohydrates; stress complex-carbohydrate, high-fiber foods; minimize fats; encourage legumes, onions and garlic.

● **Supplements:**

— chromium: 200–400 µg q.d.

— vitamin C: > 2,000 mg q.d.

— biotin: 16 mg q.d. (IDDM); 9 mg q.d. (NIDDM)

— pyridoxine: 150 mg q.d.

— vitamin E: 900 IU q.d.

— selenium: 200 µg q.d.

— magnesium: 300–500 mg q.d.

— manganese: 30 mg q.d.

— zinc (picolinate): 25 mg q.d.

— mixed flavonoids: 1,000–2,000 mg q.d.

— fiber (guar, pectin, or oat bran): 20–30 g q.d.

— lipoic acid: 300–600 mg q.d.

● **Botanical medicines:**

— *Momordica charantia*: 30–60 ml fresh juice t.i.d.

— *Gymnema sylvestre* extract: 200 mg b.i.d.

— defatted fenugreek powder: 50 g q.d.

— *Atriplex halimus*: 3 g q.d.

— green tea: two 120 ml cups q.d. or 200–300 mg of green tea polyphenols

— *Ginkgo biloba* extract (24% ginkgo flavoglycosides, 6% terpenoids): 40 mg t.i.d.

— *Panax ginseng* extract (5% ginsenosides): 100 mg q.d.–t.i.d.

● **Exercise:** graded program based on patient's fitness and interest, which elevates heart rate > 50% × 1/2 hour three times a week.

Epididymitis

DIAGNOSTIC SUMMARY

Acute or chronic, painful, tender swelling of epididymis; fever, chills, groin pain, leukocytosis; usually secondary to other infections of GU tract.

GENERAL CONSIDERATIONS

Acute epididymitis self-limited and, with immune support and medical care, resolves without complications; chronic epididymitis uncommon and generally seen as irreversible end stage of severe acute attack untreated or unresponsive, and followed by frequent mild attacks; pain in epididymitis caused by pressure against inelastic casing of tunica albuginea; as inflammation spreads up vas deferens, pain intensified by constricting action of external inguinal ring, which, by not allowing swelling, increases pressure; infection may spread through lumen of ducts, lymphatics, and blood vessels or directly through tissues and along membranes; ligation of vas deferens, but not lymphatics, does not prevent epididymitis; rows of tight junctions form blood –testis barrier; large molecules prevent access while smaller molecules freely permeate lumen, although much of transport stereospecific.

DIAGNOSIS

Differential diagnosis of the acute scrotum.

- **Epididymitis:** sudden onset of severe scrotal pain and swelling; possible history of gradual onset of swelling and pain; pain may radiate along spermatic cord and can become flank pain; visible swelling follows pain; early stage, epididymis can be distinguished within scrotal sac, but within hours testis can double in size and epididymis become one mass; tenderness over groin or lower abdominal quadrant of same side; if epididymis palpable, structure indurated, enlarged and painful; inflammation unilateral, left and right sides equally represented; slight elevation in temperature in only half of patients; urinalysis (UA) recommended, but frequently negative; follow with culture if bacteriuria; pyuria is most frequent finding; to improve sensitivity, do prostatic massage and collect first 20–30 ml of urine; cleanse penis before massage and urine collection; i.v. urography has been employed diagnostically, but not recommended – findings do not alter method of care, is expensive, risky, and is poor choice unless TB suspected and abnormal chest films obtained.

● **Intrascrotal torsion:** in children, suspect torsion; intrascrotal torsion is rotational twisting of vascular pedicle causing venous and arterial insufficiency; damage in proportion to duration of ischemia; duration ≤ 8 h – usually 100% recovery; 24 h of ischemia – only 50% chance of total recovery; three types of torsion:

— *extravaginal torsion*: newborns present as asymptomatic, firm, discolored mass;

— *intravaginal torsion*: most common in children (also in post-teen young adults); congenital problem with abnormal testicular suspension; pain is the presenting complaint with acute scrotal inflammation, N&V;

— *torsion from twisting of testicular appendage*: point tenderness on superior aspect of testis; sometimes a palpable firm, pea-sized nodule; precipitated by human chorionic gonadotropin in puberty; appendage enlarges and infarcts.

● **Procedures differentiating torsion from epididymitis:** spermatic cord twisted in torsion – testis often elevated and rotated with epididymis out of normal position; Prehn's sign (elevation of testis) gives relief in epididymitis, but not torsion; epididymitis – skin adheres to epididymis on affected side, but no skin adherence in torsion; cremasteric reflex (elicited by stroking medial thigh and observing testicular retraction) usually absent in torsion; if pyuria, diagnosis of torsion more difficult; normal UA in a child makes epididymitis unlikely; Doppler reveals reduced sounds with torsion – less spermatic blood flow; epididymitis has sounds of increased blood flow.

● **Mumps:** Epididymo-orchitis occurs in 20% of postpubertal males with mumps; usually unilateral; parotitis makes diagnosis simple; parotitis absent – other associated syndromes of obscure etiology (aseptic meningitis, encephalitis, pancreatitis, arthritis) may help diagnosis.

● **Tubercular epididymitis:** rarely associated with pain or fever; beading of vas and induration of prostate; TB involvement suspected if no sexual contact or STD unlikely and no bacteriuria or pyuria (bacteriuria or pyuria plus sexual contact, suspect link to non-gonococcal urethritis [NGU] rather than TB); when TB suspected, order chest film before more elaborate testing; TB of testis and epididymis is usually secondary to infection elsewhere in body, most often GU tract.

● **Scrotal tumors:** swelling painless, but hemorrhage causes painful distension against tunica albuginea; prostate UA normal; diagnosis via ultrasonography and lab tests for tumor marker glycoproteins (alpha-fetoprotein and human chorionic gonadotropin); biopsy should never be performed – greatly increases risk of lymphatic spread; testicular cancer is most common CA in young men; neoplasm suspected when epididymitis fails to respond to adequate treatment.

- **Trauma:** rare cause of epididymitis – scrotum will "roll away" from injuries; etiology reserved for cases with objective evidence of trauma and absence of infection of urine or prostate; trauma displays discoloration, while infection does not; scrotal trauma obvious from history.

- **Henoch–Schönlein purpura:** presents with scrotal involvement in 15–38% of cases; tends to mimic torsion more than epididymitis; associated with diffuse systemic vasculitis; rarely presents with only scrotal symptoms.

- **Inguinal hernia:** inguinal hernia or hydrocele does not look like acute scrotum, except when hernia is incarcerated; focus – above scrotum; palpable spermatic thickening between vas and inguinal ring.

- **Idiopathic scrotal edema:** generally seen in children; scrotal enlargement bilateral and symmetrical; etiology may be allergy and redness can extend beyond scrotum to perineum or inguinal region; no deep tenderness – pain coming from skin or subcutaneous layers.

- **Spermatoceles:** arise from the epididymis; translucent – sufficient to differentiate them from epididymitis.

- **Chemical epididymitis:** controversial non-pathogenic basis; triggered by reflux of sterile urine into epididymis; induced in lab models but such research has not eliminated controversy; many researchers insist reflux is impossible; if reflux is occurring, urine follows urethra back through ejaculatory ducts into vas deferens; studies demonstrate idiopathic epididymitis with sterile cultures of epididymal washings; strenuous exercise or straining with full bladder may cause "retrograde urination" into vas.

- **Sexually transmitted diseases:** always consider STDs with suspected epididymitis; urethral discharge and sexual exposure are important parts of the history; *Chlamydia trachomatis* is a major cause of acute epididymitis in men under 35 in Seattle; epididymitis from STD generally presents with urethritis – urethral culture more useful than urine culture; in older men, epididymitis is due to urinary tract abnormalities or sequelae from instrumentation rather than STDs; epididymitis not arising from STD and in elderly men usually from Enterobacteriacea or *Pseudomonas*; chlamydial epididymitis – more discharge and inguinal pain; coliforms – prominent scrotal edema and erythema; homosexual men with acute epididymitis – coliforms rather than *Chlamydia* – prevalence of *E. coli* due to urethral exposure to enteric bacteria during anal intercourse; heterosexual men performing unprotected anal intercourse on women are subject to same exposure.

THERAPEUTIC CONSIDERATIONS

- **Bromelain:** good all-purpose therapy for epididymitis; kinins and prostaglandins inhibited by bromelain, decreased inflammation reduces recovery time; combine antibacterial agents with bromelain except when trauma clearly involved; with trauma, bromelain, bedrest, ice and support

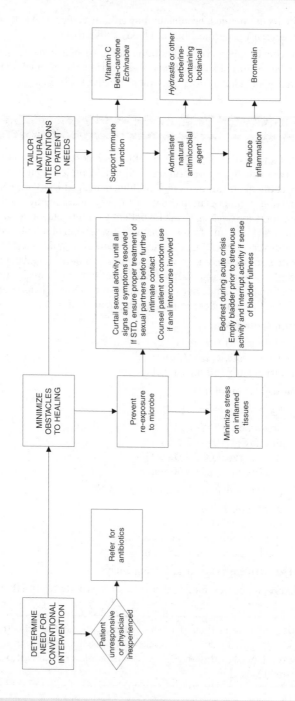

EPIDIDYMITIS

DETERMINE NEED FOR CONVENTIONAL INTERVENTION

Patient unresponsive or physician inexperienced

Refer for antibiotics

MINIMIZE OBSTACLES TO HEALING

Prevent re-exposure to microbe

Curtail sexual activity until all signs and symptoms resolved
If STD, ensure proper treatment of sexual partners before further intimate contact
Counsel patient on condom use if anal intercourse involved

Minimize stress on inflamed tissues

Bedrest during acute crisis
Empty bladder prior to strenuous activity and interrupt activity if sense of bladder fullness

TAILOR NATURAL INTERVENTIONS TO PATIENT NEEDS

Support immune function

Vitamin C
Beta-carotene
Echinacea

Administer natural antimicrobial agent

Hydrastis or other berberine-containing botanical

Reduce inflammation

Bromelain

are recommended; bromelain may enhance efficacy of antibacterial herbs by increasing permeability of blood–testis barrier.

● **Berberine:** berberine-containing herbs are effective antibacterial agents; berberine inhibits *C. trachomatis* – berberine with bromelain is an excellent choice for "idiopathic epididymitis" (*Textbook*, Ch. 91).

THERAPEUTIC APPROACH

Bedrest and local ice for first 48 h; athletic supporter relieves pain once normal activity resumed; positive urine culture with identified organism mandates specific treatment and immune support; for a man aged 18–37 or is sexually active in new or non-monogamous relationship, *Chlamydia* highly suspected; test sexual partners for *Chlamydia*; advise patient to empty bladder prior to strenuous activity and interrupt strenuous activity if sensation of full bladder; pain of epididymitis very motivating and patients follow clear guidelines; instruct patient to return immediately if recurring signs/symptoms of epididymitis; pain and swelling can be relieved within 2 weeks, but typically 4 weeks; up to 3 months for scrotum to return to normal size; all treatments (except ice and bedrest) continued for 1+ week after scrotum returns to normal size.

● **Supplements:**
   — vitamin C: 1,000 mg q.i.d.
   — beta-carotene: 200,000 IU q.d.
   — bromelain: 250 mg q.i.d. (between meals).

● **Botanical medicines:**
   — *Hydrastis canadensis* (t.i.d.):
      dried root: 0.5–1.0 g
      tincture (1:10): 6–12 ml
      fluid extract (1:1): 1.0–2.0 ml
      solid extract (4:1): 250 mg
   — *Echinacea angustifolia* (t.i.d.):
      dried root: 1–2 g
      tincture (1:10): 8–12 ml
      fluid extract: 1.5–3.0 ml
      solid extract (6.5:1): 250 mg

● **Hydrotherapy:** ice packs for first 2 days.

● **Exercise:** Bedrest for first 2 days; restricted activity until there is no pain.

Note: men, and their partners, with STDs must be effectively treated ASAP; if patient does not immediately respond to therapy, or physician inexperienced in this area, refer for antibiotics; repeat cultures needed to ensure resolution.

Epilepsy

DIAGNOSTIC SUMMARY

Recurrent seizures; characteristic EEG changes accompanying seizures; mental status abnormalities or focal neurologic symptoms may persist for hours postictally.

GENERAL CONSIDERATIONS

Epilepsy is not a disease in itself, but a symptom of disease; epilepsies are a group of disorders characterized by sudden, recurrent, and episodic changes in neurologic function caused by abnormalities in electrical activity of the brain; an episode of neurologic dysfunction is called a "seizure"; seizures are termed "convulsive" when accompanied by motor manifestations and "non-convulsive" when accompanied by sensory, cognitive, or emotional events; epilepsy can result from abnormalities (neural injuries, structural brain lesions, systemic diseases); "idiopathic" when there is neither history of neural insult nor other apparent neural dysfunction; common denominator is the epileptic attack or seizure.

Epidemiology: prevalence of chronic, recurrent epilepsy = 10 per 1,000; 2–5% of population will have non-febrile seizure at some point in life; additional 2–5% of children have febrile convulsions during first several years of life; 10% of these children, especially prolonged febrile seizures, develop epilepsy later in life; genetic factors – prevalence of seizures in close relatives is three times that of overall population.

Etiology: classified etiologically as "symptomatic" or "idiopathic"; symptomatic – probable cause identified; 70–80% of cases idiopathic.

Probable causes determined by age of onset

Age of onset	Presumptive causes
Birth to 2 years	Birth injury, degenerative brain disease
2–19 years	Congenital birth injury, febrile thrombosis, head trauma, infection (meningitis or encephalitis)
20–34 years	Head trauma, brain neoplasm
35–54 years	Brain neoplasm, head trauma, stroke
55 years and over	Stroke, brain neoplasm

Common causes of seizures

- Brain damage before or at birth (congenital malformations, anemia, fetal infection)
- Head trauma injuring brain and gliosis
- CNS infections (meningitis, encephalitis, brain abscess, neurosyphilis, rabies, tetanus, falciparum malaria, toxoplasmosis, cysticercosis of brain)
- Metabolic disorders (hypocalcemia, hypoglycemia, hypoparathyroidism, phenylketonuria, withdrawal from ETOH and drugs)
- Brain tumors and other space-occupying lesions
- Stroke and other vascular disorders
- Degenerative brain disease
- Genetic disease
- Toxic conditions
- Idiopathic

Classification: based on clinical and EEG criteria (International League Against Epilepsy)

Partial (focal, local) seizures

- Simple partial seizures (consciousness not impaired)
    — motor signs
    — somatosensory or special sensory symptoms
    — autonomic symptoms or signs
    — psychic symptoms
- Complex partial (consciousness impaired)
    — simple partial onset followed by impaired consciousness
    — consciousness impaired at onset
- Partial seizures evolving to generalized seizures (tonic, clonic, or tonic-clonic)
    — simple partial seizures evolving to generalized seizures
    — complex partial seizures evolving to generalized seizures
    — simple partial seizures evolving to partial seizures evolving to generalized seizures

Generalized seizures (convulsive or non-convulsive)

- Absence seizures
    — typical (brief stare, eye flickering, no emotion)
    — atypical (associated with movement)
- Myoclonic seizures
- Clonic seizures
- Tonic seizures
- Tonic-clonic seizures
- Atonic seizures
- *Unclassified seizures*

DIAGNOSIS

Differentiating between partial or focal seizures and generalized seizures is of great clinical significance; partial seizures begin focally – specific sensory, motor, or psychic aberration reflecting affected part of cerebrum; these seizures may remain localized; generalized seizures affect consciousness and motor function; partial seizures are indicative of focal brain disorders (tumors, gliosis); generalized seizures rarely have definable etiology (perhaps metabolic disorders); eyewitness account of typical attack is valuable in classifying seizure; explore past trauma, infections, drugs, ETOH, family history; complete neurological exam is a preliminary screen for neoplasms.

● **Lab work:** serum glucose and Ca, CBC, liver and kidney function tests, syphilis serology, skull X-rays, EEG, CT scan (all adult onset seizures); cerebrospinal fluid exam indicated if infection or meningeal neoplasm suspected.

Epilepsy not diagnosed from solitary seizure; recurrence rate after single seizure = 27% over 3 years.

PATHOPHYSIOLOGY

Hallmark of altered physiologic state of epilepsy is rhythmic and repetitive, synchronous discharge of many neurons in localized brain area; discharge pattern recorded on EEG during attack; cause of abnormal discharges unknown; synchronous depolarization of masses of neurons due to combination of increased excitation and decreased inhibition; GABA blockers are potent convulsants; anti-epileptic drugs enhance GABA; in some forms of chronic focal epilepsy, inhibitory terminals on neurons in areas around cortical gliotic lesions are diminished; nerve cell membranes in epileptics are unstable – during seizures, stored intracellular Ca^{2+} is released and moves towards inner cell membranes, binding to Ca^{2+}-receptive proteins, causing protein conformational changes; these changes trigger transmembranal Ca^{2+}, K^+, and Na^+ channels to remain open, potentiating excitation; earliest symptomatology (aura) – generated by focal discharge = best clue to localization and characterization of responsible lesion.

THERAPEUTIC CONSIDERATIONS

Environmental toxins

● **Heavy metals:** Pb, Hg, Cd, Al induce seizures by disrupting neural function; rule out heavy metal toxicity; hair mineral analysis is the most cost-effective screening method (*Textbook*, Chs 17 and 18).

- **Neurotoxic chemicals:** many neuron-, axon-, and myelin-toxic chemicals released into ecosystem; explore possible exposure during detailed history-taking (*Textbook*, Ch. 37).

Dietary considerations

- **Hypoglycemia:** important metabolic cause of seizures – serum glucose unusually low prior to seizure; 50–90% of epileptics have constant or periodic hypoglycemia; 70% of epileptics have abnormal glucose tolerance tests; correlation of glucose abnormalities and epilepsy is well documented, but mechanism unknown; hypoglycemia may impair ATP production in neurons, reducing efficacy of Na-ATPase pump; defective Na pump increases intracellular Na, depolarizing cell membrane, lowering firing threshold; single measurements of serum glucose are inadequate to determine glycemic status – extended glucose tolerance test required.

- **Ketogenic diet:** long history of use to reduce seizure activity; large amounts of fat and minimal protein and carbohydrate; low carbohydrate inhibits fat metabolism, causing production of excess ketone bodies (acetone, aceto-acetic acid, beta-hydroxybutyric acid), which are intermediary oxidation products; beneficial effects are due to metabolic acidosis, which corrects underlying tendency of epileptics towards spontaneous alkalosis; acidosis may normalize nerve conductivity, irritability, and membrane permeability; 40% of 27 children aged 1–16 years experienced seizure reduction of > 50%, with 25% becoming seizure-free; 35% discontinued diet due to difficulty following rigorous guidelines; ketogenic diet's success rate exceeds that of medications and is cheaper; there are long-term risks associated with a high-fat diet and it is unhealthy for a growing child; children should not be allowed to eat very large meals – predispose them to seizures.

- **Food allergy:** little research into correlation between food allergy and epilepsy; epileptic patients may have allergic reactions in brain similar to swelling, anoxia, and inflammatory chemical reactions of local allergic reactions; suspect allergy in epileptics suffering from multiple other symptoms of food allergy (*Textbook*, Chs 15 and 51); folic acid deficiency is a common side-effect of most anti-epileptic drugs; link between celiac disease, epilepsy, and cerebral calcifications – rule out celiac disease in all cases of epilepsy and cerebral calcifications of unexplained origin, especially when epilepsy characterized by occipital seizures and calcification located bilaterally in posterior regions.

Nutritional considerations

- **Pyridoxine:** two types of vitamin B_6-related seizures in newborns and infants < 18 months old: B_6-deficient and B_6-dependent – similar

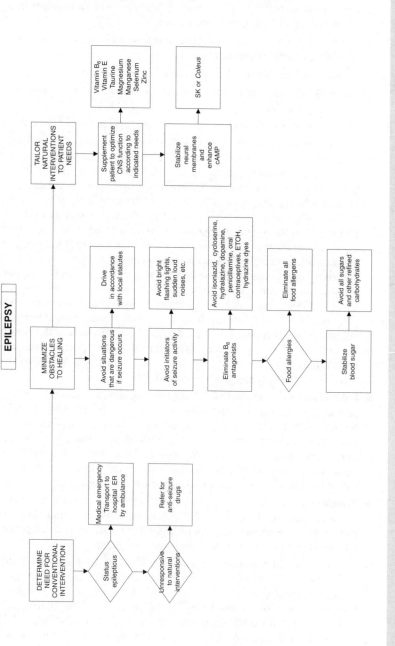

EPILEPSY

DETERMINE NEED FOR CONVENTIONAL INTERVENTION

Status epilepticus → Medical emergency Transport to hospital ER by ambulance

Unresponsive to natural interventions → Refer for anti-seizure drugs

MINIMIZE OBSTACLES TO HEALING

Avoid situations that are dangerous if seizure occurs → Drive in accordance with local statutes

Avoid initiators of seizure activity → Avoid bright flashing lights, sudden loud noises, etc.

Eliminate B$_6$ antagonists → Avoid isoniazid, cycloserine, hydralazine, dopamine, penicillamine, oral contraceptives, ETOH, hydrazine dyes

Food allergies → Eliminate all food allergens

Stabilize blood sugar → Avoid all sugars and other refined carbohydrates

TAILOR NATURAL INTERVENTIONS TO PATIENT NEEDS

Supplement patient to optimize CNS function according to indicated needs → Vitamin B$_6$ Vitamin E Taurine Magnesium Manganese Selenium Zinc

Stabilize neural membranes and enhance cAMP → SK or Coleus

neurological symptoms, EEG abnormalities, and prognosis of mental retardation if untreated; B_6 responsiveness to be suspected if convulsions in first 18 months of life with these clinical features:

— seizures of unknown origin in previously normal infant without abnormal gestational or perinatal history

— history of severe convulsive disorders

— long-lasting focal or unilateral seizures, often with partial preservation of consciousness

— irritability, restlessness, crying, and vomiting preceding actual seizure.

Atypical presentations of B_6-responsive seizures suggests empiric trial of parenteral B_6 for neonate or infant with long-lasting convulsions, especially with no clear-cut etiology; dose = 100–200 mg i.v. dose or 20 mg dose every 5 min to total of 200 mg; if seizures stop, child has B_6-responsive seizures; diagnosis of B_6-responsiveness lost if B_6 given together with, or after, anticonvulsant drugs; B_6 deficiency responds to dietary amounts, but B_6 dependency requires continuous high-dose supplementing at 25–50 mg q.d.; mechanism not fully understood, but it is related to B_6 as cofactor in synthesis of neurotransmitters dependent on amino acid decarboxylation; absorbed B_6 is phosphorylated to pyridoxal-5-phosphate, a coenzyme in converting glutamic acid to gamma-aminobutyric acid (GABA); GABA is an inhibitory neurotransmitter; proposed mechanism: pyridoxal phosphate does not bind with usual affinity to glutamic acid decarboxylase, reducing GABA production – higher levels of B_6 required for activity of this enzyme; administering B_6 to epileptics must be strictly monitored; improvements noted, but daily doses of 80–400 mg interfere with commonly used anticonvulsants.

● **Folic acid:** low blood and CSF folic acid are common in patients using anticonvulsants phenytoin, primidone, and phenobarbital – drugs interfere with intestinal uptake of folate by mucosa; folic acid supplements may exacerbate seizure in some individuals; folate metabolism may be involved in epileptic process; supplementing folic acid does not lead to significant clinical improvement and can decrease serum vitamin B_{12} – folic acid is contraindicated in the absence of demonstrated deficiency.

● **Thiamin:** deficiency may promote epileptic episodes in those with subclinical predisposition for seizures; significant role in nerve conduction; deficiency may accompany low concentrations of GABA; in patients with late-onset epilepsy, thiamin deficiency may be a cause.

● **Taurine:** one of the most abundant amino acids in brain; involved in hyperpolarizing neurons by changing ion permeability; may mimic effects of GABA and glycine; anticonvulsive activity – mode of action = membrane-stabilizing effects (normalize flow of Na^+, K^+, and Ca^{2+} into and out of the cell; acts as GABA-like neurotransmitter – may also help inhibit seizure by increasing GABA levels by enhancing action of glutamic acid decarboxylase; epileptics have much lower taurine in platelets than controls; there are demonstrated anticonvulsant effects, but rate of efficacy is far below the level warranting recommendation as standard "drug" treatment; daily dose = 0.05–0.3 g/kg in one study and 750 mg in another – effective in some cases of intractable epilepsy, decreasing seizures by > 30% in one-third of subjects unresponsive to any other anticonvulsants; partial epilepsy – best results, those achieving highest taurine concentrations showing best response; monitoring platelet or plasma taurine levels is useful.

- **Magnesium:** epileptics have much lower serum Mg compared with normals; seizure severity correlates with level of hypomagnesemia; mechanism not fully understood; Mg beneficial in control of seizures; Mg deficiency induces muscle tremors and convulsive seizures; dose = 450 mg q.d.

- **Manganese:** low whole blood and hair Mn in epileptics; those with lowest levels have highest seizure activity; Mn is a critical cofactor for glucose utilization within neuron, adenylate cyclase activity, and neurotransmitter control; optimal CNS function requires sufficient Mn; supplements may help control seizure activity in some patients.

- **Zinc:** children with epilepsy have much lower serum Zn, especially in West or Lennox syndromes; epileptics may have elevated copper-to-zinc ratio; seizures may be triggered when Zn levels fall, as in absence of adequate taurine; exact role of Zn or Cu:Zn ratio is unclear; may involve storage or binding of GABA; anticonvulsants may cause Zn deficiency.

- **Choline, betaine (N,N,N,-trimethylglycine), dimethylglycine (DMG), and sarcosine:** anticonvulsant activity in human and animal studies; choline converted to betaine when acting as methyl donor; betaine converted to DMG when donating methyl group to homocysteine to produce methionine; supplemental betaine is very effective in alleviating seizures in humans with homocystinuria; DMG strikingly decreased seizure frequency in a patient with long-standing mental retardation at dose of 90 mg b.i.d.; glycine and betaine may act indirectly on glycine metabolism and glycine-mediated neuronal inhibition, enhance GABA activity, or simply have non-specific effect on biological membranes.

- **Vitamin D:** anticonvulsant drugs are linked to disorders of mineral metabolism (hypocalcemia, rickets, osteomalacia); studies of serum levels of vitamin D in epilepsy are conflicting; supplemental vitamin D is recommended when climate or lifestyle do not allow adequate exposure to sunlight; supplementing epileptics with 4,000–16,000 IU vitamin D has significantly decreased the number of seizures, but that large dosage can be quite toxic, requiring careful monitoring.

- **Vitamin E and selenium:** function synergistically; vitamin E deficiency produces seizures; anti-epileptic drugs decrease vitamin E levels; both nutrients are low in epileptics; supplements may improve control of seizures; selenium is helpful in children with reduced glutathione peroxidase activity, intractable seizures, multiple infections and resistance to anticonvulsants.

Botanical medicines

● **Chinese herbal medicine:** Chinese herbal combination, Saiko-Keishi-To (SK), demonstrated dramatic therapeutic effects on some difficult cases unresponsive to anticonvulsives; SK is a combination of nine botanicals:

— *Bupleuri radix*: 5.0 g

— *Scutellaria radix*: 3.0 g

— *Pinelliae tuber*: 5.0 g

— *Paeoniae radix*: 6.0 g

— *Cinnamon cortex*: 2.0 g

— *Zizyphi fructus*: 4.0 g

— *Ginseng radix*: 30.0 g

— *Glycyrrhizae radix*: 1.5 g

— *Zingiber rhizoma*: 2.0 g.

SK inhibits intracellular shift of Ca^{2+} towards cell membrane; inhibits binding of Ca^{2+} to Ca^{2+}-receptive membrane proteins and Ca^{2+}-calmodulin complex; inhibits conformational changes of Ca^{2+}-receptive membrane proteins; inhibits pathologic transmembrane current of Na^+, K^+, and Ca^{2+}; attempts to isolate purified chemicals from component herbs failed to match crude drug's efficacy – synergistic effect among herbal agents.

● *Coleus forskohlii:* cyclic nucleotides are involved in pathophysiology of seizures – possible mechanism of action of several botanicals; cyclic AMP depresses electrical activity in animal models; cGMP can produce seizure-like discharge in same tissues; cAMP inhibits Ca^{2+} binding to intracellular proteins (calmodulin), decreasing extrusion of neurotransmitters into synapse; *Coleus* is an Ayurvedic herb that activates adenylate cyclase, increasing cAMP; the constituent forskolin, a diterpine, increases adenylate cyclase activity by 530%; seven – *Bupleuri radix, Cinnamon cortex, Glycyrrhizae radix, Paeoniae radix, Ginseng radix, Scutellaria radix, and Zingiber rhizoma* – of the nine botanicals in SK also increase cAMP by enhancing adenylate cyclase or inhibiting cAMP phosphodiesterase.

THERAPEUTIC APPROACH

Avoid situations that could be dangerous if seizures occur; be aware of state laws regarding epilepsy and driving; avoid known initiators of seizure activity (bright flashing lights, sudden loud sounds); continue therapy at full dosages until patient is seizure-free for 2+ years; dosage reduction then gradual over several months; epileptics not controlled with natural therapies require drug therapy; eliminate pyridoxine antagonists (isoniazid, cycloserine, hydralazine, dopamine, penicillamine, oral contraceptives, ETOH, hydrazine dyes [FD&C yellow #5]).

> **Note.** Status epilepticus is a medical emergency causing serious neurological damage or death if untreated; immediate hospitalization is mandatory, preferably with EMT transport to maintain airway, assist ventilation, and administer i.v. glucose and anticonvulsants.

- **Diet:** eliminate all sugar and refined carbohydrates; moderate protein; identify and eliminate food allergens; if ketotic effect desired, strictly limit all carbohydrates and increase fat (use this diet sparingly and rarely for children).
- **Nutritional supplements** (adult doses; reduce proportionately for children):
  — vitamin B_6: 50 mg t.i.d.
  — vitamin E: 400 IU q.d.
  — taurine: 500 mg t.i.d.
  — magnesium: 300 mg t.i.d.
  — manganese: 10 mg t.i.d.
  — selenium: 100 µg q.d.
  — zinc: 25 mg q.d.
- **Botanical medicine:** Saiko-Keishi-To: 300 ml before bedtime.

Erythema multiforme

DIAGNOSTIC SUMMARY

- Sudden onset of symmetric, erythematous, edematous, macular, papular, urticarial, bullous or purpuric skin lesions.
- Evolves into "target lesions" (lesions with clear centers and concentric erythematous rings).
- Characteristic first site: dorsum of hand.
- Characteristic distribution: extensor surfaces of extremities with relative sparing of head and trunk.
- Tendency to recur in spring and fall.

GENERAL CONSIDERATIONS

Erythema multiforme (EM) can occur as primary skin disorder or as skin manifestation of systemic infection or chronic inflammatory disease; often a manifestation of hypersensitivity to drugs (penicillin, sulfonamides, barbiturates); vaccinia, BCG, and poliomyelitis vaccines, herpes simplex, food allergens, and infectious organisms can induce EM; hypersensitivity is a common factor; tissue damage caused by release of highly reactive, PMN-derived, oxygen intermediates.

THERAPEUTIC CONSIDERATIONS

- **Potassium iodide:** historically used to treat a variety of erythematous disorders, including erythema multiforme, erythema nodosum, nodular vasculitis, acute febrile neutrophilic dermatosis, subacute nodular migratory panniculitis; documented dramatic success; mechanism related to suppression of generation of oxygen intermediates (hydrogen peroxide, hydroxyl radical) by stimulated PMNs; iodine therapy occasionally associated with adverse skin reactions and GI discomfort – never utilized in pregnant women in last trimester due to suppression of fetal thyroid.
- **Zinc:** zinc sulfate (0.025–0.05%) is used locally at site of herpetic infection and to prevent relapse of post-herpetic erythema multiforme.

ERYTHEMA MULTIFORME

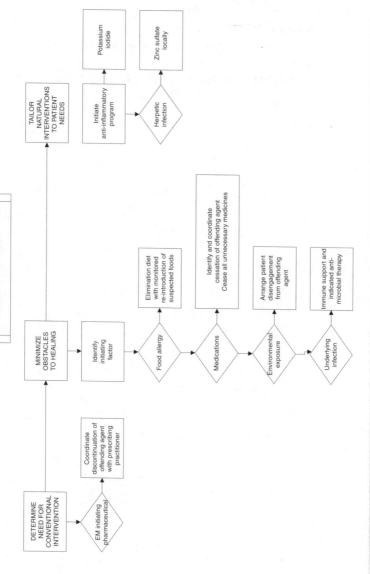

THERAPEUTIC APPROACH

Careful search to determine initiating factor; treat underlying infections; cease all unnecessary medications; initiate anti-inflammatory program.

● **Supplements:**
  — potassium iodide: 100 mg t.i.d. for 4–6 weeks; discontinue if adverse reactions
  — zinc sulfate: 0.025–0.05% solution locally if post-herpetic.

Fibrocystic breast disease

DIAGNOSTIC SUMMARY

- Very common: 20–40% of premenopausal women.
- Pain or premenstrual breast pain and tenderness common, although the condition is often asymptomatic.
- Cyclic and bilateral with multiple cysts of varying sizes giving breast nodular consistency.

GENERAL CONSIDERATIONS

Benign fibrocystic breast disease (FBD) ("cystic mastitis") is a component of premenstrual syndrome (PMS); risk factor for breast cancer, but not as significant as family history, early menarche, and late or no first pregnancy.

- **Pathogenesis:** increased estrogen-to-progesterone ratio; during menstrual cycle there is a recurring biphasic stimulation of the breast – (1) proliferation of breast tissue by estrogens, (2) alveolar secretory activity by progesterone – followed by period of involution; in many women these changes are slight and clinically signs are asymptomatic; in others, significant inflammation occurs.

- **Histology:** proliferation and hyperplasia of alveolar epithelium, increased secretory activity, ectasia of milk ducts, and periductal fibrosis – elevated prolactin in women with FBD, but insufficient to cause amenorrhea; estrogen (endogenous and exogenous) causes increase in prolactin; prolactin inhibits luteal function.

DIFFERENTIAL DIAGNOSIS

Fibrocystic breast disease cannot be definitively differentiated from breast cancer or breast fibroadenoma on clinical criteria alone; pain, cyclic variations in size, high mobility, and multiplicity of nodules – indicative of FBD; non-invasive procedures (ultrasonography and thermography) are helpful, but definitive procedure is biopsy.

THERAPEUTIC CONSIDERATIONS (see PMS chapter)

● **Methylxanthines:** caffeine, theophylline and theobromine inhibit action of cAMP and cGMP phosphodiesterase and elevate their levels in breast tissue; increased cyclic nucleotides excessively stimulate protein-kinase, causing overproduction of cellular products (fibrous tissue, cyst fluid); an excess of cyclic nucleotides in breast is one of the biochemical findings in breast cancer; caffeine promotes carcinogenesis in mammary gland of rats; limiting dietary methylxanthines (coffee, tea, cola, chocolate, caffeinated medications) improved 97.5% of 45 women who completely abstained, and 75% of 28 who limited consumption; women may have varying thresholds of response to methylxanthines; stress plays a role – fibrocystic breasts are more responsive to epinephrine, which increases adenylate cyclase activity and cAMP.

● **Vitamin E:** alpha-tocopherol may relieve FBD symptoms in some patients; mode of action is obscure – normalizes circulating hormones in PMS and FBD patients; 600 IU q.d. normalizes elevated FSH and LH in FBD.

● **Vitamin A:** 150,000 IU q.d. for 3 months caused complete or partial remission of FBD in five of the nine patients who completed the study; some developed mild side-effects, causing two of the original 12 to withdraw due to HA, and one patient had dosage reduced; beta-carotene may be a better source of retinol – much less toxic and similar activity in ovarian and inflammatory disorders (*Textbook*, Chs 122 and 183).

● **Thyroid and iodine:** hypothyroidism and/or iodine deficiency are linked to higher incidence of breast cancer; thyroid hormone replacement in hypothyroid (and some euthyroid) patients may give improvement; thyroid supplement (0.1 mg q.d. Synthroid) decreases mastodynia, serum prolactin, and breast nodules in euthyroid patients – subclinical hypothyroidism and/or iodine deficiency may be etiological factors in FBD; iodine caseinate may be effective treatment for FBD; theory: absence of iodine renders epithelium more sensitive to estrogen stimulation; hypersensitivity produces excess secretions, distending ducts and producing cysts and later fibrosis; in animal models, iodides correct cystic spaces and partially correct excess cellular reproduction; elemental iodine corrects entire disease process; oral iodine has acute and chronic anti-inflammatory and antifibrotic effects; human studies: iodides effective in 70% of subjects, but with high rate of side-effects (altered thyroid function in 4%, iodinism in 3%, and acne in 15%); elemental iodine gives same benefits but no significant side-effects – short-term increased breast pain corresponding to softening of breast and disappearance of fibrous tissue plaques; dosage of molecular iodine = 70–90 µg/kg body weight (iodine caseinate or liquid iodine).

● **Liver function:** primary site for estrogen clearance; any factor (cholestasis, "toxic liver syndrome", environmental pollution) compromising liver

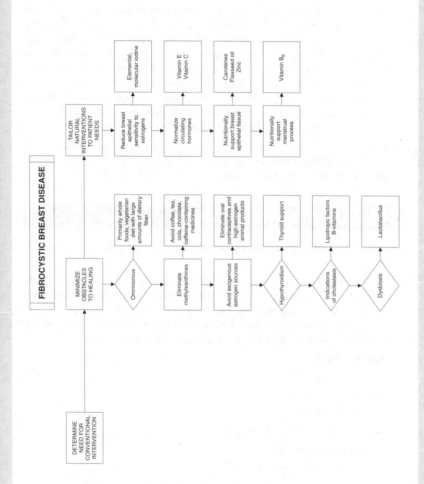

can cause estrogen excess; lipotropic factors and B vitamins are necessary for estrogen conjugation.

● **Colon function:** breast disease is linked to a Western diet and bowel function; epithelial dysplasia in nipple aspirates of breast fluid and frequency of bowel movements (BMs) are also linked; women having < 3 BMs per week have 4.5-fold greater risk of FBD compared with women having 1+ BM q.d.; link = colon bacteria transforming endogenous and exogenous sterols and fatty acids into toxic metabolites (polycyclic carcinogens and mutagens); fecal microbes can synthesize estrogens and metabolize estrogen sulfate and glucuronate conjugates; the result is absorption of bacteria-derived and previously conjugated estrogens; diet influences microflora, transit time, and concentration of absorbable metabolites; vegetarian women excrete two to three times more conjugated estrogens than omnivores; omnivorous women have 50% higher unconjugated estrogens; *Lactobacillus* supplements lower fecal beta-glucuronidase.

● **Fiber:** inverse correlation between dietary fiber and risk of benign, proliferative, epithelial breast disorders; increasing dietary fiber may reduce risk for benign disease and breast cancer.

THERAPEUTIC APPROACH

Unless a woman has pure FBD, the approach outlined in the PMS chapter is indicated.

● **Diet:** primarily vegetarian with large amounts of dietary fiber; eliminate all methylxanthines until symptoms alleviated, then reintroduce in small amounts; avoid exogenous estrogens (oral contraceptives, high-estrogen animal products); emphasize whole, unprocessed foods (whole grains, legumes, vegetables, fruits, nuts, and seeds); drink 48+ oz water q.d.

● **Supplements:**
  — B-complex: $10 \times$ RDA
  — lipotropic factors:
    choline: 500–1,000 mg q.d.
    methionine: 500–1,000 mg q.d.
  — vitamin B_6: 25–50 mg t.i.d.
  — vitamin C: 500 mg t.i.d.
  — vitamin E: 400–800 IU q.d. D-alpha tocopherol
  — beta-carotene: 50,000–300,000 IU q.d.
  — iodine (molecular iodine): 70–90 μg of iodine/kg body weight
  — zinc: 15 mg q.d.
  — flaxseed oil: 1 tbsp q.d.
  — *Lactobacillus acidophilus*: 1–2 billion live organisms q.d.

Food allergies

Introduction: Food allergies (FA) cause the immune system to release cytokines, lymphokines, and interferons influencing all tissue physiology; toxins initiate similar reactions: food allergy and toxicity are intimately connected (*Textbook*, Ch. 50); FA is the culprit behind "mysterious" un-diagnosable symptoms; allergy testing (*Textbook*, Ch. 15) uncovers causes of illness, reveals unsuspected food sensitivities in asymptomatic patients; bronchial hypersensitivities doubled in the last decade; atopic dermatitis in 10–15% of population, provoked by food antigens; adverse food reactions in 25% of younger children; the leading cause of most undiagnosed symptoms.

Causes and development

- **Increased incidence:** regular consumption of a limited number of foods; hidden ingredients in processed foods; food additives; medicinal drugs (e.g. penicillin) added to foods; environmental pollution; early weaning and solid foods given to infants; genetic manipulation of food components which cross-react with normal tissues; impaired digestion; less dietary diversity.

- FA is an expression of genetic predisposition: allergic histories in both parents and siblings; if both parents are allergic, 67% of children are allergic; if one parent allergic, 33% of children are allergic.

- **Maldigestion:** hypochlorhydria and/or pancreatic enzyme deficiency; undigested proteins retain antigenicity, are exposed to immune system or absorbed through a "leaky gut", and create chronic hypersensitivity.

Signs and symptoms

System	Symptoms and diseases
Gastrointestinal	Canker sores, celiac disease, chronic diarrhea, duodenal ulcer, gastritis, irritable colon, malabsorption, ulcerative colitis
Genitourinary	Bed-wetting, chronic bladder infections, nephrosis
Immune	Chronic infections, frequent ear infections
Mental/emotional	Anxiety, depression, hyperactivity, inability to concentrate, insomnia, irritability, mental confusion, personality change, seizures

(continued over)

(continued)

System	Symptoms and diseases
Musculoskeletal	Bursitis, joint pain, low back pain
Respiratory	Asthma, chronic bronchitis, wheezing
Skin	Acne, eczema, hives, itching, skin rash
Miscellaneous	Arrhythmia, edema, fainting, fatigue, headache, hypoglycemia, itchy nose or throat, migraines, sinusitis

Types of immune reactions

● **Type I – immediate hypersensitivity:** < 2 h after contact; antigens bind to pre-formed IgE mast cells and basophils, release histamine and eosinophilic chemotactic factor; symptoms vary with tissue location of mast cells.

● **Type II – cytotoxic reactions:** binding of IgG or IgM to cell-bound antigen; antigen–antibody binding activates complement and destruction of cell bound to antigen.

● **Type III – immune complex-mediated reactions:** antigens bound to antibodies; usually cleared via phagocytosis; deposition in tissues/vascular endothelium causes tissue injury; vasoactive amines increase vascular permeability and deposition of more complexes; delayed hours or days after exposure; involve both IgG and IgM.

● **Type IV – T-cell-dependent:** delayed reaction by T-lymphocytes after allergen makes contact with mucosal surface; sensitized T-cells may induce inflammation within 36–72 h; does not involve antibodies.

The allergic reaction: antigens are proteins or large polysaccharides > 8,000 Da; food is the largest antigenic challenge to immune system; food hypersensitivity is a result of interactions among food antigens, GI tract, tissue mast cells and circulating basophils, and food antigen-specific immunoglobulins.

Role of IgE and IgG$_4$

● Repeated antigen exposure produces hypersensitivities: IgE antibodies cross-link on GI mast cells, stimulate the release of histamine, proteoglycans, and leukotrienes, instigating mucosal permeability and allowing food antigens into blood; other organs may be involved, causing perpetual autoimmune response.

● Most severe, immediate allergy symptoms are IgE-mediated; but IgG and IgG complex involved in 80% of all food allergies; 60% of patients exhibit delayed reactions to provoking foods; primarily mediated by IgG.

● Specific IgE has half-life in circulation = 1–2 days, and on the mast cell = 14 days; IgG circulating half-life = 21 days, and on mast cells = 2–3 months; IgG assay is essential for "hidden" allergies undetected by IgE RAST or skin testing.

- IgG$_4$ subclass: associated with high antigen levels, particularly food antigens; increases with increasing antigens; higher levels than other IgG subclasses; IgG$_4$ is the only IgG subclass inducing basophil degranulation, triggering histamine release.
- IgG increases GI permeability, due to selective transport mediated by Fc receptors on mucosa; this increases exposure to antigens.
- Production of IgG$_4$ and IgE is controlled by interleukin-4 (IL-4) and interferon-γ (IFN-γ); there is increased synthesis of IgG$_4$ and IgE from decreased inhibitory effect of IFN-γ; postulate: defective immunoregulation involving IL-4 and IFN-γ support synthesis of IgG$_4$ and IgE.

FOOD ALLERGY AND RELATED TESTING

- **Oral challenge test:** most accurate for immediate hypersensitivities, but costly, time-consuming, and potentially dangerous; not easily applicable to delayed sensitivities.
- **Food-specific IgE and IgG$_4$:** correspond more closely with patient history than challenge test.
- **RAST and skin testing:** only measure IgE reactions, not delayed non-IgE reactions; skin testing is sometimes unfeasible and may trigger life-threatening reactions (*Textbook*, Ch. 15).
- **Follow-up testing necessary:** monitors changing sensitivities from changes in eating habits; helps modify therapy, as needed.
- **Intestinal permeability:** evaluates GI effectiveness as macromolecule barrier, and determines causes of systemic problems linked to GI function (*Textbook*, Ch. 21).
- **Comprehensive digestive stool analysis (CDSA):** maldigestion is a significant cause of food allergy; examines digestion and absorption status of GI tract.
- **Fecal secretory IgA:** sIgA is the predominant immunoglobulin in intestinal secretions and saliva; first-line defender against microbes and toxins; forms immune complexes with pathogens preventing binding to mucosa; fecal sIgA evaluates status of mucosal immunity.
- **Adrenocortex and melatonin profiles:** many sensitized individuals have endocrine dysfunctions; severity of symptoms often follows chronobiotic pattern influenced by circadian hormone rhythms.

THERAPEUTIC CONSIDERATIONS

Five essential components: avoid identified allergens; rotate diet until sensitivity decreases; re-establish proper microbial milieu; heal damaged intestinal mucosa; correct causative factors, such as maldigestion.

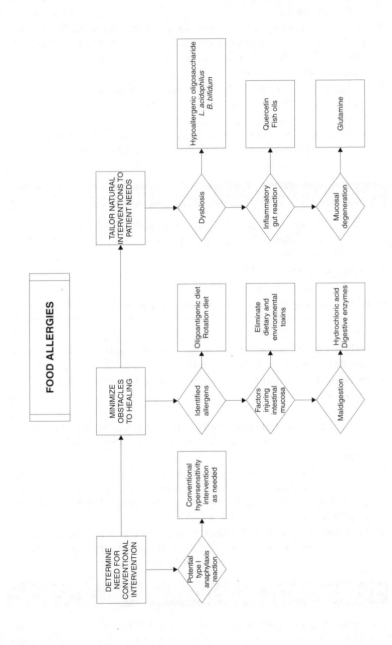

- **Evaluate each case carefully using variety of criteria:** antibody tests, detailed medical history, thorough physical exam, challenge tests once certain antigens have been ruled out by preliminary tests.

- **Oligoantigenic diet:** highly effective in treating food allergies; ADD children show improved hyperactivity; 93% of children with migraine recover, even when migraines are provoked by other factors (blows to head, exercise, flashing lights); reduces colic in infants and chronic urticaria with arthralgia in adults.

- **Rotation diet:** prevents new allergies, gives immune system rest, and intestines a chance to heal (*Textbook*, Ch. 58); infrequent consumption of tolerated foods not likely to induce new sensitivities or worsen old ones.

- **Re-establish healthy bowel microflora:** suppresses toxic microbes; probiotics are normal bacteria in healthy intestines (*Lactobacillus* and *Bifidobacteria*); prebiotics are enzymatically indigestible substrates selective for healthful bacteria; increase intestinal sIgA with oligosaccharides, especially fructo-oligosaccharides (onions, asparagus, bananas, maple syrup).

- **Healing damaged gut:** eliminate all factors injuring mucosa; re-establish microflora, remove intestinal toxins; improve digestion; decrease inflammation; promote metabolism, repair of mucosa.

- **Decrease inflammatory gut reaction:** *quercetin* is a natural flavonoid which inhibits mast cell histamine release, scavenges free radicals, inhibits intestinal smooth muscle irritability; also reduces damage by food allergens – dose = 250 mg t.i.d. with vitamin C; *fish oils:* polyunsaturated N-3 fatty acids, EPA, DHA; they reduce inflammation, PAF, neutrophil chemotaxis, and cell adherence to endothelium; dosage: 1–3 g q.d. EPA.

- **Stimulating regeneration of gut mucosa:** glutamine is the most abundant amino acid in blood, and a substrate for mucosa cells (35% of their energy production); supplementation stimulates regeneration, prevents mucosal damage, decreases bacterial leakage across mucosa after damage; dosage = 100 mg t.i.d. (*Textbook*, Ch. 54).

- **Re-establishing normal digestion:** use Heidelberg gastric analysis test if achlorhydria or hypochlorhydria suspected (*Textbook*, Ch. 19); oral betaine HCl (*Textbook*, App. 7); pancreatic insufficiency: treat with pork or beef pancreatin (*Textbook*, Ch. 101) or microbial-derived digestive enzymes (*Aspergillus oryzae*) (*Textbook*, Ch. 66).

Gallstones

DIAGNOSTIC SUMMARY

Asymptomatic or biliary colic with irregular pain-free intervals of days or months; real-time ultrasonography provides definitive diagnosis.

GENERAL CONSIDERATIONS

"Western diet"-induced disease; 20% of women and 8% of men over age 40; 20 million Americans have gallstones; each year 1 million more develop gallstones; > 300,000 cholecystectomies annually due to gallstones; bile components = bile salts, bilirubin, cholesterol, phospholipids, fatty acids, water, electrolytes, other organic and inorganic substances; gallstones arise when solubilized bile components become supersaturated and precipitate.

● **Four categories:** (1) pure cholesterol, (2) pure pigment (calcium bilirubinate), (3) mixed – containing cholesterol and derivatives plus bile salts, pigments, inorganic calcium salts, (4) stones composed entirely of minerals.

Pure stones (cholesterol or calcium bilirubinate) are rare in the US, where 80% are mixed and 20% exclusively minerals (calcium salts, oxides of silicon and aluminum).

PATHOGENESIS

Three steps: (1) bile supersaturation, (2) nucleation and initiation of stone formation, (3) enlargement of gallstone by accretion.

Cholesterol and mixed stones: requisite step is cholesterol supersaturation of bile within gall bladder; bile solubility and supersaturation based on relative molar concentrations of cholesterol, bile acids, phosphatidylcholine (lecithin), and water; free cholesterol is water-insoluble – must be in lecithin-bile salt micelle; increased cholesterol secretion or decreased bile acid or lecithin secretion induces supersaturation; stone formation initiated by biliary stasis, infection or mucin; radius increases at 2.6 mm/year, eventually reaching size of a few millimeters to over a centimeter; symptomatic 8 years after formation begins; cholelithiasis in 95% of patients with cholecystitis.

Risk factors for cholesterol and mixed stones: diet, sex, race, obesity, high caloric intake, estrogens, GI diseases (Crohn's disease, cystic fibrosis), drugs, age.

● **Sex:** frequency two to four times greater in women than in men; women predisposed – either increased cholesterol synthesis or suppression of bile acids by estrogens; pregnancy, oral contraceptives or other causes of elevated estrogen increase incidence.

● **Genetic and ethnic:** most common in Native American women over age 30; only 10% of black women over 30; differences reflect extent of cholesterol saturation of bile; dietary factors outweigh genetic factors.

● **Obesity:** causes increased secretion of cholesterol in bile from increased cholesterol synthesis; obesity linked to much increased incidence – biliary cholesterol saturation; during active weight reduction, biliary cholesterol saturation initially increases; secretion of biliary lipids is reduced during weight loss, but secretion of bile acids decreases more than cholesterol; when weight is stabilized, bile acid output returns to normal and cholesterol output remains low; net effect is a significant reduction in cholesterol saturation.

● **Gastrointestinal tract diseases:** malabsorption of bile acids from terminal ileum disturbs enterohepatic circulation – reducing bile acid pool and rate of bile secretion (Crohn's disease and cystic fibrosis).

● **Drugs:** oral contraceptives, other estrogens, clofibrate and possibly other lipid-lowering drugs.

● **Age:** average patient 40–50 years old; incidence increases with age.

Risk factors for pigmented gallstones: not related to diet as much as geography, sun exposure and severe diseases; more common in Asia – higher incidence of liver and gall bladder parasites – liver fluke *Clonorchis sinensis*; bacteria and protozoa cause stasis or act as nucleating agents; in US, pigmented stones are caused by chronic hemolysis or ETOH liver cirrhosis.

THERAPEUTIC CONSIDERATIONS

Easier to prevent than reverse; primary treatment is to reduce controllable risk factors; therapeutic intervention – avoid aggravating foods and increase solubility of cholesterol in bile; if symptoms persist or worsen, cholecystectomy is indicated; eliminate foods producing symptoms; increase dietary fiber; eliminate food allergens; reduce animal protein; use nutritional lipotropic compounds and herbal choleretics to increase solubility of bile; biliary cholesterol concentration and serum cholesterol do not correlate, but increased serum triglycerides are linked to bile saturation.

> **Asymptomatic gallstones:** natural history of silent/asymptomatic gallstones suggests elective cholecystectomy is not warranted; cumulative chance for developing symptoms – 10% at 5 years, 15% at 10 years, and 18% at 15 years; if controllable risk factors eliminated or reduced, patient remains asymptomatic.

Diet

- **Dietary fiber:** diet high in refined carbohydrates and fat, low in fiber reduces liver synthesis of bile acids and lowers bile acids in gall bladder; fiber reduces absorption of deoxycholic acid, produced from bile acids by gut bacteria, which lessens solubility of cholesterol in bile; fiber decreases formation of deoxycholic acid and binds deoxycholic acid for fecal excretion; prefer water-soluble fibers: vegetables, fruits, pectin, oat bran, and guar gum; diets rich in legumes with water-soluble fiber (Native Americans) are linked to risk for gallstones; legumes increase biliary cholesterol saturation due to saponin content – restrict legume intake with gallstones.

- **Vegetarian diet:** protective against gallstones – fiber content of vegetarian diet; animal proteins (casein from dairy) increase formation of gallstones in animals; vegetable proteins (soy) are preventive against gallstones.

- **Food allergies:** food allergies may cause gall bladder pain; foods inducing symptoms, in decreasing order of occurrence are: egg, pork, onion, fowl, milk, coffee, citrus, corn, beans, nuts; ingestion of allergy-causing substances may cause swelling of bile ducts, resulting in impairment of bile flow from gall bladder.

- **Sugar:** increased risk of biliary tract cancer; increased cholesterol saturation of bile and gallstones linked to sugar intake – monosaccharides or disaccharides, independent of other energy sources.

- **Caloric restriction:** total calorie and carbohydrate intake and serum triglycerides are higher in gallstone patients than in controls; refined carbohydrate intake is higher in female gallstone patients; fat intake is higher in male gallstone patients; caloric restriction must be instituted carefully – rapid weight loss and fasting increase risk of gallstones.

- **Coffee:** avoid coffee until stones are resolved: coffee (regular and decaf) induces gall bladder contractions.

Nutritional factors

- **Lecithin (phosphatidylcholine):** low lecithin in bile may be a causative factor; a pure bile salt micelle requires 50 molecules to enclose a single molecule of cholesterol; a mixed bile salt/phospholipid micelle requires only seven molecules; taking only 100 mg lecithin t.i.d. increases lecithin in bile and larger doses (up to 10 g) provide greater increases; increased lecithin content of bile usually increases solubility of cholesterol; no significant effects on gallstone dissolution obtained using lecithin alone.

- **Nutrient deficiencies:** deficiencies of either vitamins E or C cause gallstones in animal studies.
- **Olive oil:** olive oil liver flush is undesirable for patients with gallstones: consuming large quantities of any oil will induce contraction of gall bladder, increasing risk of stone blocking bile duct = surgical emergency; oleic acid increases development of gallstones in lab animals by increasing cholesterol in gall bladder.
- **Fish oils:** in animal studies, fish oil reduces cholesterol concentration in gall bladder and rate of gallstone formation; omega-3 eicosapentaenoic and docosahexaenoic acids inhibit gallstone formation and decrease biliary calcium and total protein; omega-3 fatty acids enhance stability of biliary phospholipid-cholesterol vesicles.
- **Lipotropic factors and botanical choleretics:** lipotropic factors are substances hastening removal or decrease deposit of fat in liver by interaction with fat metabolism; lipotropic agents: choline, methionine, betaine, folic acid, and vitamin B_{12} – used with herbal cholagogues and choleretics; cholagogues stimulate gall bladder, while choleretics increase bile secretion by liver; herbal choleretics have favorable effect on solubility of bile; choleretics appropriate to gallstones are *Taraxacum officinale*, silymarin from *Silybum marianum*, *Cynara scolymus*, *Curcuma longa*, and *Peumus boldo*.

Chemical dissolution of gallstones

Use complex of plant terpenes alone or, preferably, in combination with oral bile acids; decreasing gall bladder cholesterol and/or increasing bile acids or lecithin should result in dissolution of stone; chemical dissolution is especially indicated for gallstones in the elderly who cannot withstand stress of surgery and in others for whom surgery is contraindicated.

- **Bile acids:** increase cholesterol solubility; oral chenodeoxycholic acid alone (750 mg q.d.) has completely dissolved gallstones in 13.5% and partially dissolved in 27% of patients in one study, but often takes several years with mild diarrhea and possible liver damage; ursodeoxycholic acid is more effective with fewer side-effects.
- **Terpenes:** natural terpene combination (menthol, menthone, pinene, borneol, cineol, camphene) is effective alternative to surgery; safe even when consumed up to 4 years.
- **Combined therapy:** terpenes are effective alone, but best results come from combining plant terpenes and bile acid; lower dose of bile acid needed reduces risk of side-effects and cost of bile acid therapy; menthol is major component of formula – peppermint oil, especially enteric-coated, may offer similar results.

Lifestyle

Sunbathing: almost all cholesterol gallstones contain central, pigmented nucleus with radial or lamellar pigmented bands, alternating with layers of crystalline cholesterol; activation of pigmentary system by UV light may increase concentrations of indole metabolites in bile, triggering their polymerization; positive attitude towards sunbathing is linked to twice the risk of cholelithiasis compared with those with negative attitude; association almost entirely restricted to those who always burn after long sunbathing.

THERAPEUTIC APPROACH

Healthy diet rich in dietary fiber gives adequate prevention; after development of stones, require measures to avoid gall bladder attacks and increase bile solubility; limit incidence of symptoms – intolerant/allergic foods and fatty foods must be avoided; increase solubility of bile – follow dietary guidelines plus nutritional and herbal supplements below.

● **Diet:** increase vegetables, fruits and dietary fiber, especially gel-forming/mucilaginous fibers (flaxseed, oat bran, guar gum, pectin); reduce saturated fats, cholesterol, sugar, animal proteins; avoid all fried foods; allergy elimination diet reduces gall bladder attacks (*Textbook*, Ch. 51).

● **Water:** six to eight glasses water q.d. to optimize water content of bile.

● **Nutritional supplements:**
   — vitamin C: 1–3 g q.d.
   — vitamin E: 200–400 IU q.d.
   — phosphatidylcholine: 500 mg q.d.
   — choline: 1 g q.d.
   — L-methionine: 1 g q.d.
   — fiber supplement (guar gum, pectin, psyllium, or oat bran): minimum of 5 g q.d.

● **Botanical medicines:**
   — *Taraxacum officinale* (t.i.d.):
      dried root: 4 g
      fluid extract (1:1): 4–8 ml
      solid extract (4:1): 250–500 mg
   — *Peumus boldo* (t.i.d.):
      dried leaves (or by infusion): 250–500 mg
      tincture (1:10): 2–4 ml
      fluid extract (1:1): 0.5–1.0 ml
   — *Silybum marianum*: sufficient dosage according to form to yield 70–210 mg of silymarin t.i.d.

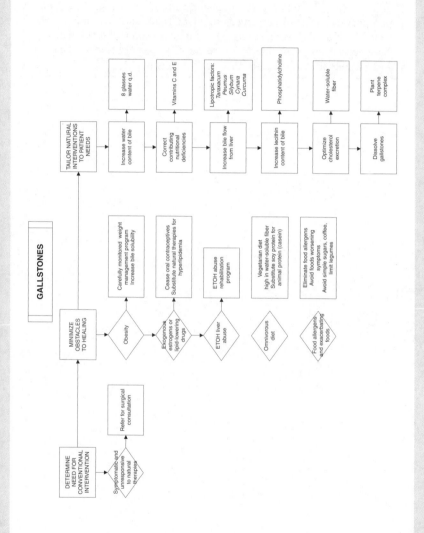

GALLSTONES

DETERMINE NEED FOR CONVENTIONAL INTERVENTION

Symptomatic and unresponsive to natural therapies → Refer for surgical consultation

MINIMIZE OBSTACLES TO HEALING

Obesity → Carefully monitored weight management program / Increase bile solubility

Exogenous estrogens or lipid-lowering drugs → Cease oral contraceptives / Substitute natural therapies for hyperlipidemia

ETOH liver abuse → ETOH abuse rehabilitation program

Omnivorous diet → Vegetarian diet high in water-soluble fiber / Substitute soy protein for animal protein (casein)

Food allergens and exacerbating foods → Eliminate food allergens / Avoid foods worsening symptoms / Avoid simple sugars, coffee, limit legumes

TAILOR NATURAL INTERVENTIONS TO PATIENT NEEDS

Increase water content of bile → 8 glasses water q.d.

Correct contributing nutritional deficiencies → Vitamins C and E

Increase bile flow from liver → Lipotropic factors: Taraxacum / Peumus / Silybum / Cynara / Curcuma

Increase lecithin content of bile → Phosphatidylcholine

Optimize cholesterol excretion → Water-soluble fiber

Dissolve gallstones → Plant terpene complex

— *Cynara scolymus*: extract (15% cynarin): 500 mg t.i.d.

— *Curcuma longa*: use liberally as a spice; curcumin: 300 mg t.i.d.

Gallstone dissolving formula: menthol 30 mg; menthone 5 mg; pinene 15 mg; borneol 5 mg; camphene 5 mg; cineol 2 mg; citral 5 mg; phosphatidylcholine 50 mg; medium-chain triglycerides 125 mg; chenodeoxycholic acid 750 mg. *Dosage:* t.i.d. if used in combination with meals. *Note:* peppermint oil in enteric-coated capsule can substitute at dosage of 1–2 capsules (0.2 ml/capsule) t.i.d. between meals.

Glaucoma: acute (angle closure) and chronic (open-angle)

DIAGNOSTIC SUMMARY

Acute glaucoma
- Increased intraocular pressure, usually unilateral.
- Severe throbbing pain in eye with markedly blurred vision.
- Pupil moderately dilated and fixed.
- Absence of pupillary light response.
- Nausea and vomiting common.

Chronic glaucoma
- Persistent elevation of intraocular pressure is associated with pathological cupping of optic discs.
- Asymptomatic in early stages.
- Gradual loss of peripheral vision resulting in tunnel vision.
- Insidious onset in older individuals.

GENERAL CONSIDERATIONS

- Increased intraocular pressure (IOP) from imbalance between production and outflow of aqueous humor; obstruction to outflow is the main factor in closed-angle glaucoma; acute glaucoma occurs only with closure of pre-existing narrow anterior chamber angle; in chronic open-angle glaucoma, anterior chamber appears normal.
- Two million cases in US – 25% undetected, 90% chronic open-angle type (no consistent anatomical basis for condition); strong correlation between content and composition of collagen and glaucomatous eye.
- Collagen is the most abundant protein in body, including eye – provides tissue strength and integrity of cornea, sclera, lamina cribosa, trabecular meshwork, vitreous; inborn errors of collagen metabolism (osteogenesis

imperfecta, Ehlers–Danlos syndrome, Marfan's syndrome) have ocular complications: glaucoma, myopia, retinal detachment, ectopia lentis, and blue sclera; morphological changes in lamina cribosa (scleral area pierced by optic nerve and blood vessels), trabecular meshwork (connective tissue network aqueous humor must traverse to reach canal of Schlemm), and papillary blood vessels found in glaucomatous eyes; changes may elevate IOP or lead to progressive loss of peripheral vision.

● Collagen structure changes may explain: similar peripheral vision loss in patients with normal and elevated IOP, cupping of optic disc even at low IOP, no apparent anatomical reason for decreased aqueous outflow.

DIAGNOSIS

Open-angle glaucoma initially asymptomatic – insidious; may reveal slight cupping of optic disc and narrowing of visual fields; tonometry is the key to confirming diagnosis; early recognition critical – delayed surgical intervention increases risk of blindness.

THERAPEUTIC CONSIDERATIONS

● Dependent upon reducing IOP and improving collagen metabolism in optic disc and trabecular meshwork.

● Optic disc composed of lamina cribosa, optic nerve fibers, and blood vessels; lamina cribosa is a mesh-like network rich in collagen traversed by optic nerves and blood vessels; collagen changes in lamina cribosa, papillary vessels, and trabecular meshwork precede pressure changes – prevention of ground substance and collagen breakdown important here.

● **Corticosteroids:** use should be discouraged in glaucoma – inhibit biosynthesis of collagen and glycosaminoglycans, causing glaucoma to develop.

Nutrition

● **Vitamin C:** achieving collagen integrity requires optimal tissue ascorbic acid (AA); AA lowers IOP in clinical studies; daily dose of 0.5 g/kg body weight (single or divided doses) reduces IOP by 16 mmHg; near normal tension achieved in some patients unresponsive to acetazolamide and 2% pilocarpine; hypotonic action of AA on eye is long-lasting if supplement continued; i.v. administration gives greater initial reduction in IOP; patient monitoring necessary to determine required individual dose (2–35 g q.d.); abdominal discomfort using high doses is common, but resolves after 3–4 days; proposed mechanisms – increased blood osmolarity, diminished production of aqueous fluid by ciliary epithelium, and improved aqueous fluid outflow; AA role in collagen formation may be key.

- **Bioflavonoids:** anthocyanosides (blue-red pigments in berries) elicit AA-sparing effect, improve capillary integrity, and stabilize collagen matrix by preventing free radical damage, inhibiting enzymatic cleavage of collagen matrix, and by cross-linking with collagen fibers directly to form more stable collagen matrix; *Vaccinium myrtillus* (European bilberry) is rich in these compounds – used in Europe to reduce myopia, improve nocturnal vision, and reverse diabetic retinopathy; rutin lowers IOP when used as an adjunct in patients unresponsive to miotics alone.

- **Allergy:** chronic glaucoma successfully treated by anti-allergy measures; immediate rise in IOP of up to 20 mm (plus other allergic symptoms) in patients challenged with appropriate allergen; allergic responses of altered vascular permeability and vasospasm may cause congestion and edema characteristic of glaucoma.

- **Magnesium:** channel-blocking drugs benefit some glaucoma patients; Mg is "nature's physiological calcium-channel blocker"; demonstrates improvement of peripheral circulation and visual field in patients with glaucoma.

- **Chromium**: primary open-angle glaucoma strongly linked to deficiency of RBC Cr and AA and elevated RBC vanadium (chromium's principal antagonist); AA and Cr potentiate insulin receptors that help sustain strong ciliary-muscle eye-focusing activity; AA or Cr deficiency linked with elevated IOP, which stretches normal eye, reducing capacity for focusing power.

- **Fish oil:** cod liver oil reduces IOP dramatically in lab animals in a dose-dependent fashion.

THERAPEUTIC APPROACH

Acute closed-angle glaucoma is an ocular emergency – refer immediately to ophthalmologist – unless treated within 12–48 h, patient will be permanently blinded within 2–5 days; asymptomatic eye with narrow anterior chamber angle may convert spontaneously to angle-closure glaucoma; process can be precipitated by anything dilating pupil (atropine, epinephrine-like drugs); agents which dilate pupils must be strictly avoided if glaucoma suspected.

- **Supplements:**
  - vitamin C: 0.1–0.5 g/kg q.d. in divided doses
  - bioflavonoids (mixed): 1,000 mg q.d.
  - magnesium: 200 mg q.d.
  - chromium: 100 μg q.d.
- **Botanical medicines:**
  - *Vaccinium myrtillus* extract (25% anthocyanidin): 80 mg t.i.d.

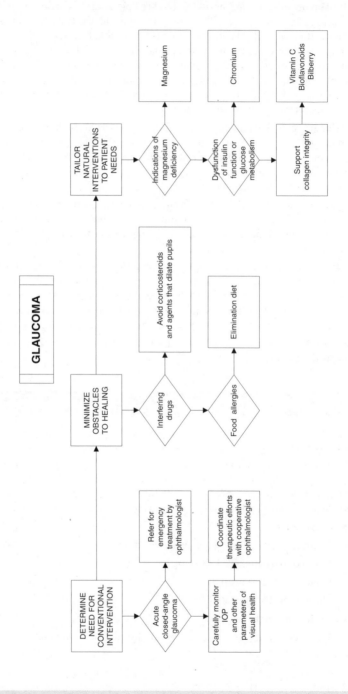

Differential diagnosis of the inflamed eye

	Acute conjunctivitis	Acute iritis	Acute glaucoma	Corneal trauma or infection
Incidence	Very common	Common	Uncommon	Common
Discharge	Moderate to copious	None	None	Watery or purulent
Vision	No effect	Slightly blurred	Markedly blurred	Usually blurred
Pain	None	Moderate	Severe	Moderate to severe
Conjunctival injection	Diffuse, mostly fornices	Circumcorneal	Diffuse	Diffuse
Cornea	Clear	Usually clear	Steamy	Clarity may change
Pupil size	Normal	Small	Dilated and fixed	Normal
Pupil light response	Normal	Poor	None	Normal
Intraocular pressure	Normal	Normal	Elevated	Normal
Anterior chamber	Normal depth	Very shallow	Normal depth	Normal unless infected
Iris	Normal	Dull, swollen	Congested and bulging	Normal unless infected
Smear	Causative organisms	No organisms	No organisms	Causative organisms if there is infection
Cornea	Clear	Usually clear	Steamy	Clarity may change
Pupil size	Normal	Small	Dilated and fixed	Normal
Pupil light response	Normal	Poor	None	Normal
Intraocular pressure	Normal	Normal	Elevated	Normal
Anterior chamber	Normal depth	Normal depth	Very shallow	Normal depth
Iris	Normal	Dull, swollen	Congested and bulging	Normal unless infected
Smear	Causative organisms	No organisms	No organisms	Causative organisms if there is infection

Gout

DIAGNOSTIC SUMMARY

- Acute onset, frequently nocturnal, of typically monarticular joint pain, involving metatarsophalangeal joint of big toe in about 50% of cases.
- Elevated serum uric acid level.
- Asymptomatic periods between acute attacks.
- Identification of urate crystals in joint fluid.
- Aggregated deposits of monosodium urate monohydrate (tophi) chiefly in and around the joints of extremities, but also in subcutaneous tissue, bone, cartilage, and other tissues.
- Uric acid kidney stones.
- Familial disease; 95% males.

GENERAL CONSIDERATIONS

Gout is a common arthritis caused by increased uric acid (final breakdown product of purine metabolism) in biological fluid; in gout, uric acid crystals (monosodium urate) deposit in joints, tendons, kidneys, and other tissues, causing inflammation and damage.

- Characterized biochemically by increased serum uric acid, leukotrienes, and neutrophil accumulation; may debilitate due to tophaceous deposits around joints and tendons; renal involvement may cause kidney failure via parenchymal disease or urinary tract obstruction.
- Associated with affluence ("rich man's disease"); meats (organ meats) high in purines; ETOH inhibits uric acid secretion by kidneys; primarily a disease of adult men (95% of cases – men over age 30); incidence = 3 adults in 1,000; 10–20% of adult population have hyperuricemia.

Causes of gout

Two major categories – (1) primary gout: 90% of all cases; usually idiopathic, but several genetic defects in which exact cause of elevated uric acid known; (2) secondary gout: 10% of cases; elevated uric acid secondary to some other disorder (excessive breakdown of cells or renal disease); diuretics for hypertension and low-dose aspirin are causes because they decrease uric acid excretion.

- Hyperuricemia of primary idiopathic gout – three categories: (1) increased synthesis of uric acid (majority of cases); (2) reduced ability to excrete uric acid (30% of cases); (3) overproduction of uric acid and underexcretion of uric acid (small %).

- Exact metabolic defect unknown in most cases, but gout is a controllable metabolic disease; causes of gout are summarized at the end of the chapter.

- 200–600 mg uric acid excreted daily in urine of adult male, two-thirds of the amount produced; remainder is excreted in bile and other GI secretions; dietary component of uric acid = 10–20%; in hyperuricemia, 1 mg/ 100 ml added to serum, enough to precipitate into tissues if individual near saturation threshold.

- Almost all plasma urate filtered at glomerulus: only a small amount bound to protein is not filtered; renal excretion is peculiar – 80% of filtered uric acid is reabsorbed in proximal tubule of nephron; distal tubule secretes most uric acid in urine; distal to this site, post-secondary reabsorption occurs; uric acid highly insoluble; at pH 7.4 and body temperature, serum saturated at 6.4–7.0 mg/100 ml; unknown factor in serum inhibits urate precipitation; chance of acute attack is 90% when level > 9 mg/100 ml; lower temperatures decrease saturation point – urate deposits form in areas (e.g. pinna of ear) where temperature is lower than mean body temperature; uric acid is insoluble below pH 6.0 and can precipitate as urine is concentrated in collecting ducts and passes to renal pelvis.

Signs and symptoms

First attack – intense pain, usually involving only one joint; first joint of big toe affected in 50% of first attacks and involved in 90% of cases; if attack progresses, fever and chills appear; first attacks usually occur at night preceded by specific event (dietary excess, ETOH, trauma, certain drugs, or surgery); subsequent attacks are common, majority having another attack within 1 year; but 7% never have a second attack; chronic gout is extremely rare, dietary therapy and drugs lowering urate; some kidney dysfunction occurs in 90% of subjects with gout, plus higher risk of kidney stones.

THERAPEUTIC CONSIDERATIONS

- **Conventional treatment** is colchicine, an anti-inflammatory drug originally isolated from plant *Colchicum autumnale* (autumn crocus, meadow saffron); colchicine has no effect on uric acid levels – it stops inflammation by inhibiting neutrophil migration into areas of inflammation; 75% of patients improve within the first 12 h of taking colchicine, but 80% of patients are unable to tolerate optimal dose – GI side-effects preceding or coinciding with improvement; colchicine may cause bone marrow depression, hair loss, liver damage, depression, seizures, respiratory depression, and even death; other anti-inflammatory agents are also used (indomethacin, phenylbutazone, naproxen, fenoprofen).

- **Post-acute episode measures to reduce risk of recurrence:** drugs to normalize urate levels; controlled weight loss in obese patients; avoiding known precipitating factors (ETOH excess or diet rich in purines); low-dose colchicine to prevent attacks.

- **Dietary factors exacerbating gout:** ETOH, high-purine foods (organ meats, meat, yeast, poultry), fats, refined carbohydrates, caloric excess; gout patients are typically obese, hypertensive, prone to diabetes, greater risk for cardiovascular disease; obesity is the most important dietary factor.

- **Naturopathic approach** for chronic gout similar to conventional approach: dietary and herbal measures instead of drugs to maintain normal urates; weight management to reduce obesity; control of known precipitating factors; nutritional substances to prevent acute attacks.

- **Lead toxicity:** a secondary type of gout ("saturnine gout") results from Pb toxicity; source = leaded crystal (port wine elutes Pb when stored in crystal decanter); Pb increases with storage time – toxic after several months; even a few minutes in crystal glass produces measurable increases of Pb in wine; mechanism of action – decrease in renal urate excretion.

Dietary guidelines

Eliminate ETOH, low-purine diet, achieve ideal body weight, abundant complex carbohydrates, low fat, low protein, abundant fluids.

- **Alcohol:** increases urate production by accelerating purine nucleotide degradation; reduces urate excretion by increasing lactate (from EROH oxidation), impairing kidney function; ETOH intake often initiates acute attack; abstinence can be only change needed to prevent attacks in some patients.

- **Low-purine diet:** reduces metabolic stress; omit high-purine foods (organ meats, meats, shellfish, yeast – brewer's and baker's – herring, sardines, mackerel, anchovies); curtail foods with moderate protein (dried legumes, spinach, asparagus, fish, poultry, mushrooms).

- **Weight reduction:** obesity linked to increased rate of gout; weight reduction in obese persons reduces serum urate; use high-fiber, low-fat diet to manage elevated cholesterol and triglycerides common in obesity; this diet = alkaline ash diet – alkaline pH increases urate solubility.

- **Carbohydrates, fats, and protein:** refined carbohydrates increase urate production; saturated fats increase urate retention; avoid excess protein (> 0.8 g/kg body weight) – high protein intake may accelerate urate synthesis in normal and gouty patients; adequate protein (0.8 g/kg body weight) necessary – amino acids decrease resorption of urate in renal tubules, increasing urate excretion and reducing serum urate.

● **Fluid intake:** liberal fluid intake keeps urine dilute to promote urate excretion and reduce risk of kidney stones.

Nutritional supplements

● **Eicosapentaenoic acid:** EPA supplements are very useful for gout; EPA limits production of proinflammatory leukotrienes, mediators of inflammation and tissue damage in gout.

● **Vitamin E:** mildly inhibits production of leukotrienes; acts as antioxidant; selenium functions synergistically with vitamin E.

● **Folic acid:** inhibits xanthine oxidase, enzyme producing uric acid; drug allopurinol is a potent inhibitor of enzyme; derivative of folic acid is an even greater inhibitor of xanthine oxidase than allopurinol; folic acid at pharmacological doses may be effective treatment; positive results reported, but data incomplete and uncontrolled.

● **Bromelain:** proteolytic enzyme of pineapple is an effective anti-inflammatory; suitable alternative to stronger prescription anti-inflammatory agents; take between meals (*Textbook*, Ch. 83).

● **Quercetin:** bioflavonoid may offer significant protection by inhibiting: xanthine oxidase in similar fashion to drug allopurinol, leukotriene synthesis and release, neutrophil accumulation and enzyme release; take with bromelain between meals (bromelain may enhance absorption of quercetin and other medications).

● **Alanine, aspartic acid, glutamic acid, and glycine:** these amino acids lower serum uric acid, presumably by decreasing uric acid resorption in renal tubule, increasing uric acid excretion.

● **Vitamin C:** megadose vitamin C contraindicated in gout – vitamin C may increase urate in small number of individuals.

● **Niacin:** high-dose niacin (> 50 mg q.d.) contraindicated in gout – niacin competes with urate for excretion.

Botanical medicines

● **Cherries:** Consuming 0.25 kg fresh or canned cherries q.d. is effective in lowering uric acid and preventing gout attacks; cherries, hawthorn berries, blueberries, and other dark red-blue berries are rich sources of anthocyanidins and proanthocyanidins; these flavonoids give fruits deep red-blue color and prevent collagen destruction; effects of anthocyanidins and other flavonoids are to cross-link collagen fibers, reinforcing natural cross-linking of collagen matrix of connective tissue; prevent free radical damage via potent antioxidant and free radical scavenging action; inhibit cleavage of collagen by enzymes secreted by leukocytes during inflammation; prevent synthesis and release of compounds promoting inflammation (histamine, serine proteases, prostaglandins, leukotrienes).

● *Harpagophytum procumbens* **(Devil's claw):** relieves joint pain, reduces serum cholesterol and uric acid levels; equivocal research results concerning anti-inflammatory and analgesic effects; may be useful in short-term management of gout; use of Devil's claw in long-term management is probably unnecessary due to efficacy of dietary regimen.

THERAPEUTIC APPROACH

● **Basic approach:**
  — dietary and herbal measures which maintain normal uric acid levels
  — controlled weight loss for obesity
  — avoidance of known precipitating factors (ETOH abuse, high-purine diet)
  — nutritional substances to prevent acute attacks
  — herbal and nutritional substances to inhibit inflammation.

● **Diet:** eliminate ETOH; low-purine diet; increase complex carbohydrates; decrease simple carbohydrates; low fat intake; optimize protein (0.8 g/kg body weight); liberal quantities of fluid; monitor dietary compliance with urinary 24-h uric acid (maintain below 0.8 g/day); liberal amounts (250–500 g q.d.) cherries, blueberries, other anthocyanoside-rich red-blue berries (or extracts).

● **Nutritional supplements:**
  — EPA: 1.8 g q.d.
  — vitamin E: 400–800 IU q.d.
  — folic acid: 10–40 mg q.d.
  — bromelain: 125–250 mg t.i.d. between meals
  — quercetin: 125–250 mg t.i.d. between meals.

● **Botanical medicine:**
  — *Harpagophytum procumbens*:
    dried powdered root: 1–2 g t.i.d.
    tincture (1:5): 4–5 ml t.i.d.
    dry solid extract (3:1): 400 mg t.i.d.
  — anthocyanoside extracts (e.g. *Vaccinium myrtillus*): equivalent to 80 mg anthocyanoside content q.d.

Causes of hyperuricemia

Metabolic
● Increased production of purine (primary)
● Idiopathic
● Specific enzyme defects (e.g. Lesch–Nyhan syndrome, glycogen storage disease)

(continued on p.208)

GOUT

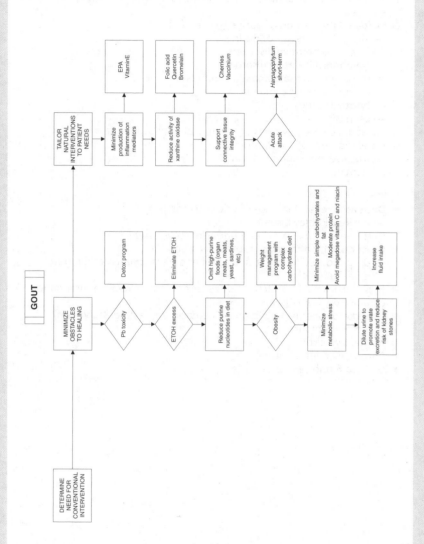

DETERMINE NEED FOR CONVENTIONAL INTERVENTION

MINIMIZE OBSTACLES TO HEALING

Pb toxicity → Detox program

ETOH excess → Eliminate ETOH

Reduce purine nucleotides in diet → Omit high-purine foods (organ meats, meats, yeast, sardines, etc)

Obesity → Weight management program with complex carbohydrate diet

Minimize metabolic stress → Minimize simple carbohydrates and fat / Moderate protein / Avoid megadose vitamin C and niacin

Dilute urine to promote urate excretion and reduce risk of kidney stones → Increase fluid intake

TAILOR NATURAL INTERVENTIONS TO PATIENT NEEDS

Minimize production of inflammation mediators → EPA / Vitamin E

Reduce activity of xanthine oxidase → Folic acid / Quercetin / Bromelain

Support connective tissue integrity → Cherries / *Vaccinium*

Acute attack → *Harpagophytum* short-term

Causes of hyperuricemia (continued)

- Decreased enzyme activity (e.g. hypoxanthine-guanine phosphoribosyl-transferase is decreased in 1–2% of adult gouty individuals)
- Increased enzyme activity (e.g. phosphoribosylpyrophosphate synthetase)
- Increased production of purine (secondary)
  — increased turnover of purines
  — myeloproliferative disorders
  — lymphoproliferative disorders
  — carcinoma and sarcoma (disseminated)
  — chronic hemolytic anemia
  — cytotoxic drugs
  — psoriasis
- Increased de novo synthesis (e.g. glucose-6-phosphatase deficiency)
- Increased catabolism of purines
  — fructose ingestion or infusion
  — exercise

Renal

- Decreased renal clearance of uric acid (primary)
  — intrinsic kidney disease
- Decreased renal clearance of uric acid (secondary)
- Functional impairment of tubular secretion
  — drug-induced (e.g. thiazides, probenecid, salicylates, ethambutol, pyrazinamide)
- Hyperlacticemia (e.g. lactic acidosis, alcoholism, toxemia of pregnancy, chronic beryllium disease)
- Hyperketoacidemia (e.g. diabetic ketoacidosis, fasting, starvation)
- Diabetes insipidus
- Bartter's syndrome
- Chronic lead intoxication
- Glucose-6-phosphatase deficiency

Hemorrhoids

DIAGNOSTIC SUMMARY

- Abnormally large or symptomatic varices of vessels or conglomerates of supporting tissues and overlying mucous membrane or skin of anorectal area.
- Bright red bleeding on surface of stool, on toilet tissue, and/or in toilet bowl.
- Anemia an uncommon complication.

GENERAL CONSIDERATIONS

Extremely common in industrialized countries; most individuals may begin developing hemorrhoids in their 20s, but symptoms usually not evident until 30s; 50% of persons over age 50 have symptomatic hemorrhoids and one-third of total US population have hemorrhoids to some degree.

Etiology: similar to those of varicose veins: genetic weakness of veins, excessive venous pressure, pregnancy, long periods of standing or sitting, and heavy lifting; portal venous system contains no valves – factors increasing venous congestion in perianal region can induce hemorrhoid formation, including increasing intra-abdominal pressure (defecation, pregnancy, coughing, sneezing, vomiting, physical exertion, portal hypertension due to cirrhosis), low-fiber diet-induced straining on defecation, and standing or sitting for prolonged periods.

Classification of hemorrhoids: classified according to location and degree of severity.

- **External hemorrhoids:** occur below anorectal line, the point in 3 cm long anal canal at which skin lining changes to mucous membrane; may be thrombotic or cutaneous; *thrombotic* – produced when hemorrhoidal vessel ruptures and forms thrombus; *cutaneous* – fibrous connective tissue covered by anal skin, located at any point on circumference of anus and caused by resolution of thrombotic hemorrhoid (thrombus becomes organized and replaced by connective tissue).
- **Internal hemorrhoids**: occur above anorectal line; may enlarge and prolapse, descending below anal sphincter.
- **Internal-external hemorrhoids:** mixed hemorrhoids = combination of contiguous external and internal hemorrhoids appearing as baggy

swellings; types: *without prolapse* (bleeding possible, but no pain), *prolapsed* (pain and possibly bleeding), *strangulated* (prolapsed to a degree and for so long that blood supply is occluded by anal sphincter constriction) – very painful and usually become thrombosed.

Clinical symptoms: itching, burning, pain, inflammation, irritation, swelling, bleeding, seepage.

- **Itching** rarely due to hemorrhoids, except when mucous discharge from prolapsing internal hemorrhoids; causes of pruritus ani – tissue trauma from harsh toilet paper, *Candida albicans*, parasites, and allergies.

- **Pain:** only with acute inflammation of external hemorrhoids; no sensory nerves ending above anorectal line – uncomplicated internal hemorrhoids rarely cause pain.

- **Bleeding:** linked to internal hemorrhoids; may occur before, during or after defecation; bleeding from external hemorrhoid due to rupture of acute thrombotic hemorrhoid; bleeding can produce severe anemia.

- Large hemorrhoids of long duration may have associated *anal fissures* and *hypertrophied papillae*; internal hemorrhoids are not palpable unless thrombosed, fibrosed (long-standing), and/or recently injected with sclerosing agent.

> **Note:** serious lesions (cancer) must be ruled out by sigmoidoscopy.

THERAPEUTIC CONSIDERATIONS

Nutrition

- **Diet:** high-fiber diet is the most important component in preventing hemorrhoids; vegetables, fruits, legumes, and grains promote peristalsis; fiber attracts water and forms gelatinous mass, keeping feces soft, bulky, and easy to pass; breakfast effect: 7.5-fold increase in odds of suffering hemorrhoids or anal fissures in persons who do not eat breakfast.

- **Fiber supplements:** used to reduce fecal straining; psyllium seed and guar gum – mild laxatives due to attraction of water forming gelatinous mass; less irritating than wheat bran and other cellulose fibers; reduce hemorrhoid symptoms (bleeding, pain, pruritus, prolapse) and improve bowel habits; reduce number of bleeding episodes, number of congested hemorrhoids, and friability of hemorrhoidal tissue.

- **Flavonoids:** prevent and treat hemorrhoids by strengthening venous tissues; rutin and hydroxyethylrutosides (HERs) have documented benefit (*Textbook*, Ch. 87); HER (1,000 mg q.d. for 4 weeks) relieves signs and symptoms in pregnant women; similar results in hemorrhoids not associated with pregnancy; micronized flavonoid combination (diosmin 90% and hesperidin 10%) for 8 weeks before delivery and

4 weeks after delivery – very successful; treatment well accepted and did not affect pregnancy, fetal development, birth weight, infant growth or feeding.

Topical therapy: will only provide temporary relief; types – suppositories, ointments, and anorectal pads; many OTC products contain primarily natural ingredients: witch hazel (*Hamamelis* water), shark liver oil, cod liver oil, cocoa butter, Peruvian balsam, zinc oxide, live yeast cell derivative, allantoin.

Botanical medicines: *Centella asiatica, Aesculus hippocastanum,* and *Ruscus aculeatus* are useful for enhancing integrity of venous structures of rectum.

Hydrotherapy: warm Sitz bath (*Textbook*, Ch. 42) is effective non-invasive treatment for uncomplicated hemorrhoids.

Surgical treatments: injection of sclerosing agents, rubber band ligation, dilation of anal canal and lower rectum, cryosurgery, hemorrhoidectomy, infrared coagulation.

Monopolar direct current therapy (inverse galvanism): painless outpatient treatment of all grades of hemorrhoids; effective and safe; may be treatment of choice of hemorrhoidal disease; relieves chronic anal pain within two treatments and anal fissures heal in nine within 4 weeks; purely an office procedure; no anesthetic needed, except local anesthetic for hypersensitive or nervous patient (2% procaine solution injected directly into hemorrhoid); no reported cases of stricture or metastatic abscesses; mechanism of action – when introduced into interior of hemorrhoid, negative pole of galvanic current makes contact with water of blood and generates hydrogen gas and hydroxide ions; hydroxide destroys organized structure of hemorrhoid and capillary circulation, producing first hydrolysis and then hardening of hemorrhoid; final disappearance – either absorbed as would a bodily contusion, or, if hemorrhoid is large, it ruptures, causing discharge of contents into rectum, followed by contraction of residual tissues; physician must be thoroughly familiar with anatomy/physiology of rectum and surrounding structures; no preoperative preparation necessary. (See *Textbook*, Ch. 155, for detailed description of this technique.)

THERAPEUTIC APPROACH

Primary treatment of hemorrhoids is prevention; reduce factors responsible for increasing pelvic congestion: straining during defecation, sitting or standing for prolonged periods, or underlying liver disease; high-fiber diet for proper bowel activity; nutrients and botanicals which enhance integrity of venous structures; warm Sitz baths and topical preparations useful to ameliorate discomfort; when indicated, monopolar direct current method will give permanent results – especially useful in advanced hemorrhoidal disease.

HEMORRHOIDS

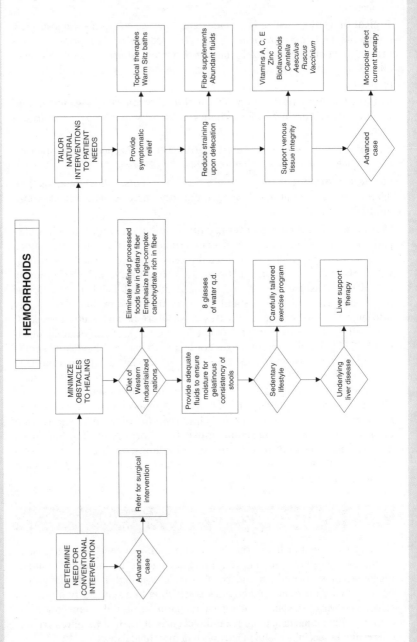

- **Diet:** high-complex carbohydrate diet rich in dietary fiber; liberal amounts of proanthocyanidin- and anthocyanidin-rich foods (blackberries, cherries, blueberries to strengthen vein structures).
- **Supplements:**
  — vitamin A: 10,000 IU q.d.
  — vitamin B-complex: 10–100 mg q.d.
  — vitamin C: 500–3,000 mg q.d.
  — vitamin E: 200–600 IU q.d.
  — bioflavonoids: 100–1,000 mg q.d.
  — zinc: 15–30 mg q.d.
- **Botanical medicines** (see chapter on varicose veins)
- **Physical medicine:**
  — monopolar direct current therapy
  — hydrotherapy: warm Sitz baths to relieve uncomplicated hemorrhoids.

Hepatitis

DIAGNOSTIC SUMMARY

- Prodrome of anorexia, nausea, vomiting, fatigue, flu-like symptoms 2 weeks to 1 month before liver involvement depending upon incubation period of virus.
- Symptoms may occur abruptly or rather insidiously.
- Fever, headaches, abdominal discomfort, light stools, diarrhea, myalgia, arthralgia, drowsiness, enlarged, tender liver, jaundice, itching.
- Dark urine.
- Normal to low WBC count, markedly elevated aminotransaminases, elevated bilirubin.

GENERAL CONSIDERATIONS

Hepatitis caused by drugs and toxic chemicals, but most often by virus; types A, B, and C most common.

- **Hepatitis A:** occurs sporadically or in epidemics; transmitted primarily via fecal contamination.
- **Hepatitis B:** 50% of viral cases in US; transmitted via infected blood or blood products or sexual contact (virus shed in saliva, semen, vaginal secretion).
- **Hepatitis C (hepatitis non-A, non-B):** transmission via blood transfusion; responsible for 90% of all cases of hepatitis via blood transfusions (10% of people receiving blood transfusions in past developed hepatitis C); only 4% of cases of hepatitis C result from transfusions; most cases are due to i.v. drug use; in other cases, source unclear; mortality rate (1–12%) much higher than other forms.
- **Other viral causes of hepatitis:** hepatitis viruses D, E, and G, herpes simplex, cytomegalovirus, and Epstein–Barr virus.
- **Acute viral hepatitis** extremely debilitating, requiring bedrest and 2–16 weeks for recovery; most patients recover completely (9 weeks for type A and 16 weeks for B, C, D, and G); 1 in 100 will die; 10% of hepatitis B and 10–40% of hepatitis C cases develop chronicity (hepatitis C from transfusion has 70–80% rate of chronicity).

- **Symptoms of chronic hepatitis** vary from virtually non-existent to chronic fatigue, serious liver damage, and even death.

DIAGNOSTIC CONSIDERATIONS

Suspected when typical signs and symptoms present; confirmed by blood tests for elevated liver enzymes and presence of viral antigens or virus-specific antibodies; type of virus determined by identifying specific viral antigens or antibodies; in chronic hepatitis B or C, use serology to monitor progression or clearance; hepatitis C is monitored by liver enzymes plus hepatitis C viral RNA (HCV-RNA) by polymerase chain reaction (PCR); hepatitis B serological findings and their interpretation are as follows:

Serological patterns and their interpretations in hepatitis B

HbsAg	Anti-HBS	Anti-HBc	HBeAg	Anti-HBe	Interpretation
+	−	IgM	+	−	Acute hepatitis B
+	−	IgG	+	−	Chronic active hepatitis B
+	−	IgG	−	+	Chronic non-active hepatitis B
+	+	IgG	+ or −	+ or −	Chronic hepatitis B
−	−	IgM	+ or −	+ or −	Acute hepatitis B
−	+	IgG	−	+ or −	Recovery from hepatitis B
−	+	−	−	−	Vaccinated against hepatitis B
−	−	IgG	−	−	False positive or infection in remote past

HBsAG, hepatitis surface antigen; HBc, hepatitis B core antigen; HbeAg, hepatitis B secretory antigen; IgG, immunoglobulin G; IgM, immunoglobulin M.

THERAPEUTIC CONSIDERATIONS

Hepatitis greatly benefited by natural therapies – nutrients and herbs to inhibit viral reproduction, improve immune function, stimulate regeneration of damaged liver cells (*Textbook*, Ch. 50); in chronic hepatitis, be aggressive in treatment – increased risk for hepatocellular carcinoma and cirrhosis (if cirrhosis present in chronic hepatitis B, 5-year survival rate only 50–60%).

Prevention of hepatitis B

Vaccination for high-risk occupations (health care professionals); acute exposure to HBV – hyperimmune globulin (HBIG) administered i.m. – confers immediate, but short-lived, passive immunity lasting 3 months; two doses

HBIG given within 2 weeks of exposure provides adequate protective immunity in 75% of exposed individuals; HBIG recommended for persons exposed to HBV surface antigen-contaminated material via mucous secretions or through breaks in skin; newborns with HBsAG-positive mothers should receive vaccine (0.5 ml shortly after birth and at ages 3 and 6 months).

Nutritional considerations

- **Diet:** *acute phase* – focus on replacing fluids: vegetable broths, diluted vegetable juices (diluted with 50% water), and herbal teas; restrict solid foods to brown rice, steamed vegetables, and moderate lean protein; *chronic cases* – low in saturated fats, simple carbohydrates (sugar, white flour, fruit juice, honey), oxidized fatty acids (fried oils), and animal products; diet focused on plant foods (high-fiber diet) increases elimination of bile acids, drugs and toxic bile substances.

- **Vitamin C:** high dosages of vitamin C (40–100 g p.o. or i.v.) may greatly improve acute viral hepatitis in 2–4 days and clear jaundice within 6 days; 2 g q.d. or more vitamin C dramatically prevents hepatitis B in hospitalized patients.

- **Liver extracts:** promote hepatic regeneration; effective in treating chronic liver disease, including chronic active hepatitis; placebo-controlled study: 70 mg liver extract for 3 months greatly lowered liver enzymes (aminotransaminases); blood liver enzymes reflect damage to liver – liver extract effective in chronic hepatitis via ability to improve function of damaged liver cells and prevent further liver damage.

- **Thymus extracts:** oral bovine thymus extracts are effective in acute and chronic viral hepatitis (*Textbook*, Ch. 53); provide broad-spectrum immune enhancement mediated by improved thymus function; double-blind studies: therapeutic effect noted by accelerated decreases of liver enzymes (transaminases), elimination of virus, and higher rate of seroconversion to anti-HBe, signifying clinical remission.

Botanical medicines

Licorice (*Glycyrrhiza glabra* and silymarin (flavonoid complex from milk thistle [*Silybum marianum*]) best documented; catechin (from *Uncaria gambir*) is effective but associated with potentially serious side-effects in rare cases (*Textbook*, Ch. 73).

- ***Glycyrrhiza glabra*:** effects of licorice beneficial in hepatitis – antihepatotoxic effects, immune-enhancing actions, potentiation of interferon, antiviral effects, actions as choleretic; goal – achieve a high level of glycyrrhizin in blood without producing side-effects; main hazard of licorice is its aldosterone-like effects (at doses > 3 g q.d. for 6+ weeks) or glycyrrhizin acid (> 100 mg q.d.) may cause Na^+ and water retention, hypertension, hypokalemia, and suppression of renin-aldosterone system; monitor BP

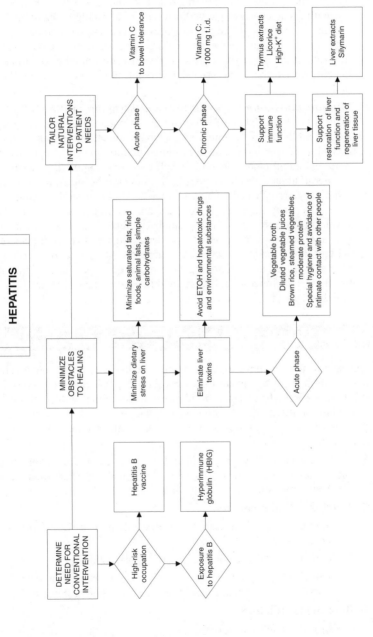

and electrolytes and increasing dietary K⁺ suggested; great individual variation in susceptibility to symptom-producing effects of glycyrrhizin; adverse effects rare below 100 mg q.d., but common above 400 mg q.d.; preventing side-effects of glycyrrhizin is possible via high-potassium, low-sodium diet; no formal trial performed, but patients who consume high-K⁺ foods and restrict Na⁺ – even those with hypertension and angina – are free from aldosterone-like side-effects of glycyrrhizin; nonetheless, avoid for patients with history of hypertension or renal failure, or current use of digitalis.

● ***Silybum marianum***: milk thistle contains silymarin, mixture of flavanolignans (silybin, silidianin, silichristine) – a potent liver-protecting substance; inhibits hepatic damage by acting as direct antioxidant and free radical scavenger, increasing intracellular glutathione and superoxide dismutase, inhibiting formation of leukotrienes, and stimulating hepatocyte regeneration; effective in acute and chronic viral hepatitis; reverses liver cell damage (confirmed by biopsy), increases protein level in blood, and lowers liver enzymes while improving symptoms in chronic cases; binding silymarin to phosphatidylcholine (silymarin phytosome) improves absorption and clinical results; very low toxicity and well tolerated; choleretic activity may produce looser stool – increases bile flow and secretion at higher doses – bile-sequestering fiber (guar gum, pectin, psyllium, oat bran) prevents mucosal irritation and loose stools' lack of toxicity allows long-term use (*Textbook*, Ch. 111).

THERAPEUTIC APPROACH

Bedrest during acute phase of viral hepatitis, with slow resumption of activities as health improves; avoid strenuous exertion, ETOH and other liver-toxic substances; careful hygiene and avoidance of close contact with others during contagious phase (2–3 weeks before symptoms appear to 3 weeks after); once diagnosis made, work in day-care center, restaurant, or other similar occupations are not recommended.

● **Diet:** natural diet, low in natural and synthetically saturated fats, simple carbohydrates (sugar, white flour, fruit juice, honey), oxidized fatty acids (fried oils), and animal fat; high in fiber.

● **Nutritional supplements:**
— vitamin C: to bowel tolerance (10–50 g q.d.) in acute cases; 1,000 mg t.i.d. in chronic cases
— liver extracts: 500–1,000 mg q.d. crude polypeptides
— thymus extracts: equivalent to 120 mg pure polypeptides with molecular weights < 10,000 or roughly 750 mg crude polypeptide fractions.

● **Botanical medicines:**
— *Glycyrrhiza glabra* (licorice):

powdered root: 1–2 g t.i.d.

fluid extract (1:1): 2–4 ml (1–2 g) t.i.d.

solid (dry powdered) extract (5% glycyrrhetinic acid content): 250–500 mg t.i.d.

— *Silybum marianum* (milk thistle): standard dose based on silymarin content (70–210 mg t.i.d.); prefer standardized extracts; best results at higher dosages: 140–210 mg silymarin t.i.d.; dosage for silybin bound to phosphatidylcholine = 120 mg b.i.d.-t.i.d. between meals.

(Note: if licorice to be used over a long period of time, increase intake of potassium-rich foods and monitor carefully for signs of hypertension.)

Herpes simplex

DIAGNOSTIC SUMMARY

- Recurrent viral infection of skin or mucous membranes characterized by single or multiple clusters of small vesicles on erythematous base frequently occurring about the mouth (herpes gingivostomatitis), lips (herpes labialis), genitals (herpes genitalis), and conjunctiva and cornea (herpes keratoconjunctivitis).

- Incubation period 2–12 days, averaging 6–7 days.

- Vesicle scraping stained with Giemsa's stain gives positive Tzanck's test.

- Regional lymph nodes may be tender and swollen.

- Outbreak may follow minor infections, trauma, stress (emotional, dietary, environmental), and sun exposure.

GENERAL CONSIDERATIONS

More than 70 viruses compose herpes viradae; of these, four are in human disease: herpes simplex (HSV), varicella zoster (VZV), Epstein–Barr (EBV), and cytomegalovirus (CMV); serology distinguishes two types of HSV: HSV-1 and HSV-2; 20–40% of US population have recurrent HSV infections; 30–100% of adults have been infected with one or both HSV types; greatest incidence among lower socioeconomic groups; HSV-1 is mainly from extragenital sites; genital infections mainly by HSV-2 (10–40% due to HSV-1).

- **Recurrence rate:** genital HSV-1 lesions – recurrence rate of 14%; HSV-2 recurrence rate = 60%; men are more susceptible to recurrences; after primary infection resolves, HSV is a dormant inhabitant in sensory and/or autonomic ganglia; recurrences develop at or near site of primary infection; precipitated by sunburn, sexual activity, menses, stress, food allergy, drugs, certain foods; risk of infection after sexual contact with partner with active lesions = 75%.

- **Immunological aspects:** host defense is paramount in protecting against HSV infection; persistent genital infections are seen in immunosuppressed individuals; cell-mediated immunity is the major factor determining outcome of herpes exposure: resistance, latent infection, or clinical disease; HSV-neutralizing antibody found in saliva is decreased during active

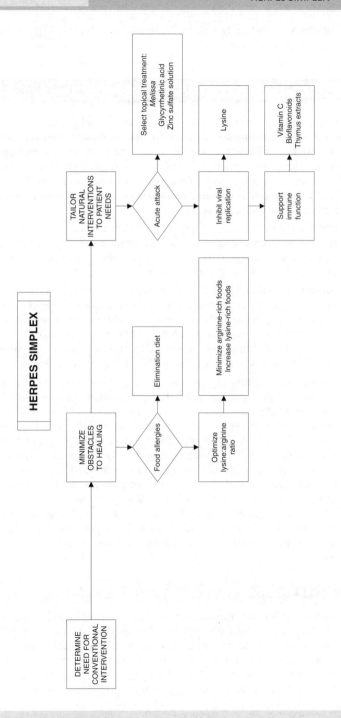

recurrence, and is IgG form – significant, since IgA is the major immunoglobulin in saliva.

THERAPEUTIC CONSIDERATIONS

Enhancing host immune status is the key to controlling herpes infection; defect of specific cell-mediated immunity may be present even in apparently normal subjects with recurrent HSV; key natural measure to strengthen cell-mediated immunity = bovine thymus extracts; benefits of thymus extracts – reduce number and severity of recurrent infections in immune-suppressed persons and increase lymphoproliferative response to HSV, natural killer cell activity, and interferon production.

- **Zinc:** oral zinc (50 mg q.d.) is effective in clinical studies; inhibitor of HSV replication in vitro; effect in vivo is to enhance cell-mediated immunity; topical application of 0.01–0.025% zinc sulfate solutions is effective in ameliorating symptoms and inhibiting recurrence.

- **Vitamin C:** oral and topical application of vitamin C increase rate of healing of herpes ulcers; topical ascorbic acid reduces number of days with scabs, number of cases of worsening of symptoms, and frequency of culturing HSV from lesions; oral ascorbate–bioflavonoid complex reduces outbreak of vesiculation and prevents disruption of vesicular membranes; therapy most beneficial when initiated at the beginning of disease.

- **Lysine and arginine:** lysine has antiviral activity in vitro due to antagonism of arginine metabolism; HSV replication requires synthesis of arginine-rich proteins; arginine may be an operon coordinate inducer; preponderance of lysine over arginine may act as either allosteric enzyme inhibitor or operon coordinate repressor; lysine at 1 g t.i.d. with dietary restriction of nuts, chocolate, and gelatin for 6 months – lysine rated much better than placebo; lysine and arginine are dibasic amino acids that compete with each other for intestinal transport; rats fed lysine-rich diet show 60% decrease in brain arginine, although no change in serum levels; HSV resides in ganglia during latency; supplemental lysine and arginine avoidance is warranted but not curative – only inhibits recurrences; in some patients, withdrawal from lysine followed by relapse within 1–4 weeks.

Topical preparations

- ***Melissa officinalis* (lemon balm):** concentrated extract (70:1) contains several components that work together to prevent virus from infecting human cells; dramatically reduces recurrence – many patients never again have a recurrence; rapidly interrupts infection and reduces healing time from 10 to 5 days; applied fairly thickly (1–2 mm) to lesions q.i.d. during active recurrence; extremely safe and suitable for long-term use.

- *Glycyrrhiza glabra* **(licorice root):** preparations containing glycyrrhetinic acid (triterpenoid) – inhibits growth and cytopathic effects of herpes simplex, vaccinia, Newcastle's disease, and vesicular stomatitis viruses; topical glycyrrhetinic acid is quite helpful in reducing healing time and pain of cold sores and genital herpes.

THERAPEUTIC APPROACH

Goal is to shorten current attack and prevent recurrences; support immune system – control food allergens and optimize nutrients necessary for cell-mediated immunity; inhibit HSV replication by manipulating dietary lysine:arginine ratio; no curative methodology known, but strengthening immune system is very effective in reducing frequency, duration, and severity of recurrences.

- **Diet:** develop diet which avoids food allergens and arginine-rich foods while promoting lysine-rich foods (*Textbook*, App. 5); foods with worst arginine:lysine ratio are chocolate, peanuts, and almonds.

- **Supplements:**
  — vitamin C: 2,000 mg q.d.
  — bioflavonoids: 1,000 mg q.d.
  — zinc: 25 mg q.d.
  — lysine: 1,000 mg t.i.d.
  — thymus extract: equivalent to 120 mg pure polypeptides with molecular weights < 10,000 or roughly 500 mg crude polypeptide fraction.

- **Topical treatment:**
  — ice: 10 min on, 5 min off during prodrome
  — zinc sulfate solution: 0.025% solution t.i.d.
  — melissa cream: apply b.i.d.
  — glycyrrhetinic acid: apply b.i.d.

HIV/AIDS

DIAGNOSTIC SUMMARY

- Positive test for antibody against human immunodeficiency virus.
- Onset sudden or insidious, or may present first as opportunistic infection (thrush [oral candidiasis] or *Pneumocystis carinii* pneumonia).
- Sudden onset (duration of up to 14 days) of fevers, sweats, malaise, fatigability, joint and muscle pain, headaches, sore throat, diarrhea, generalized swelling of lymph glands, and/or rash on trunk.
- Insidious onset may present as unexplained progressive fatigue, weight loss, fever, diarrhea, and/or generalized swelling of lymph glands.
- Advanced stages show neurological changes, including dementia and loss of nerve function (e.g. partial paralysis, vertigo, visual disturbances, etc.).

GENERAL CONSIDERATIONS

Acquired immune deficiency (AIDS) is a complex multifactorial disease of immunodeficiency and autoimmune inflammation involving multiple systems of the body (immune, GI, GU, endocrine, dermatologic, nervous).

Conventional medical management: there are two treatment principles:

- inactivate or slow replication of HIV
- provide antibiotic prophylaxis for patients with abnormally low CD4 lymphocyte counts.

Naturopathic medical management: nine treatment principles to optimize health, slow disease progression, improve quality of life, and possibly improve immune function:

1. Reduce oxidative stress using antioxidants.
2. Optimize nutritional status by improving GI nutrient absorption and mucosal immunity, eliminating food allergens; optimize GI ecology health, remove GI parasites and provide optimal therapeutic and dietary nutrition.
3. Eliminate cofactors (STDs and their residual, miasmatic effects, yeast, and viral cofactors).

4. Botanical and hydrotherapeutic antiviral therapy.
5. Immunomodulation through botanical medicine and exercise.
6. Increase oxidation of tissues through exercise.
7. Opportunistic infection prophylaxis.
8. Psychoneuroimmunological support.
9. Support patients receiving pharmaceutical drugs (prophylactic antibiotics and anti-retroviral drugs).

DIAGNOSIS

History: standard medical history plus additional information.

Additional historic information required

- History of sexually transmitted diseases in chronological order, e.g. syphilis, gonorrhea, hepatitis B, human papilloma virus
- History of mononucleosis
- History of antibiotic courses for childhood and adult infections including STDs
- Vaccination history and adverse reactions to vaccines
- History of cofactor viruses in chronological order (EBV; herpes I, II, 6 and 8; hepatitis A, B, C or E; HPV; CMV)
- History of vaginal and GI yeast infections
- History of genital or anal warts and abnormal Pap smears
- Detailed 24-h diet history ("Choose a typical day and tell me exactly what you ate and drank.")
- Exercise pattern
- History of psychoemotional trauma and issues (abuse history, anxiety, depression)
- Nature of the patient's spiritual life, if any, and the felt purpose of the patient's life

Lab assessment: tests that are essential for a full naturopathic evaluation of each HIV+ patient.

Essential laboratory assessments

- CBC with platelet count and ESR
- Full fasting chemistry and lipid panel (triglycerides, HDL, LDL)
- T/B/NK cell subsets (immune panel that includes CD3, CD4, CD8, CD19 and CD56 subsets)
- HIV RNA viral load
- DHEA (serum)

(continued over)

Essential laboratory assessments (continued)

● Urinalysis with microscopic analysis (especially important in patients who are taking certain protease inhibitors)
● Serum *Candida* antibodies (IgA, IgG, IgM) and *Candida* antigen when available
● For women, a recent Pap read by a thorough cytopathologist, i.e. in addition to the standard classification of cervical cells, the pathologist should look for and report koilocytotic changes as well as assessment of bacterial dysbiosis

Tests recommended if history indicates problems in associated area

● Complete digestive stool analysis
● Serum and antibody titers of cofactor viruses present in the history
● Serum food allergy panels that evaluate the IgE and IgG reactivity against panels of common foods. This is especially helpful in evaluating chronic sinusitis
● Thyroid panel
● Ferritin if anemia is present
● Serum vitamin B_{12} and folate
● Toxoplasmosis IgG
● *Mycobacterium avian* intracellular (MAI) blood culture if CD4 count is lower than 100 cells/ml

THERAPEUTIC CONSIDERATIONS

Individualize treatment.

Core protocol

● Beta-carotene: 150,000 IU q.d.
● Vitamin C: 2,000 mg t.i.d.
● Vitamin E: 400 IU b.i.d.
● Cod liver oil: 1 tbsp q.d.
● Multiple vitamin-mineral supplement: 2 capsules b.i.d. with breakfast and lunch; if HIV viral load is high, vitamin supplement without iron
● Aerobic exercise: minimum 20 min three times/week
● Coenzyme Q_{10}: 30 mg t.i.d. between meals
● SPV-30: one capsule t.i.d. if HIV viral load is detectable and/or patient has refused anti-retroviral therapy
● Maitake mushroom extract: 10 drops b.i.d.
● *Glycyrrhiza glabra* (licorice) solid extract: 0.25–0.5 tsp b.i.d. between meals.

Treatment principle 1: antioxidant therapy to reduce oxidative stress

Oxidative stress may contribute to HIV disease pathogenesis and progression via viral replication, inflammation, decreased immune cell proliferation, loss of immune function, apoptosis, weight loss, and increased drug toxicities; goal of antioxidant therapy – quench free radicals or reactive oxygen intermediates produced by inflammation.

- **Beta-carotene:** dosage = 150,000 IU b.i.d. in natural form.
- **Coenzyme Q_{10}:** dosage = 30–100 mg t.i.d.
- **Vitamin C:** 2,000 mg t.i.d. between meals – some antiviral protease inhibitors (Indinavir) can induce nephrolithiasis; no specific studies addressing whether vitamin C adds to risk of kidney stones in patients taking Indinavir, but there is concern that a nutrient–drug interaction exists; patients with dysbiosis will experience diarrhea from even the lowest dose recommended; perform complete digestive stool test to assess GI candidiasis and/or inflammation.
- **Vitamin E:** 400 IU q.d.
- **Selenium:** 200–600 μg q.d.
- **N-acetylcysteine:** 1,000 mg b.i.d.
- **Lipoic acid** (lipoate, alpha-lipoic acid, dihydrolipoic acid, thioctic acid) – alpha-lipoic acid was originally classified as a vitamin, but later found to be synthesized by animals and humans.

Treatment principle 2: improve nutritional status (GI nutrient absorption and mucosal immunity)

- *Lactobacillus acidophilus*: 2 capsules b.i.d. away from food.
- **Nystatin:** 500,000 units t.i.d. × 30 days – prescribe if *Candida* antigen-positive and/or abnormally high *Candida* antibodies, even if patient asymptomatic; *Candida* is both the result and cause of HIV-related health problems; nystatin is safe – not absorbed into circulation from gut.
- **Capryllic acid:** swish and swallow for thrush.
- **Phytostan:** 2 tablets t.i.d. (NF formula – capryllic acid, grapefruit seed extract, beta-carotene, rosemary, thymus vulgaris, glutamic acid).
- **Butyric acid:** 2 caps t.i.d. with meals.
- **Digestive enzymes:** 1–2 t.i.d. with major meals (*Textbook*, Ch. 5) – digestive stool analyses detect poor pancreatic output in many patients with digestive complaints, including HIV+ patients; digestive enzymes with meals can assist degradation of foods for absorption.
- **Garlic:** 2 capsules b.i.d. (600–1,000 mg b.i.d.).
- **Glutamine**

- **Carnitine:** 2,000 mg q.d. in wasting and high serum triglycerides.
- **Permeability factors:** 2 caps t.i.d. away from food (Tyler – 1, 500 mg L-glutamine, 750 mg n-acetyl-D-glycosamine, 400 mg gamma-linolenic acid, 200 mg oryzanol).
- **Saccharomyces boulardii:** 2 capsules t.i.d. away from food.
- **Ultra Clear Sustain:** 2 scoops b.i.d. as fruit smoothie or in water, rice, or soy milk (Metagenics and HealthComm).

Treatment principle 2: improve nutritional status (therapeutic and dietary nutrition)

Assume food sensitivities; try therapeutic trial of elimination diet – eliminate all gluten/gliadin grains, milk and dairy, and food allergies/sensitivities for at least 2 weeks to observe change in symptoms.

- **Whole foods:** reduce simple sugars; ensure essential fatty acids; emphasize protein; clean fresh fruits and vegetables; increase variety; eliminate caffeine and alcohol.
- **Protein powder smoothie:** 2 scoops protein powder with 1 cup of nuts/nut butter (not peanuts), 1 cup yogurt, 1 cup fresh fruit/berries, 1 tbsp honey, 1 tbsp flaxseed oil; thin with rice milk/juice to make 24 fluid ounces; drink 8 oz t.i.d.
- **Flaxseed oil or cod liver oil:** 1 tbsp q.d.–b.i.d.
- **Oat bran:** add 1–2 tbsp to other foods.
- **Multiple vitamin-mineral with or without iron:** 2 caps b.i.d. (pediatric liquids useful in wasting and malabsorption – 1 tbsp b.i.d.).
- **Copper:** may be excessively low or elevated.
- **Folate:** 400 µg q.d. if there is macrocytic anemia or after folate antagonist drugs have been used.
- **Vitamin B_1 (thiamin):** up to 50 mg b.i.d.
- **Vitamin B_{12} (hydroxycobalamin):** 1,000 µg i.m. one-two times/week in macrocytic anemia, peripheral neuropathy, and depression.
- **High dilutional IGF-1 (200C):** orally administered high dilutional IGF-1 was hypothesized to be the high dilutional growth factor responsible for weight gain observed in those HIV+ patients receiving IGF-1 200C.
- **DHEA**
- **Testosterone:** androgen deficiency plus classical growth hormone resistance may contribute to loss of lean body and muscle mass in hypogonadal men with AIDS wasting syndrome.
- **Intravenous nutrition:** if wasting, consider i.v. nutrition (e.g. vitamin C, cachexia formula, Myers cocktail, and/or total parenteral nutrition).

Cachexia formula – *administer over 2–4 h:*
— total volume: 558.6 ml
— sterile water: 35 ml
— ACE: 6 ml
— boron: 2 mg
— calcium gluconate: 4 g
— chromium: 200 µg
— copper: 1 mg
— Freamine or Travasol: 100 ml
— lithium: 5 mg
— manganese: 1 mg
— magnesium sulfate: 2 g
— molybdenum: 200 µg
— potassium: 20 meq
— rubidium: 100 µg
— selenium: 200 µg
— strontium: 1 mg
— vanadium: 5 µg
— vitamin A: 10,000 IU
— vitamin B_6: 300 µg
— vitamin B_{12}: 3000 µg
— vitamin B-complex: 3 ml
— zinc: 0.5 mg.

Myers cocktail – *draw up cocktail into one syringe, add 10–20 ml sterile water to reduce hypertonicity, and inject slowly over 5–15 min through a 25G butterfly needle:*
— magnesium chloride hexahydrate (20%): 2–5 ml
— calcium gluconate (10%): 2–4 ml
— hydroxycobalamin (1,000 µg/ml): 1 ml
— pyridoxine hydrochloride (100 mg/ml): 1 ml
— dexpanthenol (250 mg/ml): 1 ml
— B-complex 100: 1 ml
— vitamin C (222 mg/ml): 1–20 ml.

Treatment principle 3: clear drug, STDs, yeast, and viral cofactors

● **Acupuncture** detoxification auricular program.
● **Homeopathy:** helpful tips for classical homeopathic prescribing:

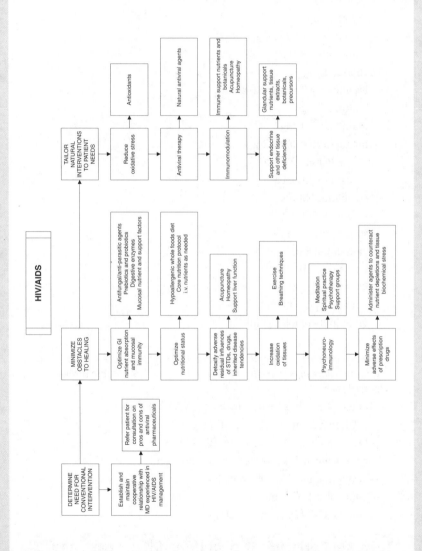

— clear concurrent viral cofactors (HSV, HHV-6, HZ, EBV, CMV, HPV) with nosodes (Staufen Pharma)

— homeopathic marijuana, cocaine, amphetamines, LSD, heroin, amyl nitrate, etc.

— consider homeopathic miasmatic polychrests (sulfur, *Psorinum*, *Medorrhinum*, *Syphilinum*, *Mercurius*, HIV when available; also phosphorus, *Lycopodium*, *Calcarea*, *Baryta*, etc.)

— when skin symptoms predominate, consider: sulfur, *Psorinum*, HSV nosode (for herpes infection)

— if growths (warts or condylomata) are predominant symptoms, consider: *Thuja*, nitric acid, *Medorrhinum*

— when GI symptoms predominate, consider: *Lycopodium*, including *Hepar sulph.*, *Mercurius* (for liver symptoms)

— when neurological symptoms predominate, consider: *Arsenicum alba*, *Aurum metallicum*, *Bufo*, *Calcarea c.*, *Cannabis i.*, *Causticum*, *Kali phosphorus*, *Lachesis*, *Lycopodium*, *Mercurius sol.*, *Nux vomica*, *Natrum muriaticum*, opium, phosphorus, *Phosphoricum ac.*, *Silicea*, *Staphysagria*, *Stramonium*, sulfur, *Syphilinum*, *Tarentual c.*, *Thuja occ.*, *Thyroidinum*

— when respiratory and wasting symptoms predominate, consider: *Aurum m.*, *Arsenicum a.*, *Tuburculinum*, *Iodum*, *Arsenicum iod.*, *Phosphoricum ac.*

— STD-related AIDS cases, consider using *Medorrhinum* and *Mercurius sol.* intercurrently

— for harmful effects of chemotherapy, steroids, AZT, combination drugs, consider X-ray.

● ***Glycyrrhiza glabra* (licorice root):** broad-spectrum antiviral botanical.

● **Herpes tincture** (*Hydrastis canadensis*, 2; *Lomatium dissectum*, 2; *Passiflora incarnata*, 1; *Taraxacum officinale*, 2; *Astragulus membranous*, 1; *Gelsemium*, 15): tincture 30–60 gtt q 2 hours during prodrome; q.i.d. during outbreak.

● **HPV tincture**: *Lomatium dissectum* and *Thuja occidentalis*.

● **Silymarin** (in milk thistle and artichoke): 160 mg t.i.d – drug addictions can be related to deficiencies in amino acids essential for optimal neurochemical function; consider combination amino acid supplementation when a history of drug use is present.

Treatment principle 4: provide antiviral therapy

Note: pharmaceutical antiretroviral therapy (ART) is effective in lowering HIV viral load and, in many patients, modestly increasing CD+ cells. Others recommend waiting until HIV viral load rises to moderate levels (depending on the clinician 5,000–30,000 copies/ml). At this time there exists no highly effective natural antiviral therapy for HIV/AIDS. Botanical and nutritional therapies may contribute to slowing viral replication. None of these natural therapies has been thoroughly evaluated in clinical trial. Refer to MDs experienced in HIV care for consultation regarding initiation of ART. For patients who wish to try natural antiviral approaches, we recommend getting a baseline HIV RNA viral load, then prescribing concurrent multiple naturopathic antiviral medicines at adequate doses. A follow-up HIV RNA viral load should be repeated at 1–3 months after initiation of natural antiviral therapy. If viral load has not dropped by a factor of 5 (or 0.3 log units) you may conclude that the natural antiviral combination has not produced the intended benefit. You should then reintroduce the decision to initiate ART.

- *Glycyrrhiza glabra* **(licorice root):** 2 caps t.i.d. or 0.25–0.5 tsp solid extract as tea q.d. or b.i.d. (monitor blood pressure) – also helpful for adrenal fatigue as indicated by low DHEA (< 250 ng/dl).

- *Hypericum perforatum* **(St John's wort):** 3 capsules (300 mg each) q.i.d. MandT, or 2–10 mg q.d. "HY" (Pacific Biologics) – it is difficult to achieve sufficiently high blood levels of *Hypericum* via oral administration to produce antiviral activity; it is highly recommended, however, as an antidepressant for HIV+ patients; be aware that *Hypericum* can produce photosensitivity; patients will tan and burn more rapidly; recommend sun block; caution is imperative if patient is using pharmaceutical drugs; there is new evidence that the hyperforin constituent of *Hypericum* may accelerate liver metabolism of drugs, diminishing their clinical efficacy.

- *Buxus sepervirens* **(evergreen boxwood):** 100 mg t.i.d. (SPV-30).

- *Curcuma longa* (curcumin)

- **Whole-body hyperthermia:** core temperature increased to 102°F for 20 min, two times/week for 3 weeks.

- *Momordica charantia* (bitter melon)

- **N-acetylcysteine** (NAC)

- *Aloe vera*: 1 oz b.i.d. or Acemannan capsules (Carrington Labs).

- *Allium sativa* (garlic)

- **Quercetin (derived from yellow onion):** 2,000 mg q.d.

- **Vitamin A:** 25,000–100,000 IU q.d. – watch carefully for vitamin A toxicity symptoms, such as headaches, body aches, excessively dry skin.

- **Vitamin B$_3$** (niacin): up to 250 mg b.i.d.

- **Vitamin C:** to bowel tolerance.

- **Vitamin E:** 400 IU b.i.d.

- **Substances to be further investigated:**
  — ozone: rectal insufflation.
  — *Olea* (olive leaf): 1 capsule t.i.d. to q.i.d. (Allergy Research).

Treatment principle 5: immunomodulation

- **Adrenal glandular:** 2 caps b.i.d. – use caution when employing glandular products in the age of prions and cross-species viral contamination (see also "*Eleutherococcus senticosus*" and "*Glycyrrhiza glabra*", both of which are purported to help in "adrenal fatigue").

- **Astragulus membranous**
- **Coenzyme Q$_{10}$:** 30–100 mg t.i.d.
- **Constitutional acupuncture:** acupuncture may help with depression and other symptoms.
- **Constitutional homeopathy**
- **Constitutional hydrotherapy**
- **DHEA:** 5–10 p.o. mg q.d. in women, and 15–50 mg q.d. in men; supplement if serum levels are low; note that the adrenal steroid hormone, dehydroepiandrosterone (DHEA), is an intermediate compound in the synthesis of testosterone and other steroid reproductive hormones; use with caution in women who are at risk for hormone-sensitive malignancies such as breast cancer.
- **Echinacea sp.:** 0.5 tsp tincture q.i.d. for acute viral symptoms; not for chronic use.
- **Eleutherococcus senticosus:** 10 gtt b.i.d. (Maxim-L from Omega) – it is helpful in cases of adrenal fatigue.
- **Lentinus edodes (shiitake mushroom):** 3 caps t.i.d. (Lentinan active constituent).
- **Corifola frondosa (maitake mushroom):** 3 caps t.i.d.
- **N-acetylcysteine**
- **Thymic fractions:** 2 caps b.i.d. (use caution when using glandular products in the age of prions and cross-species viral contamination).
- **Vitamin B$_6$ (pyridoxine):** up to 100 mg b.i.d.
- **Zinc:** not generally recommended; recommend foods high in zinc (pumpkin seeds, oysters, etc.) instead of supplements.
- **Promising substances to be further investigated:**
  - melatonin: not only regulates neuroendocrine functions but also has immunoenhancing and antitumor effects
  - testosterone: 5–10 mg q.d. for women; 50–100 mg q.d. for men – supplement if levels are low
  - *Ganoderma lucidum* mushrooms (reishi)
  - amino acids: deficiency of cysteine, methionine, phenylalanine, threonine, tryptophan, tyrosine, or valine may result in reduced humoral antibody response.

Treatment principle 6: increase oxidation of tissues through exercise and breathing disciplines

Physical fitness program.

Treatment principle 7: opportunistic infection: prophylaxis and treatment – viral/bacterial/protozoal/yeast

● **Bacterial infections:**
— zinc: hypozincemia in 228 HIV+ patients was associated with an increased incidence of concomitant systemic bacterial infections, but not PCP, viral, or fungal infections.

● **CMV, *Candida, Cryptococcus,* herpes, *Mycobacteria, Mycoplasma,* tuberculosis:**
— garlic: 4 caps q.d.
— colloidal silver: 1 tsp b.i.d. of 3 ppm solution
— SSKI (supersaturated potassium iodide): 8 gtt q.d.
— vitamin D_3: supplements are not recommended for most patients, unless they have TB, MAI or psoriasis (exposure of skin to sunlight produces vitamin D, and in moderation is a healthy source).

● **Fungal infections:**
— *Thuja occidentalis* (cedar), *Melaleuca alternafolia* (tea tree oil), *Calendula officinalis*: ointment applied locally.

● **Kaposi's sarcoma:**
— unsaturated fatty acids: essential fatty acids formulated to increase the tissue levels of dihomo-gamma-linolenic acid (DGLA) relative to arachidonic acid (AA) cause a regression in early Kaposi's sarcoma
— *Chelidonium majus*: extract given as 10 mg i.v. every other day for 10 injections made KS lesions diminish in size, thickness, and color, and no new lesions were noted; experimental group did significantly better compared with controls
— vitamin A: this may be useful in treating KS.

● **Parasites:**
— pancreatin: two 1,400 mg tablets after meals
— *Artemesia absiunthium* (worm wood): anecdotally reported to be useful in treating GI parasites.

● ***Pneumocystis carinii* pneumonia:**
— *Ginkgo biloba*: 2 caps b.i.d.–t.i.d.
— zinc.

● **Crytosporidiosis:**
— hyperimmune bovine colostrum: colostrum from cows immunized against cyptosporidium is lyophilized and given orally in 10 g doses reconstituted in water four times a day.

Treatment principle 8: psychoneuroimmunology

- **Cranioelectrical stimulation (CES):** 0.1 mA, 100 Hz, 20 min b.i.d.; or Alpha Stim.
- **Individual psychotherapy**, support groups.
- *Hypericum* **(St John's wort)** – caution is imperative if patient is using pharmaceutical drugs; there is new evidence that the hyperforin constituent of *Hypericum* may accelerate liver metabolism of drugs, diminishing their clinical efficacy.
- **Magnesium:** slowly increase dose up to 1,000 mg q.d.
- **Meditation**
- **Spiritual practice**
- **Vitamin B_6 (pyridoxine) and tryptophan**
- **Vitamin B_1 (thiamin)**
- **Vitamin B_{12}:** oral dosing or 1,000 µg i.m./week for a course of 6 weeks.
- **Yoga, qi gong**
- **Promising substances to be further investigated**
  - methyl donors (*N*-dimethylglycine [betaine], methionine, and *S*-adenosylmethionine [SAMe]); note that betaine is found in beet, and is similar to choline, but instead of CH_3 at A, it is at the B position.

Treatment principle 9: support for patients taking pharmaceutical drugs

- **AZT-induced myopathy and immune suppression:**
  - carnitine
  - vitamin B_{12}.
- **AZT-induced bone marrow suppression:**
  - vitamin E: tocopherol partially reverses the myelosuppressive action of AZT in HIV-positive patients
  - zinc.
- **Crixivan/Indinavir:**
  - kidney tonic tea should be given to those on Indinavir to prevent kidney stones (decoction of *Arctostaphylus uva ursi, Zea mays, Eupatorium perfoliatum, Equisetum arvense, Symphytum radix, Verbascum thapsus, Barosma betulina* in equal proportions).
- **ddI and isoniazid:**
  - omega-3 oils may be helpful in mitigating the inflammation associated with neuropathy (GLA 500 mg b.i.d.).

- **Hepatoprotection:**
  — silymarin
  — lipoic acid.
- **Hypersensitivity reaction to sulfa drugs** (e.g. TMP or Bactrim or Septra):
  — Alka Seltzer gold: take as directed on package
  — quercetin: 2 capsules four to five times/day
  — vitamin C: 2 g q. 2 h.
- **Peripheral neuropathy:** lower limb and feet tingling, burning or numbness, usually bilateral, can be a side-effect of several pharmaceutical antiretroviral drugs and can also appear in the absence of causative drug treatment:
  — vitamin B_{12}: 1 ml (1,000 µg/ml) two times/week for 6 weeks
  — cod liver oil: 1 tbsp b.i.d.
  — sphingomyelin: myelin basic protein 1,000 mg t.i.d. (Sphingolin is the trade name; made by Cardiovascular Research).
  — acupuncture: one to three treatments/week for 6 weeks.

Hypertension

DIAGNOSTIC SUMMARY

- Borderline high blood pressure: 120–160/90–94 mmHg.
- Mild high blood pressure: 140–160/95–104 mmHg.
- Moderate high blood pressure: 140–180/105–114 mmHg.
- Severe high blood pressure: 160+/115+ mmHg.

GENERAL CONSIDERATIONS

Hypertension is a major risk factor for MI or stroke; most significant risk factor for stroke; 60+ million Americans have hypertension, including 54.3% of all Americans age 65–74 and 71.8% of all American Blacks in same age group; persons with normal diastolic pressure (< 82 mmHg) but elevated systolic (> 158 mmHg) (increased pulse pressure) have twofold cardiovascular death rates compared with those with normal systolic pressures (< 130 mmHg).

THERAPEUTIC CONSIDERATIONS

Eighty per cent of patients with hypertension are in the borderline to moderate range – most cases can be brought under control via diet and lifestyle; many non-drug therapies (diet, exercise, relaxation therapies) are superior to drugs in cases of borderline to mild hypertension.

Conventional antihypertensive drugs

May be doing more harm than good; antihypertensive drugs (diuretics and/or beta-blockers) have side-effects, including increased risk for heart disease; virtually every medical authority recommends non-drug therapies for borderline to mild hypertension.

Lifestyle and dietary factors

Lifestyle factors: coffee, alcohol, lack of exercise, stress, smoking.
Dietary factors: obesity; high Na-to-K ratio; low-fiber, high-sugar diet; high saturated fat and low essential fatty acids; low calcium, magnesium and vitamin C.

- **Diet:** attain ideal body weight; increase proportion of plant foods in diet; vegetarians have lower BP and lower incidence of hypertension and other cardiovascular diseases than non-vegetarians; dietary levels of sodium do not differ between these two groups, but vegetarian diet contains more K^+, complex carbohydrates, essential fatty acids, fiber, Ca, Mg, and vitamin C, and less saturated fat and refined carbohydrate; most useful foods for hypertensives are celery, garlic and onions, nuts and seeds or their oils (EFAs), cold-water ocean fish (salmon, mackerel, etc.), green leafy vegetables (Ca and Mg), whole grains and legumes (fiber), foods rich in vitamin C (broccoli and citrus fruits).

- **Potassium and sodium:** diet low in K^+ and high in Na^+ is linked to hypertension; total K^+ content of food plus Na-to-K ratio; low-K, high-Na diet linked to cancer and cardiovascular disease; diet high in K^+ and low in Na^+ is protective against these diseases and therapeutic for hypertension; most Americans have K:Na ratio < 1:2; studies indicate a K:Na ratio > 5:1 is necessary to maintain health; natural diet rich in fruits and vegetables provides K:Na ratio > 100:1 (most fruits and vegetables have K:Na ratio of 50:1); increasing dietary potassium can lower BP; K supplements alone can reduce BP in hypertensives at dosage = 2.5–5.0 g q.d. of potassium; supplements useful in persons over age 65; relatively safe, except for patients with kidney disease – inability to maintain K^+ homeostasis may cause heart arrhythmias and other consequences of K^+ toxicity; K^+ supplements are also contraindicated when using some drugs (digitalis, K-sparing diuretics, and angiotensin-converting enzyme inhibitor antihypertensive drugs).

- **Magnesium:** K^+ interacts in many body systems with Mg; low intracellular K^+ may result from low Mg intake; Mg lowers BP by activating cellular membrane Na/K pump which pumps Na out of, and K into, cells; high intake of Mg is linked to lower BP; water high in minerals like Mg is called "hard water" – inverse correlation between water hardness and high BP; hypertensive patients who respond to Mg supplements are those taking diuretics, with high level of renin, with low RBC Mg, and/or with elevated intracellular Na^+ or decreased intracellular K^+; ideal Mg intake = 6 mg/kg body weight; therapeutic dose is twice as high; Mg bound to aspartate or Krebs cycle intermediates (malate, succinate, fumarate, citrate) preferred; supplements very well tolerated, sometimes cause looser stool (Mg sulfate [Epsom salts], hydroxide, or chloride); supplements must be used with great care in kidney disease or severe heart disease (high-grade atrioventricular block).

- **Stress:** causative factor of hypertension in many patients; relaxation techniques (deep breathing exercises, biofeedback, autogenics, transcendental meditation, yoga, progressive muscle relaxation, hypnosis) are useful in lowering BP; effect modest, but stress reduction technique is a necessary component in natural BP-lowering program; diaphragm breathing helpful – shallow breathing increases Na^+ retention of sodium.

- **Vitamin C:** the higher the intake of vitamin C, the lower the BP; modest blood pressure-lowering effect (drop of 5 mmHg) in people with mild hypertension; promotes excretion of Pb, which is linked to hypertension and increased cardiovascular mortality; soft water supplies have increased Pb in drinking water due to increased acidity of water (soft water also low in Ca and Mg, minerals protective against hypertension).

- **Vitamin B$_6$:** supplements lower BP; oral dosage of 5 mg/kg body weight for 4 weeks reduced systolic and diastolic BPs and serum norepinephrine; mean systolic dropped from 167 to 153 mmHg and diastolic dropped from 108 to 98 mmHg.

- **Calcium:** hypertension linked to low intake of calcium; association is not as strong as for Mg and K; Ca supplements can lower BP in hypertension, but results are inconsistent; Ca supplements reduce BP in Blacks and salt-sensitive patients, but not patients with salt-resistant hypertension; better results with calcium citrate vs. calcium carbonate; elderly hypertensives respond to Ca.

- **Coenzyme Q$_{10}$ (CoQ$_{10}$) (ubiquinone):** synthesized within body, but deficiency in 39% of hypertensive patients; lowers BP hypertensives; effect not seen until after 4–12 weeks of therapy; not typical BP-lowering drug; corrects metabolic abnormality, favorably influencing BP; reductions in systolic and diastolic BP = 10% (*Textbook*, Ch. 129); mechanism in hypertension is unknown – no changes in renin, Na, or aldosterone levels; improves cholesterol levels and peripheral vascular resistance in arteries of arms and legs.

- **Omega-3 oils:** increased intake can lower BP; fish oil and flaxseed oil very effective; fish oils produce more pronounced effect than flaxseed oil; dosage of fish oils used quite high (10 fish oil caps q.d.); prefer fish oil lab-certified against peroxides, mercury, and other undesirable substances; compare effective dose pricing with flax oil to find better value; reduce saturated fat; use 1 tbsp q.d. flaxseed oil – reduces systolic and diastolic by up to 9 mmHg; study – for every absolute 1% increase in body alpha-linolenic acid content, there is decrease of 5 mmHg in systolic, diastolic, and mean BPs.

Botanical medicines

- ***Crataegus* species:** extracts of hawthorn berries and flowering tops lower BP and improve heart function; BP-lowering effect of hawthorn very mild; requires at least 2–4 weeks before effect apparent.

- ***Allium sativum* and *Allium cepa*:** antihypertensive additions to diet; reduce systolic BP in hypertensives by 3.1% (*Textbook*, Chs 62 and 63).

- ***Viscum album* (mistletoe):** hypotensive action in animal studies; mechanism of action not fully understood; inhibits excitability of vasomotor center in medulla oblongata; possesses cholinomimetic activity; hypoten-

HYPERTENSION

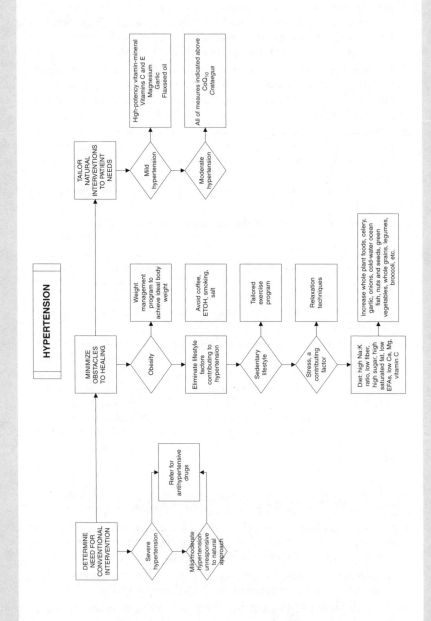

sive activity may be dependent on form in which mistletoe is administered and host tree from which it was collected; aqueous extracts more effective; highest hypotensive activity – macerate of leaves of mistletoe parasitizing on willow and gathered in January (*Textbook*, Ch. 120).

THERAPEUTIC APPROACH

Mild hypertension (140–160/90–104)

- Reduce excessive weight.
- Eliminate salt (sodium chloride) intake.
- Healthy lifestyle; avoid ETOH, caffeine, smoking; exercise and use stress reduction techniques.
- High-potassium diet rich in fiber and complex carbohydrates.
- Increase consumption of celery, garlic, and onions.
- Reduce/eliminate animal fats while increasing vegetable oils.
- Supplement diet with the following:
  - high-potency multiple vitamin-mineral formula
  - vitamin C: 500–1,000 mg t.i.d.
  - vitamin E: 400–800 IU q.d.
  - magnesium: 800–1,200 mg q.d. in divided doses
  - garlic: equivalent of 4,000 mg q.d. of fresh garlic
  - flaxseed oil: 1 tbsp q.d.

Treatment period = 3–6 months; if BP has not normalized, antihypertensive medications indicated; when prescription drug is necessary, calcium-channel blockers or ACE inhibitors appear to be the safest.

Moderate hypertension (140–180/105–114)

- Employ all measures above.
- Coenzyme Q_{10}: 50 mg b.i.d.–t.i.d.
- Hawthorn extract (10% procyanidins or 1.8% vitexin-4′-rhamnoside): 100–250 mg t.i.d.

Treatment period = 1–3 months; if BP has not normalized, antihypertensive medications indicated.

Severe hypertension (160+/115+)

Drug intervention required; employ all measures above; when satisfactory BP control achieved, taper off medication gradually.

Hyperthyroidism

DIAGNOSTIC SUMMARY

- Weakness, sweating, weight loss, nervousness, loose stools, and heat intolerance, irritability, fatigue.
- Tachycardia; warm, thin, moist skin; stare; and tremor.
- Diffuse, non-painful goiter.
- Increased T_4, free T_4, and free T_4 index.
- Failure of thyroid suppression with T_3 administration.
- In Graves' disease: goiter (often with bruit), ophthalmopathy.

GENERAL CONSIDERATIONS

Hyperthyroidism (thyrotoxicosis) is a group of disorders characterized by increased free thyroxine (tetraiodothyronine, T_4) and/or triiodothyronine (T_3); the autoimmune disorder Graves' disease comprises 85% of all cases of hyperthyroidism; much more common in women than in men (ratio 8:1); begins between ages 20 and 40; diffuse non-painful goiter with hyperthyroidism is the most common presentation of Graves' disease; less common signs/symptoms are exophthalmos, pretibial myxedema, nail changes (acropachy) and even paralysis in some groups; common denominator is the antibodies against thyroid-stimulating hormone (TSH) receptors; exophthalmos and skin changes can progress independently from thyroid dysfunction (euthyroid Graves' disease) – difficult to predict course of disease in a given patient.

Patterns of susceptibility in autoimmune disease (especially Graves'):

- **Gender:** female:male ratio is 7:1 to 10:1; ratio in those with ophthalmic complications is 1:1.
- **Stress:** recent stress is a precipitating factor; most common precipitating event is "actual or threatened separation from person upon whom patient is emotionally dependent"; onset of Graves' often follows emotional shock – divorce, death, or difficult separation.
- **Genetics:** Graves' is more prevalent in some HLA haplotypes (HLA-B_8 and HLA-DR_3 in Caucasians, HLA-Bw_{35} in Japanese, HLA-Bw_{46} in Chinese); HLA identical twins have a 50% chance of manifesting Graves' if one twin

is affected, and a 9% chance for fraternal twins; some haplotypes are protective against Graves'; genetic haplotype does not affect clinical course of Graves' disease or response to treatment.

- **Left-handedness:** statistical trend for left-handed people to manifest Graves' and other autoimmune diseases; 70% of male Graves' patients had some degree of left-handedness compared with 24% of controls; some evidence for higher rate of dyslexia in Graves' patients.

- **Smoking:** statistical correlation between smoking and Graves', especially with ophthalmic complications; smoking risk (1.5) less than heredity (3.6) and negative life events (6.3); the group at highest risk of increase for severe endocrine ophthalmopathy involves those with eye manifestation who continue to smoke.

- **Iodine supplementation:** dietary iodine supplementation in iodine-sufficient areas can increase incidence of thyrotoxicosis in susceptible individuals.

- **Mercury and cadmium exposure:** exposing animals to toxic levels of Cd or Hg induces immediate hyperthyroidism; confirmatory anecdotal human clinical cases have been reported.

- **Drugs:** in older patients with hyperthyroidism, consider toxic reaction to prescription drugs; most common causes of hyperthyroidism in the elderly are low iodine intake and higher use of aminodarone (antihypertensive drug); symptoms of hyperthyroidism vary in elderly – apathy, tachycardia, and weight loss are more common.

DIAGNOSIS

Clinical presentation

Graves' disease in young adult female: nervousness, irritability, sweating, palpitations, insomnia, tremor, frequent stools, weight loss despite good appetite.

- **Physical exam:** smooth, diffuse, non-tender goiter; tachycardia, especially after exercise; loud heart sounds (often systolic murmur); mild proptosis, lid retraction, lid lag, and tremor.

- **Other signs and symptoms:** muscle weakness and fatigue, anxiety, heat intolerance, pretibial myxedema.

- **Atypical cases (elderly):** above symptoms may be absent = "apathetic thyrotoxicosis"; in elderly, only symptom may be depression.

- Screening lab test for suppressed TSH.

- Increased thyroid hormone can present as worsening of already present cardiac symptoms (angina pectoris, CHF, and atrial fibrillation).

- **Characteristic skin changes:** moist, warm, and finely textured; perspiration increases in response to increased body temperature; pigment changes (vitiligo), increased pigmentation of areas (skin creases, knuckles).

- **Hair** may thin or fall out in patches or altogether (alopecia).
- **Nails** may separate prematurely from nail bed (onycholysis).
- **Localized non-pitting edema** along shins (myxedema); may occur elsewhere, on extensor surfaces; often pruritic and red.
- Osteoporosis, dyspnea, polyurea and polydipsia, myopathy, paralysis, Parkinsonian or choreoathetoid affect.

Differential diagnosis of hyperthyroidism

- **Graves' disease:** most common diagnosis of hyperthyroidism.
- **Several types of thyroiditis** cause hyperthyroidism: Hashimoto's thyroiditis (early stage), subacute thyroiditis, painless thyroiditis, and radiation thyroiditis.
- **Hyperthyroidism from exogenous causes:** iatrogenic hyperthyroidism, factitious hyperthyroidism (dieters taking thyroxine for weight loss), and iodine-induced hyperthyroidism (Jod–Basedow disease).
- **Toxic nodular goiters:** toxic adenoma and multinodular goiter.
- **Rare causes:** thyroid carcinoma, ectopic hyperthyroidism, trophoblastic tumors (hydatidiform mole, choriocarcinoma, embryonic carcinoma of testis), excess TSH (pituitary adenoma, non-neoplastic pituitary secretion of TSH), and struma ovarii.

Laboratory diagnosis

Definitive:

- Serum T_3, T_4, thyroid resin uptake, and free thyroxine usually all elevated.
- TSH assay will show low levels, except in rare cases.
- TSH receptor antibodies (TSH-R Ab) present in 80% of cases.
- Nodular goiter present – thyroid scan to rule out cancer and guide treatment.
- Serum antibodies to help rule out cancer in patients with lobular firm goiters; high antibody levels suggest chronic thyroiditis.

THERAPEUTIC CONSIDERATIONS

Chief objective of natural treatment of Graves' and hyperthyroidism is to reduce symptoms while trying to re-establish normal thyroid status; little research on natural approach.

- **Reduce risk factors:** stress, smoking, excess iodine intake; stress control is the single most important action; avoid anything that will excite patient and increase agitation; counseling to prevent return to stress-generating life strategies; increase rest – daily nap after lunch plus full night's sleep.

HYPERTHYROIDISM

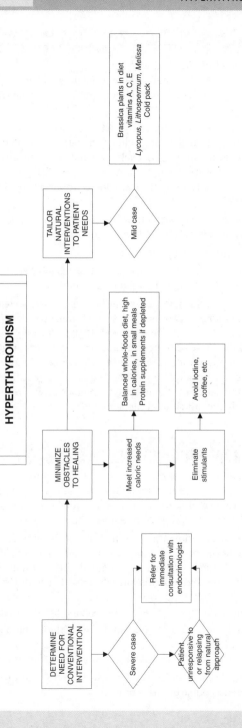

DETERMINE NEED FOR CONVENTIONAL INTERVENTION

Severe case

Patient unresponsive to or relapsing from natural approach

Refer for immediate consultation with endocrinologist

MINIMIZE OBSTACLES TO HEALING

Meet increased caloric needs

Balanced whole-foods diet, high in calories, in small meals
Protein supplements if depleted

Eliminate stimulants

Avoid iodine, coffee, etc.

TAILOR NATURAL INTERVENTIONS TO PATIENT NEEDS

Mild case

Brassica plants in diet
vitamins A, C, E
Lycopus, Lithospermum, Melissa
Cold pack

Diet

- **Balanced whole foods diet:** high in calories to compensate for increased metabolism; eaten in small, frequent meals; supplement protein if patient nutritionally depleted; avoid iodine supplements; avoid caffeine and other stimulants.

- **Dietary goitrogens:** substances which prevent utilization of iodine are isothiocyanates, which are similar in action and structure to propyl-thiouracil; found in turnips, cabbage, rutabagas, mustard, rapeseeds, cassava root, soybeans, peanuts, pine nuts and millet; goitrogens transmitted from cow's milk to humans; these foods are unreliable in treating hyperthyroidism:

  — goitrogen content quite low, compared with dosages of PTU used in hyperthyroidism (100–200 mg t.i.d.–q.i.d.)

  — cooking inactivates goitrogens

  — no documentation that natural goitrogens interfere with thyroid function significantly if dietary iodine adequate.

  Naturally occurring goitrogens may be in mild cases instead of PTU and related drugs; large amounts of these foods must be consumed in raw state, and iodine intake must be restricted; highest levels of isothiocyanates in raw soymilk (0.46–2.5 mg/dl); Brassica family: rutabagas, cabbage, and turnips have highest levels; quantity varies according to climate and soil factors; a half head of raw cabbage q.d. is a typical prescription; iodine sources are kelp, other seaweeds, vegetables grown near ocean, seafood, iodized salt, and nutritional supplements.

Nutritional supplements

- **Vitamin A:** large amounts inhibit thyroid function and ameliorate Graves' symptoms; exact mechanism unknown, but iodine metabolism is altered; animal studies: alteration in cellular uptake of thyroxin, capacity of nuclear T_3 receptors, and thyroid hormone metabolism.

- **Vitamin C:** experimental administration of thyroid, thyroxin or thyrotrophic hormone reduces ascorbate in serum, blood, liver, adrenal, thymus, and kidney; antithyroid drugs (thiourea, thiouracil) cause same effect; hyperthyroid humans have decreased excretion of ascorbate; supplemental vitamin C has no direct effect on the course of disease; supplementation is warranted to ameliorate symptoms and metabolic effects.

- **Vitamin E:** may protect patient from oxidative damage of hyperthyroidism; rat model: vitamin E prevented lipid peroxidation linked to hyperthyroidism; benefits to hyperthyroid patients are unknown.

- **Calcium:** Ca metabolism is altered in hyperthyroidism; Graves' patients are more susceptible to osteoporosis.

● **Iodine:** excess common in developed nations; sources – food additives (salt and iodine used to sterilize pipes in dairies), medical products (betadine washes, iodine-containing drugs, e.g. aminodarone, radiographic dyes); effects of iodine in patients with hyperthyroidism are:

— temporary symptom reduction by stopping hormone synthesis (Wolff–Chaikoff effect)

— thyroid can remain suppressed or resume hormone synthesis at reduced, former, or increased rate (escape from Wolff–Chaikoff)

— excess iodine can trigger hyperthyroidism (Jod–Basedow disease) in euthyroid person or trigger overactive thyroid to return to normal.

The action of iodine is unpredictable.

● **Zinc:** RBC zinc is decreased in hyperthyroid patients; antithyroid drugs normalize RBC zinc but not until 2 months after T_4 and T_3 levels normalize; zinc RBC in hyperthyroid patients reflects mean thyroid hormone level over preceding several months (HgbA1c indicates mean glucose levels in diabetics); oral zinc tolerance test (get baseline zinc level after 10-h fast followed by oral dose of 165 mg zinc sulfate heptahydrate – 37.5 mg zinc – dissolved in 20 ml deionized water with blood samples drawn at 30-min intervals over next 3 h) indicates hyperthyroid patients have basal serum zinc similar to euthyroid persons, but with greater urinary zinc excretion – suggesting zinc depletion from tissues to bloodstream caused by catabolism from hyperthyroid state; hyperthyroidism causes lower zinc assimilation by tissues after ingestion.

Botanical medicines

Medicinal plants traditionally used in the treatment of hyperthyroidism

Medicinal plant	Traditional indications
Valerian officinalis	Nervine effect
Scutellaria laterfloria	Nervine effect
Cactus grandiflora	Heart tonic; use with elevated pulse
Iris versicolor	Traditional use for hyperthyroidism
Fucus spp.	Use with caution, as a high iodine content can improve symptoms at first then later cause aggravation
Lycopus spp.	Blocks the TSH receptors; blocks peripheral conversion of T_4 to T_3
Lithospermum officinale	Blocks the TSH receptors
Melissa officinalis	Blocks the TSH receptors

Unfortunately, these plants have not been adequately evaluated in clinical studies.

Lycopus spp., Lithospermum officinale and Melissa officinalis:

● Aqueous, freeze-dried extracts of *Lycopus* spp., *Lithospermum officinale* and *Melissa officinalis* have been studied in vivo and in vitro; preliminary results support their use in Graves' disease; clinical research needed.

● Inhibit effects of exogenous TSH on rat thyroid glands; block effects of TSH on TSH receptor sites on thyroid membranes; inhibit peripheral deiodination of T_4 to T_3; and block effects of antithyroid immunoglobulins on TSH receptors.

● Oxidation products of derivatives of 3,4-dihydroxycinnamic acid are responsible for most of the effects; blocking effects of isolated compounds of TSH receptors are reversible; none of compounds combined irreversibly, damaged or altered TSH receptors in situ.

● Alcohol extract of *Lycopus europeus* given orally to rats caused long-lasting decrease in T_3 due to reduced peripheral T_4 deiodination; reduced TSH 24 h later with drop in LH and testosterone; water extracts less potent – active constituents are unoxidized alcohol-soluble phenolic compounds.

● Dosage recommendations from the British Herbal Pharmacopoeia for *Lycopus* spp. and *Melissa officinalis* (no mention is made of *Lithospermum officinale*) are given below.

Other therapies

● **Hydrotherapy:** calming hydrotherapy (neutral baths before bed) is indicated; cold compress to throat 15 min q.d. may improve symptoms; ice bag over heart reduces heart rate but should not be overused.

● **Acupuncture:** reported as effective treatment for hyperthyroidism.

THERAPEUTIC APPROACH

Acute Graves' disease is not easily treated by naturopathic methods; in severe cases, no guarantee that natural treatments will alleviate symptoms adequately; "thyroid storm" is a potentially fatal complication, which must be treated very aggressively with antithyroid drugs and/or iodine; in mild cases, natural therapeutics can manage symptoms well, but monitor carefully to avoid sudden exacerbation; relapse quite possible; treat mild cases symptomatically; allow patient to return to euthyroid status if possible; if iodine is used, ablative treatment needed – risk of escape (potential for more intense symptoms) increases with time.

● **Allopathic treatment** of Graves' disease offers three equal treatments to choose from; decision-making may be difficult for patient while in thyrotoxic state; symptomatic relief is mandatory before decision is made; antithyroid drugs can manage symptoms indefinitely while waiting for return to euthyroid status; if drugs not well tolerated, consider ablative therapies; surgery has higher rate of euthyroid results than radioactive iodine but carries greater risk of serious complications; render supportive natural treatment whatever the choice.

● **Diet:** whole-foods diet with increased calories, micronutrients, and protein to meet the increased metabolic needs; mild cases – large amounts of raw Brassica family foods and raw soy products; restrict iodine.

● **Supplements:**
   — vitamin A: 50,000 IU q.d.
   — vitamin C: 2,000 mg b.i.d.
   — vitamin E: 800 IU q.d.

● **Botanical medicines:**
   — *Lycopus* spp., *Lithospermum officinale* and/or *Melissa officinalis*:
      dried herb: 1–3 g or by infusion t.i.d.
      tincture (1:5): 2–6 ml t.i.d.
      fluid extract (1:1): 1–3 ml t.i.d.

● **Hydrotherapy:** cold packs placed over thyroid t.i.d.

Hypoglycemia

DIAGNOSTIC SUMMARY

- Blood glucose level below 50 mg/dl.
- Normal response curve during first 2–3 h of glucose tolerance test followed by decrease of 20 mg or more below fasting glucose level during final hours of test, with symptoms developing during decrease.

INTRODUCTION

Hypoglycemia is divided into two main categories:

- **Reactive hypoglycemia:** most common; symptoms of hypoglycemia 3–5 h after a meal; may also result from oral hypoglycemic drugs – these sulfa drugs (sulfonylureas) stimulate secretion of additional insulin by pancreas and enhance tissue sensitivity to insulin; some designate this category "idiopathic postprandial syndrome" (IPPS) because symptoms exist and are related to rapid glucose drops, but absolute glucose levels are not reliable indicators of syndrome; many asymptomatic controls have glucose below 50 and many symptomatic patients have normal postprandial glucose.

- **Fasting hypoglycemia:** rare – appears in severe disease states (pancreatic tumors, extensive liver damage, prolonged starvation, and various cancers, or excessive exogenous insulin in diabetics).

Glucose is the primary fuel for brain – low levels affect brain first.

Symptoms of hypoglycemia: HA, depression, anxiety, irritability, blurred vision, excessive sweating, mental confusion, incoherent speech, bizarre behavior, convulsions.

DIAGNOSTIC CONSIDERATIONS

Standard methods of diagnosing hypoglycemia – measuring blood glucose; normal fasting level = 70–105 mg/dl; levels < 140 mg/dl on 2 separate occasions = diabetes; levels < 50 mg/dl = fasting hypoglycemia.

- **Glucose tolerance test (GTT):** used to diagnose reactive hypoglycemia and diabetes, but rarely required for DM; after fasting 12+ h, measure baseline blood glucose; subject given glucose drink – amount consumed based on body weight, 1.75 g/kg body weight; measure blood sugar at 30 min, 1 h, and then hourly for up to 6 h; levels < 200 mg/dl indicate DM; levels > 50 mg/dl indicate reactive hypoglycemia.

● **Glucose-insulin tolerance test:** blood sugar levels alone are often not enough to diagnose hypoglycemia – signs and symptoms of hypoglycemia occur in persons with glucose well above 50 mg/dl plus wide overlap between symptomatic patients and asymptomatic controls; symptoms linked to hypoglycemia are the result of increases in insulin or epinephrine (adrenaline); measure insulin or epinephrine during GTT since symptoms often correlate better with hormones than glucose; glucose-insulin tolerance test (G-ITT) has greater sensitivity in diagnosing hypoglycemia and DM than GTT; standard 6-h GTT coupled with measurements of insulin; two-thirds of subjects with suspected DM or hypoglycemia with normal GTT demonstrate abnormal G-ITT; test is costly.

● **Hypoglycemic index:** aid in diagnosing borderline hypoglycemia; value determined by calculating fall in blood glucose during 90-min period before lowest point divided by value of lowest point; hypoglycemic index > 0.8 indicates reactive hypoglycemia.

● **Hypoglycemia questionnaire:** most useful and cost-effective method of diagnosing hypoglycemia is to assess symptoms; when symptoms appear 3–4 h after eating and disappear with ingestion of food, consider hypoglycemia.

GENERAL CONSIDERATIONS

Complex hormonal fluxes are largely the result of ingesting too much refined carbohydrate; "syndrome X" = cluster of abnormalities from high intake of refined carbohydrate, leading to hypoglycemia, hyperinsulinemia and glucose intolerance, followed by diminished insulin sensitivity, leading to hypertension, hypercholesterolemia, obesity, and type II diabetes; US government recommends that no more than 10% of total caloric intake is from refined sugars; average American consumes 100+ lb sucrose and 40 lb corn syrup each year.

Health impact of hypoglycemia

● **Brain:** dependent on glucose as energy source; hypoglycemia causes brain dysfunction; hypoglycemia involved in various psychological disorders; depressed individuals show high percentage of abnormal GTTs and G-ITTs.

● **Aggressive and criminal behavior:** reactive hypoglycemia is common in psychiatric patients and habitually violent and impulsive criminals; abnormal and emotionally explosive behavior is often seen during GTT; sugar-restricted diet reduced antisocial behavior among male juvenile inmates, but not female – men may react to hypoglycemia in a different manner from women; in non-criminal men, aggressiveness often coincides with hypoglycemia.

● **Premenstrual syndrome:** PMS-C is linked with increased appetite, craving for sweets, HA, fatigue, fainting spells, and heart palpitations; GTTs on PMS-C patients during 5–10 days before menses display flattening of early part of curve and reactive hypoglycemia; GTT is normal during other parts of menstrual cycle; flat early part of GTT curve implies excessive insulin secretion in response to sugar consumption; excessive secretion is hormonally regulated, but other factors are involved; NaCl ingestion enhances insulin response to sugar, and decreased Mg in pancreas increases insulin secretion.

● **Migraine headaches:** caused by excessive dilation of blood vessel in head; migraines surprisingly common (15–20% of men and 25–30% of women);>half of patients have family history of migraine; hypoglycemia is a common precipitating factor in migraine; eliminating refined sugar from diet of migraine sufferers with confirmed hypoglycemia greatly improves.

● **Atherosclerosis, intermittent claudication and angina:** reactive hypoglycemia or impaired glucose tolerance is a significant factor in atherosclerosis; high sugar intake elevates triglycerides and cholesterol; abnormal GTTs and hyperinsulinism are common in patients with heart disease; high sugar intake and reactive hypoglycemia can cause angina and intermittent claudication.

● **Syndrome X** is a set of cardiovascular risk factors (glucose or insulin disturbances, hyperlipidemia, hypertension, and android obesity); other terms: "metabolic cardiovascular risk syndrome" (MCVS), "Reaven's syndrome", "insulin resistance syndrome" and "atherothrombogenic syndrome"; underlying metabolic denominator is hyperinsulinemia from elevated intake of refined carbohydrate; development of type II diabetes is preceded by hyperinsulinemia and insulin insensitivity. In most cases, these defects presented themselves decades before the development of diabetes.

THERAPEUTIC CONSIDERATIONS

Dietary factors

High-complex carbohydrate, high-fiber, low-sugar diet; natural, simple sugars in fruits and vegetables have advantage over sucrose and other refined sugars – balanced by wide range of nutrients aiding utilization of sugars; sugars in whole unprocessed foods are more slowly absorbed due to integration within cells and fiber; refining removes all vitamins and trace minerals; > half of carbohydrates consumed in US are sugars added to processed foods.

● **A closer look at simple carbohydrates:** most diabetics and hypoglycemics can tolerate moderate amounts of fruits and fructose without loss of blood sugar control – they produce less sharp elevations in blood sugar compared with starch; fructose decreases the amount of calories and fat consumed; regular fruit consumption may help control sugar cravings and reduce obesity.

- **Glycemic index:** expresses rise of blood glucose after eating a particular food; standard value of 100 based on rise seen with ingestion of glucose; glycemic index ranges from 20 for fructose and whole barley to 98 for baked potato; insulin response to carbohydrate-containing foods is similar to rise in blood sugar; glycemic index used as guideline for diabetes or hypoglycemia; avoid foods with high values; choose foods with lower values; glycemic index should not be the only dietary guideline (high-fat foods have low glycemic index).

- **Fiber:** blood sugar disorders are related to inadequate dietary fiber; increase intake of complex carbohydrate sources rich in fiber; "dietary fiber" = components of plant cell wall plus indigestible residues from plant foods; water-soluble forms beneficial to blood sugar control – hemicelluloses, mucilages, gums, and pectin; beneficial effects:

  — slow digestion/absorption of carbohydrates, preventing rapid rises in blood sugar

  — increase cell sensitivity to insulin, preventing hyperinsulinism

  — improve uptake of glucose by liver and other tissues, preventing sustained hyperglycemia (*Textbook*, Ch. 57).

  Majority of fiber in most plant cell walls is water-soluble; good sources of water-soluble fiber are legumes, oat bran, nuts, seeds, psyllium seed husks, pears, apples, and most vegetables; daily intake of 50 g is recommended.

- **Chromium**: key constituent of "glucose tolerance factor"; chromium deficiency may be contributing factor to hypoglycemia, DM, and obesity; marginal chromium deficiency is common in the US; alleviates hypoglycemic symptoms, improves insulin binding, and increases number of insulin receptors.

Lifestyle factors

- **Alcohol** severely stresses blood sugar control; is a contributing factor to hypoglycemia; induces reactive hypoglycemia by interfering with normal glucose utilization and increases secretion of insulin; resultant drop in blood sugar produces craving for foods which quickly elevate blood sugar, plus craving for more alcohol; increased sugar consumption aggravates reactive hypoglycemia; hypoglycemia is a complication of acute and chronic alcohol abuse; hypoglycemia aggravates mental/emotional problems of withdrawing alcoholic; acute alcohol ingestion induces hypoglycemia; long-term abuse leads to hyperglycemia and diabetes; body becomes insensitive to chronic augmented insulin release caused by alcohol; alcohol causes insulin resistance even in healthy persons; alcohol intake is strongly correlated with DM – the higher the alcohol intake, the more likely a person will have DM.

- **Exercise:** important part of hypoglycemia treatment and prevention; regular exercise prevents type II diabetes; improves insulin sensitivity and glucose tolerance in existing diabetics; exercise increases tissue chromium concentrations.

THERAPEUTIC APPROACH

Use dietary therapy to stabilize blood sugar; reactive hypoglycemia is not a disease, but a complex set of symptoms caused by faulty carbohydrate metabolism induced by inappropriate diet.

- **Diet:** avoid all simple, processed and concentrated carbohydrates; emphasize complex-carbohydrate, high-fiber foods; small meals may stabilize blood sugar more easily; avoid alcohol.
- **Supplements:** high-potency vitamin-mineral, including chromium: 200–400 µg q.d.
- **Exercise:** graded exercise program appropriate to patient's fitness level and interest, yet which elevates heart rate at least 60% of maximum for 30 min three times a week.

Glucose tolerance test response criteria

Diagnosis	Response
Normal	No elevation greater than 160 mg Below 150 mg at the end of first hour Below 120 mg at the end of second hour Never lower than 20 mg below fasting
Flat	No variation more than ± 20 mg from fasting value
Pre-diabetic	Over 120 mg at the end of second hour
Diabetic	Over 180 mg during the first hour 200 mg or higher at the end of first hour 150 mg or higher at the end of second hour
Reactive hypoglycemia	A normal 2- or 3-h response curve followed by a decrease of 20 mg or more from the fasting level during the final hours
Probable reactive hypoglycemia	A normal 2- or 3-h response curve followed by a decrease of 10–20 mg from the fasting level during the final hours
Flat hypoglycemia	An elevation of 20 mg or less, followed by a decrease of 20 mg or more below the fasting level
Pre-diabetic hypoglycemia	A 2-h response identical to the pre-diabetic, but showing a hypoglycemic response during the final 3 h
Hyperinsulinism	A marked hypoglycemic response, with a value of less than 50 mg during the third, fourth or fifth hour

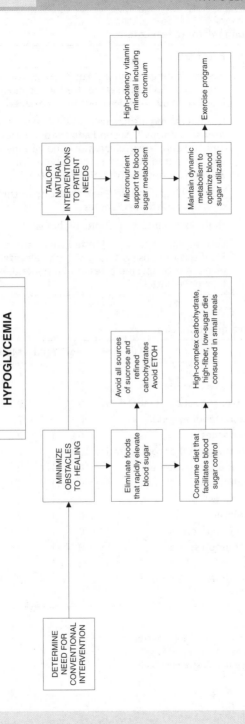

Glucose-insulin tolerance test criteria

Pattern	Response
Pattern 1	Normal fasting insulin 0–30 units. Peak insulin at 0.5–1 h. The combined insulin values for the second and third hours is less than 60 units. This pattern is considered normal
Pattern 2	Normal fasting insulin. Peak at 0.5–1 h with a "delayed return to normal". Second and third hour levels between 60 and 100 units are usually associated with hypoglycemia and are considered borderline for diabetes; values greater than 100 units considered definite diabetes
Pattern 3	Normal fasting insulin. Peak at second or third hour instead of 0.5–1 h. Definite diabetes
Pattern 4	High fasting insulin. Definite diabetes
Pattern 5	Low insulin response. All tested values for insulin less than 30. If this response is associated with elevated blood sugar levels, it probably indicates insulin-dependent diabetes ("juvenile pattern")

Hypoglycemia questionnaire

	No	Mild	Moderate	Severe
Crave sweets	0	1	2	3
Irritable if a meal is missed	0	1	2	3
Feel tired or weak if a meal is missed	0	1	2	3
Dizziness when standing suddenly	0	1	2	3
Frequent headaches	0	1	2	3
Poor memory (forgetful) or concentration	0	1	2	
Feel tired an hour or so after eating	0	1	2	3
Heart palpitations	0	1	2	3
Feel shaky at times	0	1	2	3
Afternoon fatigue	0	1	2	3
Vision blurs on occasion	0	1	2	3
Depression or mood swings	0	1	2	3
Overweight	0	1	2	3
Frequently anxious or nervous	0	1	2	3
Total				

Scoring:
< 5, hypoglycemia is not likely a factor
6–15, hypoglycemia is a likely factor
> 15, hypoglycemia is extremely likely.

Hypothyroidism

DIAGNOSTIC SUMMARY

Depression; difficulty in losing weight; dry skin; headaches; lethargy or fatigue; menstrual problems; recurrent infections; sensitivity to cold.

GENERAL CONSIDERATIONS

Hypothyroidism affects virtually all cells and body functions; severity of symptoms in adult range from mild (not detectable with standard blood tests – subclinical hypothyroidism) to severe, which can be life-threatening (myxedema).

- Low thyroid hormone and elevated TSH indicate defective thyroid hormone synthesis – "primary hypothyroidism".

- Low TSH and low thyroid hormone – pituitary gland responsible for low thyroid function = "secondary hypothyroidism".

- Normal blood thyroid hormone and TSH plus low functional thyroid activity (low basal metabolic rate) suggest cellular hypothyroidism involving impaired cellular conversion of T_4 to T_3.

Between 1 and 4% of adult population have moderate to severe hypothyroidism; another 10–12% have mild hypothyroidism; rate of hypothyroidism increases steadily with advancing age.

Causes of hypothyroidism

- **Overt hypothyroidism:** 95% of all cases of overt hypothyroidism are primary; most common cause in the past was iodine deficiency; thyroid gland adds iodine to amino acid tyrosine to create thyroid hormones; iodine deficiency leads to hypothyroidism and/or enlarged thyroid gland (goiter):
  — goiters affect 200 million people worldwide – all but 4% are caused by iodine deficiency; iodine deficiency is rare in industrialized countries due to iodized table salt; goiters in the US today are caused by excessive ingestion of goitrogens – foods which block iodine utilization: turnips, cabbage, mustard, cassava root, soybean, peanuts, pine nuts, millet; cooking usually inactivates goitrogens.

— most frequent cause of overt hypothyroidism in the US is autoimmune disorder Hashimoto's disease – antibodies are formed that bind to thyroid peroxidase enzyme, thyroglobulin, and TSH receptors and inhibit hormone synthesis; antibodies may also bind to adrenal glands, pancreas, and acid-producing cells (parietal cells) of stomach.

- **Functional hypothyroidism:** thyroid activity is measured by functional test (Broda Barnes), incidence = 25%; functional tests show greater incidence of low thyroid than blood tests – blood tests measure thyroxine (T_4), which accounts for 90% of hormone secreted; form of hormone affecting cells the most is T_3 (triiodothyronine), which cells make from T_4; T_3 has four times the activity of T_4; if cells cannot convert, the person has normal blood levels of the hormone, yet is functionally thyroid-deficient; blood tests for T_3 miss low thyroid function in 50% of patients; better to measure thyroid effects on body – measure resting metabolic rate controlled by thyroid gland; basal body temperature is a good way of assessing basal metabolic rate.

DIAGNOSTIC CONSIDERATIONS

Basal body temperature (temperature of body at rest) and Achilles reflex time (reflexes are slowed in hypothyroidism) are old indicators of dysfunction; basal body temperature is the most sensitive functional test of thyroid function.

Clinical symptomatology

- **Metabolic:** hypothyroidism decreases rate of utilization of fat, protein, and carbohydrate; moderate weight gain plus sensitivity to cold weather (cold hands or feet) are common; cholesterol and triglyceride are increased in even mildest hypothyroidism – elevation increases risk of cardiovascular disease; increased rate of heart disease due to atherosclerosis in individuals with hypothyroidism; hypothyroidism increases capillary permeability and slows lymphatic drainage – swelling of tissue (edema).

- **Endocrine:** hormonal complications are loss of libido in men and menstrual abnormalities in women – prolonged and heavy menses, with shorter menstrual cycle; infertility is problematic; miscarriages, premature deliveries, and stillbirths are common.

- **Skin, hair, and nails:** dry, rough skin covered with fine superficial scales; hair is coarse, dry, brittle; hair loss can be quite severe; nails become thin and brittle with transverse grooves.

- **Psychological:** brain sensitive to hypothyroidism; depression with weakness and fatigue are first symptoms; later – difficulty concentrating and extreme forgetfulness.

- **Muscular and skeletal:** muscle weakness and joint stiffness are predominant features; some patients experience muscle and joint pain, and tenderness.

- **Cardiovascular:** predisposition to atherosclerosis due to hyperlipidemia; hypothyroidism can also cause hypertension, reduce function of heart, and reduce heart rate.
- **Other manifestations:** SOB, constipation, and impaired kidney function; patients with dermatitis herpetiformis have significantly increased abnormalities of thyroid function tests, with significant hypothyroidism being the most common abnormality.

Laboratory evaluation

Based on results of total T_4, free T_4, T_3, and TSH levels; diagnosis is straightforward in overt cases; in subclinical cases, diagnosis is less clear; elevated TSH with normal T_4 level – subclinical; accepted normal range very broad, 0.35–5.50 μIU/ml; (conventional approach does not treat unless TSH > 10 μIU/ml); naturopathic approach: if patient does not respond to nutritional intervention, use low-dose thyroid hormone therapy if TSH > 2.5 μIU/ml – slightly higher than accepted 2.0 μIU/ml demonstrating disturbance of thyroid-pituitary axis, especially with anti-thyroid antibodies.

Functional assessment

Functional thyroid activity is estimated by measuring basal body temperature; Barnes: normal basal body temperature = 97.6–98.2°F; low basal metabolic rate can indicate nutritional deficiencies, inadequate physical activity, etc., and fever can give inaccurately high body temperature (*Textbook*, App. 8).

THERAPEUTIC CONSIDERATIONS

Nutritional considerations

Nutritionally support thyroid gland with key nutrients required in synthesis of thyroid hormone; avoid goitrogens.

- **Iodine, tyrosine, and goitrogens:** thyroid hormones are made from iodine and amino acid tyrosine; RDA for iodine in adults is quite small = 150 μg; average intake of iodine in US > 600 μg q.d.; too much iodine inhibits thyroid synthesis; the only function of iodine in the body is thyroid synthesis; dietary levels or iodine supplements should not exceed 600 μg q.d. for any length of time; goitrogens combine with iodine, making it unavailable to thyroid; cooking inactivates goitrogens; goitrogenic foods should not be eaten in excess.
- **Vitamins and minerals:**
  — zinc, vitamin E and vitamin A function together in manufacture of thyroid hormone; deficiency of any of these reduces amount of active hormone produced; low zinc is common in the elderly, as is hypothyroidism

— riboflavin (B_2), niacin (B_3), pyridoxine (B_6), and vitamin C are necessary for hormone synthesis

— zinc, copper, and selenium are required cofactors for iodothyronine iodinase enzyme converting T_4 to T_3; each form requires different trace mineral; supplementation with zinc re-establishes normal thyroid function in zinc-deficient hypothyroid patients, even though serum T_4 is normal

— areas of world where selenium is deficient have greater incidence of thyroid disease; selenium deficiency decreases conversion of T_4 to T_3 in peripheral cells of the body; people with Se deficiency have elevated T_4 and TSH; Se supplements decrease T_4 and TSH and normalize thyroid activity.

Exercise

Stimulates thyroid secretion; increases tissue sensitivity to thyroid hormone; many health benefits of exercise may result from improved thyroid function; especially important in dieting overweight hypothyroid patients; consistent effect of dieting is decreased metabolic rate as body strives to conserve fuel; exercise prevents decline in metabolic rate in response to dieting.

Thyroid hormone replacement

If more conservative measures fail, exogenous thyroid hormones are necessary; naturopathic physicians prefer desiccated natural thyroid, complete with all thyroid hormones, not just thyroxine.

● **Preparations containing only T_4 (Synthroid, Levothyroid):** advantages – consistent potency and prolonged duration of action; T_3 rarely used alone – four times more potent with shorter duration of action than T_4.

● **Desiccated thyroid:** advantage – provides T_4 and T_3, plus relevant amino acids and micronutrients; drawback – lacks consistency; by USP standard, these preparations must contain at least 85% and not more than 115% of labeled amount of T_4, and at least 90% and not more than 110% for T_3; labeled amount = 38 µg T_4 and 9 µg T_3 per grain (65 mg).

● **Synthetic mixtures of T_4 and T_3 (Liotrix, Thyrolar) in similar ratios:** provide consistency that whole, natural desiccated thyroid lacks.

● Equivalencies (1 "thyroid unit") for thyroid agents based on clinical response :

— 100 µg of T_4 (e.g. Synthroid)
— 20-25 µg T_3 (e.g. Cytomel)
— 1 grain desiccated thyroid
— 12.5 µg T_3 + 50 µg T_4 (e.g. Thyrolar)

(Note: 0.5 thyroid units would be equal to 50% of the values shown in the list.)

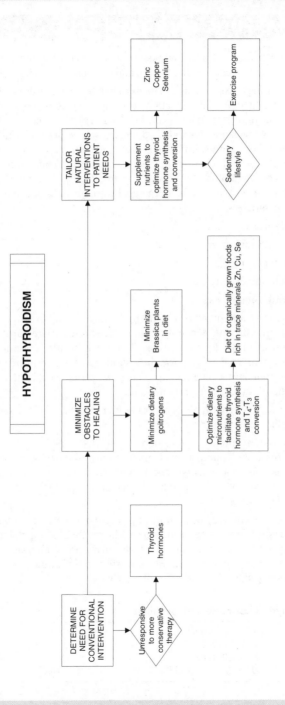

THERAPEUTIC APPROACH

Optimize nutrients needed for thyroid synthesis and cellular conversion of T_4 to T_3; if no response after a few months, thyroid hormone replacement is indicated.

● **Diet:** low in goitrogens; high in foods rich in trace minerals needed for hormone production and activation; cook goitrogens to break down constituents; sources of iodine – sea fish, sea vegetables (kelp, dulse, arame, hijiki, nori, wakame, kombu) and iodized salt; sources of zinc – seafood (oysters), beef, oatmeal, chicken, liver, spinach, nuts, and seeds; copper found in liver and other organ meats, eggs, yeast, beans, nuts, and seeds; sources of B vitamins – yeast, whole grains, and liver; source of selenium – Brazil nuts (unshelled); prefer organically grown foods due to higher levels of trace minerals.

● **Supplements:**

— zinc: 25 mg q.d.

— copper: 5 mg q.d.

— selenium: 200 µg q.d.

● **Thyroid hormones:**

— begin treatment at 0.5–2 thyroid units (see above) q.d. based on patient's size and serum hormone levels; re-evaluate basal body temperature, TSH, T_4, T_3, and free T_4 4–6 weeks after initiating therapy; treatment goal is to normalize basal body temperature and serum hormone levels; after stabilizing dosage, periodic evaluations based on patient's needs or at least once a year

— subclinical hypothyroidism: dosage no more than 0.5 thyroid units q.d. for first 3 months of treatment

— thyroid hormone replacement to be taken on empty stomach to increase absorption; avoid taking thyroid at same time as other medications and supplements (especially those containing iron) which may affect absorption; once-a-day dosage produces stable increases in thyroid hormones

— dosage of thyroid hormone during pregnancy increased due to effects of estrogens increasing serum thyroid hormone binding globulin, reducing free thyroxine; monitor carefully during pregnancy; dosage requirements increase by 30–50% during pregnancy and return to pre-pregnancy levels shortly after delivery.

Serum thyroid hormone normal values

T_4	4.8–13.2 µg/dl
Free T_4	0.9–2 ng/dl
T_3	80–220 ng/dl
TSH	0.35–5.50 µIU/ml

Inflammatory bowel disease

DIAGNOSTIC SUMMARY

Crohn's disease

- Intermittent bouts of diarrhea, low-grade fever, and right lower quadrant pain.
- Anorexia, weight loss, flatulence, and malaise.
- Abdominal tenderness, especially right lower quadrant, with signs of peritoneal irritation and an abdominal or pelvic mass.
- X-rays show abnormality of terminal ileum.

Ulcerative colitis

- Bloody diarrhea with cramps in lower abdomen.
- Mild abdominal tenderness, weight loss, and fever.
- Rectal exam may show perianal irritation, fissures, hemorrhoids, fistulas, and abscesses.
- Diagnosis confirmed by X-ray and sigmoidoscopy.

GENERAL CONSIDERATIONS

Definition

Inflammatory bowel disease (IBD) is a general term for a group of chronic inflammatory disorders of the bowel; two major categories: Crohn's disease and ulcerative colitis; IBD is characterized by recurrent inflammatory involvement of specific intestinal segments, resulting in diverse clinical manifestations.

- **Crohn's disease (CD):** granulomatous inflammatory reaction throughout entire thickness of bowel wall; 40% of cases, granulomas either poorly developed or totally absent; may involve buccal mucosa, esophagus, stomach, duodenum, jejunum, ileum, and colon; Crohn's disease of small intestine is called "regional enteritis"; colon involvement is called "Crohn's disease of the colon" or "granulomatous colitis" (only a portion of patients develop granulomatous lesions).

- **Ulcerative colitis (UC):** non-specific inflammatory response limited to colonic mucosa and submucosa; well-developed granuloma formation does not occur.

Common features shared by Crohn's disease and ulcerative colitis:

- Colon is frequently involved in Crohn's and invariably involved in UC.
- Although rare, patients with UC and total colon involvement may develop "backwash ileitis" – both conditions may cause changes in small intestine.
- Patients with CD often have close relatives with UC, and vice versa.
- When no granuloma in CD of the colon, the two lesions may resemble each other clinically and pathologically.
- There are many epidemiological similarities between CD and UC – age, race, sex, and geographic distribution.
- Both conditions are associated with similar extraintestinal manifestations.
- There are etiological parallels between the two conditions.
- Both conditions are associated with increased frequency of colonic carcinoma.

Etiology

UC more common; incidence of UC in western Europe and US = 6–8 cases per 100,000 and prevalence = 70–150 cases per 100,000; incidence of CD = 2 cases per 100,000 and prevalence = 20–40 per 100,000; incidence of CD increasing in Western cultures; IBD may occur at any age, but most often in age range 15–35; females are affected slightly more frequently than males; Caucasians are two to five times more affected than Blacks or Asians; Jews have three- to sixfold higher incidence compared with non-Jews; theories about etiology of IBD:

- **Genetic predisposition:** supported by ethnic distribution of incidence, and multiple members of a family have CD or UC in 15–40% of cases.
- **Infectious etiology:** idea that transmissible agent is responsible for IBD is a hotly debated subject; viruses (rotavirus, Epstein–Barr virus, cytomegalovirus, and an uncharacterized RNA intestinal cytopathic virus) and mycobacteria continue to be favored candidates.
- **Antibiotic exposure:** prior to 1950s, CD found in selected groups with strong genetic component; rapid climb in developed countries and countries that previously had virtually no reported cases; CD has spread like epidemic; wherever antibiotics used early and in large quantities, incidence of CD is now quite high; infectious agent may be a normal intestinal florum suddenly producing immunostimulatory toxins or becoming invasive via sublethal doses of antibiotics making flora stronger in virility and numbers.

- **Immune mechanisms:** immunologic derangements are found in IBD, but whether causal of IBD or secondary to it remains unclear; current evidence indicates that derangements are secondary to disease process.

- **Dietary factors:**
  - CD increasing in cultures consuming "Western" diet; virtually nonexistent in cultures consuming primitive diet; people who develop CD habitually eat more refined sugar and less raw fruit and vegetables and dietary fiber than healthy people (122 g sugar q.d. vs. 65 g q.d.); corn flakes have been linked to CD – high in refined carbohydrates and derived from common allergen (corn)
  - UC is not linked to refined carbohydrates; food allergy overlooked by conventional medicine
  - Reduced intake of omega-3 oils and increased intake of omega-6 oils linked to growing rise of CD in Japan; genetics of Japanese relatively homogenous – increased incidence due to incorporation of "Western" foods; increased incidence of CD strongly correlated with increased dietary total fat, animal fat, omega-6 fatty acids, animal protein, milk protein, and ratio of omega-6 to omega-3 fatty acids; less correlated with total protein; not correlated with fish protein; inversely correlated with vegetable protein; increased animal protein is the strongest independent factor followed by increased ratio of omega-6 to omega-3 fatty acids.

- **Miscellaneous factors:** emotional factors are important in modifying course of disease.

THERAPEUTIC CONSIDERATIONS

Control of causative factors

- **Natural history of Crohn's disease:** many patients will undergo spontaneous remission, 20% at 1 year and 12% at 2 years; "success" of placebo therapy rises dramatically – in patients having no history of steroid therapy, 41% remitted after 17 weeks; 23% of this group continued in remission after 2 years, compared with 4% of group with history of steroid use; once remission is achieved, 75% of patients will continue in remission at end of 1 year and up to 63% by 2 years, regardless of maintenance therapy used; key = achieving remission, which, once attained, can be maintained by conservative non-drug therapy.

- **Eicosanoid metabolism:** prostaglandins are greatly increased in colonic mucosa, serum, and stools of IBD patients; increased synthesis of lipoxygenase products, leukotrienes, and mono HETEs – produced by neutrophils and amplify inflammation and cause smooth muscle contraction; release of lipoxygenase products promoted by activation of alternative complement pathway; sulfasalazine inhibits cyclooxygenase and neutrophil lipoxygenase and inhibits degranulation of mast cells; corticosteroids inhibit phospholipase A_2, blocking release of arachidonic acid from membrane phospholipids; natural flavonoid quercetin interacts with these enzymes; formation of inflammatory compounds is decreased by reducing dietary meat and dairy while increasing omega-3 fatty acids (cold-water ocean fish) – eicosapentaenoic acid (EPA) and docosahexanoic acid (DHA); fish oil supplements (2.7–5.1 g total omega-3 oils) prevent or delay relapses in CD and UC; flaxseed oil, which contains alpha-linolenic acid, the essential omega-3 fatty acid which the body can convert to EPA, is also of value.

- **Mucin defects in ulcerative colitis:** mucins are high-molecular-weight, carbohydrate-rich glycoproteins responsible for viscous/elastic characteristics of secreted mucus; alterations in mucin composition and content in colonic mucosa noted in UC; dramatic decrease in mucous content of goblet cells (proportional to severity of disease) and decrease in major sulfomucin subfraction; these abnormalities are not found in CD; mucin content of goblet cells returns to normal during remission but sulfomucin deficiency does not; specific components of sulfomucin and cause of its lower level are unknown; mucin abnormalities are a major factor in increased risk of colon cancer in these patients.

- **Intestinal microflora** (*Textbook*, Chs 7 and 9): 400 distinct species; fecal flora of patients with IBD contain higher numbers of Gram-positive anaerobic coccoid rods and *Bacteroides vulgatus*, a Gram-negative rod; these alterations in fecal flora are not secondary to disease, and alterations in metabolic activity of bacteria are more important than alterations in number of bacteria; specific bacterial cell components may be responsible for promoting lymphocyte cytotoxic activity against colonic epithelial cells.

- **Carrageenans:** sulfated polymers of galactose and D-anhydrogalactose extracted from red seaweeds (*Eucheuma spinosum* or *Chondrus crispus*) have been used to induce IBD in animals; used by food industry as stabilizing and suspending agents (ice cream, cottage cheese, milk chocolate, etc.) due to ability to stabilize milk proteins; no correlation between human consumption of carrageenan and development of UC; differences in intestinal bacterial flora are probably responsible for discrepancy – germ-free animals do not display carrageenan-induced damage; bacteria linked to facilitating carrageenan-induced damage in animals is strain of *Bacteroides vulgatus* – found in much higher concentrations (six times as high) in fecal cultures of patients with IBD; carrageenan is metabolized into nondamaging components in most humans, and people with overgrowth of *Bacteroides vulgatus* may be at risk; avoid carrageenan.

- **Aspirin and intestinal permeability:** first-degree relatives of CD patients had 110% increase in intestinal permeability after acetylsalicylic acid vs. increase of 57% in controls; 35% were hyper-responders; familial permeability defect is a significant predisposing factor for CD – leaky gut linked to increased incidence of food allergy and absorption of intestinal toxins (*Textbook*, Ch. 21).

● **Endotoxemia and alternative complement pathway:** endotoxemia is linked to CD and UC; endotoxemia-induced activation of alternative complement pathway could explain extra-GI manifestations of IBD; whole gut irrigation significantly reduces endotoxin pool in gut and has a very beneficial anti-endotoxinemia effect; colonic irrigation may offer similar benefit; colon irrigation during acute inflammatory flare contraindicated.

Extra-gastrointestinal manifestations

Over 100 disorders are systemic complications of IBD; most common extraintestinal lesion (EIL) in adults is arthritis (25% of patients); more common form is peripheral arthritis that affects knees, ankles, and wrists; arthritis is more common in patients with colon involvement; severity of symptoms is proportional to disease activity; arthritis may affect primarily spine, with low back pain and stiffness, and eventual limitation of motion; this EIL occurs mainly in males with HLA-B$_{27}$ and resembles ankylosing spondylitis; it may antedate bowel symptoms by several years; there is probably an underlying factor in progression of ankylosing spondylitis and IBD.

● **Skin manifestations** seen in 15% of patients; lesions – erythema nodosum, pyoderma gangrenosum, and aphthous ulcerations; recurrent aphthous stomatitis in 10% of patients; serious liver disease (sclerosing cholangitis, chronic active hepatitis, cirrhosis) affects 3–7% of patients with IBD from increased endotoxin load; liver enzyme abnormalities indicate need for hepatoprotection from *Glycyrrhiza glabra*, *Silybum marianum*, catechin, and curcumin.

● **Other common EILs:** thrombophlebitis, finger clubbing, ocular manifestations (episcleritis, iritis, and uveitis), nephrolithiasis, cholelithiasis, and, in children, failure to grow, thrive, and mature normally.

Malnutrition

Nutritional complications of IBD have great influence on morbidity (and mortality).

Causes of malnutrition in inflammatory bowel disease

● Decreased oral intake
  — disease-induced (pain, diarrhea, nausea, anorexia)
  — iatrogenic (restrictive diets without supplementation)
● Malabsorption
  — decreased absorptive surface due to disease or resection
  — bile salt deficiency after resection
  — bacterial overgrowth
  — drugs (e.g. corticosteroids, sulfasalazine, cholestyramine)

(continued over)

Causes of malnutrition in inflammatory bowel disease (continued)

- Increased secretion and nutrient loss
  — protein-losing enteropathy
  — electrolyte, mineral, and trace mineral loss in diarrhea
- Increased utilization and increased requirements
  — inflammation, fever, infection
  — increased intestinal cell turnover

Weight loss prevalent in 65–75% of IBD patients; malabsorption – from extensive mucosal involvement of small intestine and resection of segments of small intestine; fat malabsorption – loss of calories and fat-soluble vitamins and minerals; ileum involvement or resection causes bile acid malabsorption – cathartic effect of bile acids on colon, causes chronic watery diarrhea; expect electrolyte and trace mineral deficiency from chronic diarrhea, plus Ca and Mg deficiency from chronic steatorrhea; loss of plasma proteins across damaged/inflamed mucosa – may exceed ability of liver to replace plasma proteins; chronic blood loss causes Fe depletion anemia; drugs used to treat IBD (corticosteroids and sulfasalazine) increase nutritional needs.

Corticosteroids are known to:

- stimulate protein catabolism
- depress protein synthesis
- decrease the absorption of calcium and phosphorus
- increase the urinary excretion of ascorbic acid, calcium, potassium, and zinc
- increase blood glucose, serum triglycerides, and serum cholesterol
- increase the requirements for vitamin B_6, ascorbic acid, folate, and vitamin D
- decrease bone formation
- impair wound healing.

Sulfasalazine has been shown to:

- inhibit the absorption and transport of folate
- decrease serum folate and iron
- increase the urinary excretion of ascorbic acid.

Nutritional consequences of chronic inflammatory and/or infectious disease – protein requirement may be increased; elevated sedimentation rate signifies increased protein breakdown and synthesis; IBD requires 25% more protein than usual recommended allowance.

Prevalence of nutritional deficiencies

Nutritional deficiencies quite high in hospitalized patients with IBD; greater prevalence of nutritional deficiencies in hospitalized patients than in outpatients (more severe condition); ambulatory CD patients also display nutrient deficiencies – Fe, B_{12}, folate, Mg, K, retinol, ascorbate, vitamin D, Zn, vitamin K, Cu, niacin, and vitamin E; assume that most patients suffer from micronutrient deficiency; often deficiency is subclinical and only detected by lab investigation; use therapeutic vitamin supplements of at least five times RDA; several minerals may need supplementing at similar levels; dietary treatment – either elemental or elimination diet.

- **Elemental diet:** effective non-toxic alternative to corticosteroids as primary treatment of acute IBD; contains all essential nutrients: protein as predigested or free-form amino acids; provides nutritional improvement, alters fecal flora, and serves as allergy elimination diet; main drawback is unpalatability, hyperosmolality (causing diarrhea); hospitalization often required for satisfactory administration, and relapse is common when patients resume normal eating; elimination diet may be acceptable alternative for acute IBD, especially for chronic IBD.

- **Elimination (oligoantigenic) diet:** elimination is the primary therapy for chronic IBD; most common offending foods are wheat and dairy; alternative approach – determine actual allergens by lab methods – measure IgG- and IgE-mediated reactions; allergens are avoided or rotary diversified diet (*Textbook*, Chs 15, 51, 58).

- **High-complex carbohydrate, high-fiber (HFC) diet:** favorable effect on course of CD, in direct contrast to allopathic dietary treatment: low-fiber diet; some foods are too "rough" to handle, but use an unrefined carbohydrate, fiber-rich diet with allergen avoidance or rotary-diversified diet; fiber has profound effect on intestinal environment and promotes optimal intestinal flora; avoid supplemental wheat bran.

Minerals

- **Zinc:** deficiency in 45% of CD patients; due to low dietary intake, poor absorption, and excess fecal losses; many complications of CD may result from Zn deficiency: poor healing of fissures and fistulas, skin lesions (acrodermatitis), hypogonadism, growth retardation, retinal dysfunction, depressed cell-mediated immunity, anorexia; many patients unresponsive to oral or i.v. Zn due to defect in tissue transport; zinc picolinate may improve intestinal absorption and tissue transport; no improvement in patients with pancreatic insufficiency; zinc citrate may also be appropriate alternative; make every attempt to ensure adequate tissue stores – disease activity correlated with zinc deficiency; use parenteral administration as needed.

- **Magnesium:** deficiency prevalent in IBD; poor correlation between serum levels (frequently normal) and intracellular levels (commonly decreased); low intracellular Mg causes: weakness, anorexia, hypotension, confusion, hyperirritability, tetany, convulsions, ECG or EEG abnormalities – responsive to parenteral Mg supplementation; daily i.v.

dose of 200–400 mg elemental Mg if patient unresponsive to oral supplements; IBD may require i.v. route due to cathartic action of Mg and poor absorption in patients with short bowel; oral supplement – Mg chelates (citrate, aspartate, etc.) rather than inorganic magnesium salts (i.e. carbonate).

- **Iron** deficiency anemia frequent in IBD from chronic gut blood loss; serum ferritin is the most useful index of Fe status; ferritin > 55 ng/ml indicates adequate Fe reserves; ferritin < 18 ng/ml indicates Fe deficiency (*Textbook*, Ch. 24); improve absorption with supplemental vitamin C rather than direct Fe supplements – Fe promotes intestinal infection.

- **Calcium:** risk of Ca deficiency due to loss of absorptive surfaces, steatorrhea, corticosteroids, vitamin D deficiency.

- **Potassium:** diarrhea linked to K^+ and other electrolyte deficiencies; symptoms of K^+ deficiency rare in IBD patients, but levels below optimum; correcting K^+ deficiency reduces rates of surgical complications.

Vitamins

- **Vitamin A:** low serum retinol in 20% of CD patients, correlated with activity of disease; vitamin A affects metabolism and differentiation of intestinal epithelial mucosa – increases number of goblet cells, production of mucins, secretion of mucus, and restores normal barrier function; vitamin A may be useful in CD, but long-term trials have (50,000 IU b.i.d.) found no benefit in majority of CD cases; certain patients may respond to vitamin A; zinc supplements often normalize vitamin A metabolism – zinc is a component of retinol-binding protein (RBP).

- **Vitamin D:** deficiency common in IBD, particularly patients with other signs of nutritional deficiency; result of decreased absorption of 25-hydroxy-vitamin D; increased risk of metabolic bone diseases (osteoporosis and osteomalacia).

- **Vitamin E:** deficiency can occur in IBD with presenting symptoms: bilateral visual field scotomata, generalized motor weakness, broad-based gait with marked ataxia, brisk reflexes, bilateral Babinski response; inhibits leukotriene formation and reduces free radical damage.

- **Vitamin K:** deficiency results in formation of abnormal prothrombin (deficient in gamma-carboxyglutamic acid), common in patients with IBD.

- **Folic acid:** low serum levels in 25–64% of cases; sulfasalazine interferes with folate-dependent enzymes and intestinal folate transport system; deficiency promotes malabsorption from altered structure of intestinal mucosa – cells have rapid turnover (1–4 days) vs. RBCs (3–4 months); deficiency affects these cells earlier than RBCs.

- **Vitamin B_{12}:** significant correlation between B_{12} absorption and terminal ileal disease and/or resection; abnormal Schilling tests in 48% of CD patients; when ileal resection exceeds 90 cm, Schilling test is abnormal in all patients and never improves; length of resection < 60 cm, or extent of inflammatory lesion < 60 cm; adequate absorption may occur.

- **Ascorbic acid:** low vitamin C intake common in IBD patients, particularly those on low-fiber diet; serum and leukocyte ascorbic acid much lower in CD patients than in matched controls; vitamin C important to prevent fistulas – patients with fistulas have lower ascorbic acid levels than those without.

Recommend a high-potency multiple vitamin and mineral formula: absolutely essential in IBD; additional antioxidants to manage increased oxidative stress and decreased antioxidant defenses in mucosa; two primary antioxidants in human body are vitamins C ("aqueous phase") and E ("lipid phase").

- vitamin E (D-alpha-tocopherol): 400–800 IU
- vitamin C (ascorbic acid): 1,000–3,000 mg.

Botanical medicines

Quercetin: plant flavonoids are natural biological response modifiers; quercetin is the most pharmacologically active flavonoid; many enzymes affected by quercetin are involved in release of histamine and other inflammatory mediators from mast cells, basophils, neutrophils, and macrophages, in the migration and infiltration of leukocytes, and in smooth muscle contraction; action of quercetin: antagonizes calmodulin; when Ca bound to calmodulin, it activates enzymes involved in cyclic nucleotide metabolism, protein phosphorylation, secretory function, muscle contraction, microtubule assembly, glycogen metabolism, and Ca flux; quercetin interacts directly with calmodulin and Ca channels; potent inhibitor of mast cell and basophil degranulation; inhibits receptor-mediated Ca influx, inhibiting primary signal for degranulation; also active when Ca-channel mechanism not operative – other mechanisms also involved; inhibits inflammatory processes of activated neutrophils via membrane stabilization, antioxidant effect (prevents production of free radicals and inflammatory leukotrienes), and inhibition of hyaluronidase (preventing breakdown of collagen); membrane-stabilizing effect – prevents mast cell and basophil degranulation and decreases neutrophil lysosomal enzyme secretion; inhibits eicosanoid metabolism – inhibits phospholipase A_2 and lipoxygenase; net result is the reduction in formation of leukotrienes; excess leukotrienes linked to asthma, psoriasis, atopic dermatitis, gout, possibly cancer, and IBD; leukotrienes C_4, D_4, and E_4 (in slow-reacting substances of anaphylaxis, SRS-A) are 1,000 times as potent as histamine in promoting inflammation; leukotrienes cause vasoconstriction (increasing vascular permeability) and other smooth muscle contraction, and promote WBC chemotaxis and aggregation; reducing leukotrienes has strong anti-inflammatory effects in IBD (*Textbook*, Ch. 87).

Bastyr's formula (modified Robert's formula):

- *Althea officinalis* (marshmallow root) – demulcent, soothing to mucous membranes
- *Baptisia tinctora* (wild indigo) – used for gastrointestinal infections
- *Echinacea angustifolia* (purple coneflower) – antibacterial that normalizes immune system (*Textbook*, Ch. 82)
- *Geranium maculatum* – a GI hemostatic
- *Hydrastis canadensis* (goldenseal) – inhibits growth of many enteropathic bacteria (*Textbook*, Ch. 91)
- *Phytolacca americana* (poke root) – used for healing ulcerations of intestinal mucosa
- *Symphytum offinale* (comfrey) – anti-inflammatory; promotes tissue growth and wound healing
- *Ulmus fulva* (slippery elm) – demulcent.

Other ingredients: cabbage powder heals GI ulcers (*Textbook*, Ch. 108); pancreatin assists digestive process (*Textbook*, Ch. 101); niacinamide has anti-inflammatory effects; and duodenal substance heals GI ulcers.

Composition of Bastyr's formula

- Eight parts *Althea officinalis*
- Four parts *Baptisia tinctora*
- Eight parts *Echinacea angustifolia*
- Eight parts *Geranium maculatum*
- Eight parts *Hydrastis canadensis*
- Eight parts *Phytolacca americana*
- Eight parts *Ulmus fulva*
- Eight parts cabbage powder
- Two parts pancreatin
- One part niacinamide
- Two parts duodenal substance

Butyrate enemas in ulcerative colitis

- **Short-chain fatty acids and colon function:** SCFAs (acetate, propionate, and butyrate) are colon end-products of bacterial carbohydrate fermentation; function as primary energy sources for luminal colon cells, especially distal segments; decreased levels or utilization of SCFAs impair cellular energetics – major role in ulcerative colitis; enemas providing SCFAs (butyrate only at 80–100 mmol/L, or SCFA combinations with acetate

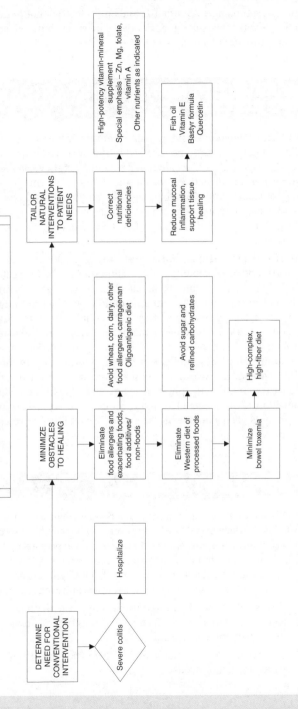

INFLAMMATORY BOWEL DISEASE

DETERMINE NEED FOR CONVENTIONAL INTERVENTION

Severe colitis

Hospitalize

MINIMIZE OBSTACLES TO HEALING

Eliminate food allergens and exacerbating foods, food additives/non-foods

Avoid wheat, corn, dairy, other food allergens, carrageenan Oligoantigenic diet

Eliminate Western diet of processed foods

Avoid sugar and refined carbohydrates

Minimize bowel toxemia

High-complex, high-fiber diet

TAILOR NATURAL INTERVENTIONS TO PATIENT NEEDS

Correct nutritional deficiencies

High-potency vitamin-mineral supplement Special emphasis – Zn, Mg, folate, vitamin A Other nutrients as indicated

Reduce mucosal inflammation, support tissue healing

Fish oil Vitamin E Bastyr formula Quercetin

60 mmol/L, propionate 25 mmol/L, and butyrate 40 mmol/L) – excellent preliminary results in well-designed double-blind study; butyrate and SCFA enemas may prove useful adjuncts for UC.

THERAPEUTIC MONITORING AND EVALUATION

● **Crohn's Disease Activity Index:** monitoring tool providing uniform clinical parameters to be assessed with consistent numerical index for recording results; CDAI calculated by adding eight variables (see below); subjective and objective information included; a form (*Textbook*, App. 3) is photocopied and given to patients for completion at home; calculation of disease activity determined; CDAI scores < 150 indicate better prognosis than higher scores; CDAI is a very useful way to monitor progress.

● **Monitoring of the pediatric patient:** very difficult to achieve normal growth and development; growth failure in 75% of CD pediatric patients and 25% in UC; evaluate at least twice yearly – pertinent history, clinical anthropometry, Tanner staging, and appropriate lab testing (see table below); use aggressive nutritional program including supplements (enteral or parenteral methods), with doses adjusted as appropriate; CDAI not as accurate in monitoring disease in children as in adults; Lloyd–Still and Green clinical scoring system for IBD in children – divided into five major divisions (maximum score is in parentheses): general activity (10), physical exam and clinical complications (30), nutrition (20), X-rays (15), lab (25); elevated score (i.e. scores in 80s) represents good status, while scores in 30s and 40s represent severe disease.

THERAPEUTIC APPROACH

● IBD is life-threatening, requiring emergency treatment in some patients; small percentage of patients with severe colitis may have severe exacerbations requiring hospitalization – more common in patients with UC – fever of 101°F or higher, profuse, constant, loose, bloody stools, anorexia, apathy and prostration; abdominal signs normal, but physical exam reveals distended abdomen, tympany, absent bowel sounds, and even rebound tenderness:

— IBD is a chronic disease requiring long-term therapy and follow-up; identify and remove all factors initiating/aggravating inflammation (food allergens, carrageenan, etc.)

— use diet maximizing macro- and micronutrients and minimizing aggravating foods/non-foods

   — broad-based individualized nutritional supplement plan; critical – Zn, Mg, folate, and vitamin A; use nutritional supplements to correct deficiencies

   — normalize inflammatory process and promote healing of damaged mucosa

   — botanical medicines to promote healing and normalize intestinal flora.

● **Diet:** eliminate all allergens, wheat, corn, dairy, carrageenan-containing foods; high in complex carbohydrates and fiber, low in sugar and refined carbohydrates.

● **Supplements:**

   — multivitamin and mineral supplement

   — magnesium: 200 mg q.d.

   — zinc picolinate: 50 mg q.d.

   — vitamin A: 50,000 IU q.d.

   — vitamin E: 200 IU q.d.

   — fish oil: 3 g q.d.

● **Botanical medicines:**

   — quercetin: 400 mg 20 min before meals

   — Bastyr's formula: two to three "00" capsules with each meal.

Independent variables and formula used to calculate the CDAI

X_1	Number of liquid or very soft stools in 1 week
X_2	Sum of seven daily abdominal pain ratings: 0 = none, 1 = mild, 2 = moderate, 3 = severe
X_3	Sum of seven daily ratings of general well-being: 0 = well, 1 = slightly below par, 2 = poor, 3 = very poor, 4 = terrible
X_4	Symptoms or findings presumed related to Crohn's disease: — arthritis or arthralgia — iritis or uveitis — erythema nodosum, pyoderma gangrenosum, aphthous stomatitis — anal fissure, fistula, or perirectal abscess — other bowel-related fistula — febrile episode > 100°F during past week Add 1 for each category corresponding to patient's symptoms
X_5	Taking Lomotil or opiates for diarrhea: 0 = no, 1 = yes
X_6	Abdominal mass: 0 = none, 0.4 = questionable, 1 = present
X_7	47 minus hematocrit, males 42 minus hematocrit, females
X_8	100 × (standard weight – body weight)/standard weight $CDAI = 2 \times X_1 + 5 \times X_2 + 7 \times X_3 + 20 \times X_4 + 30 \times X_5 + 10 \times X_6 + 6 \times X_7 + X_8$

Monitoring of the pediatric patient with IBD

History

- Appetite, extracurricular activities
- Type and duration of inflammatory bowel disease, frequency of relapses
- Severity and extent of ongoing symptoms
- Medication history

Three day diet diary
Physical examination

- Height, weight, arm circumference, triceps skinfold measurements
- Loss of subcutaneous fat, muscle wasting, edema, pallor, skin rash, hepatomegaly

Laboratory tests

- CBC and differential, reticulocyte and platelet count, sedimentation rate, urinalysis
- Serum total proteins, albumin, globulin, and retinol-binding protein
- Serum electrolytes, calcium, phosphate, ferritin, folate, carotenes, tocopherol, and B_{12}
- Leukocyte ascorbate, magnesium, and zinc
- Creatinine height index, BUN:creatinine ratio

Clinical score in chronic IBD

Measure	Score	Clinical assessment
General activity		
	10	Normal school attendance
		< 3 bowel movements per day
	5	Lacks endurance
		3–5 bowel movements per day
		Misses < 4 weeks school/year
Physical examination and complications		
Abdomen	10	Normal
	5	Mass
	1	Distension, tenderness
Proctoscope	10	Normal, no fissures
	5	Friability, one fissure
	1	Ulcers, bleeding, fistulas, multiple fissures
Arthritis	5	Nil
	3	One joint/arthralgia
	1	Multiple joints
Skin/stomatitis/eyes	5	Normal
	3	Mild stomatitis

Measure	Score	Clinical assessment
	4	Erythema nodosum, pyoderma, severe stomatitis, uveitis
Nutrition		
Height	10	> 2 in/year
	5	< optimal %
	1	No growth
X-rays	15	Normal
	10	Ileitis
	5	Total colon or ileocecal involvement
	1	Toxic megacolon or obstruction
Laboratory		
HCT	5	> 40
	3	25–35
	1	< 25
ESR	5	Normal
	3	20–40
	1	> 40
WBC	5	Normal
	3	< 20,000
	1	> 20,000
Albumin	10	Normal
	5	3.0 g/dl
	1	< 2.5 g/dl

Insomnia

DIAGNOSTIC SUMMARY

- Difficulty falling asleep (sleep-onset insomnia).
- Frequent or early awakening (maintenance insomnia).

GENERAL CONSIDERATIONS

Very common complaint; symptom with many causes.

Causes of insomnia*

Sleep-onset insomnia	Sleep-maintenance insomnia
Anxiety or tension	Depression
Environmental change	Environmental change
Emotional arousal	Sleep apnea
Fear of insomnia	Nocturnal myoclonus
Phobia of sleep	Hypoglycemia
Disruptive environment	Parasomnias
Pain or discomfort	Pain or discomfort
Caffeine	Drugs
Alcohol	Alcohol

*The boundary between the categories is not entirely distinct.

Up to 30% of population suffers; each year 4–6 million people in US receive prescriptions for sedative hypnotics; psychological factors account for 50% of insomnias evaluated in sleep labs; closely associated with affective disorders (see chapter on affective disorders); may be presenting symptom for more serious condition; thorough history and exam indicated – detailed recreational, prescription and non-prescription drug usage history plus dietary and beverage history to identify stimulants or other agents known to interfere with sleep: thyroid preparations, oral contraceptives, beta-blockers, marijuana, alcohol, coffee, tea, chocolate; consider narcolepsy and sleep apnea syndromes.

Normal sleep patterns

- Repeat themselves on a 24-h cycle, of which sleep constitutes one-third; sleep tends to decrease with age, but it is unknown whether this is normal; a 1-year-old baby requires 14 h of sleep, a 5-year-old 12 h, and adults 7–9 h; women require more sleep than men; elderly sleep less at night, but doze more during day than younger adults.

- Two distinct types of sleep (based on eye movement and EEG recordings) – REM (rapid eye movement) and non-REM sleep:

  — *REM sleep*: eyes move rapidly and dreaming takes place; when people are awakened during non-REM sleep, they will report that they were thinking about everyday matters but rarely report dreams

  — *non-REM*: four stages graded 1–4 based on level of EEG activity and ease of arousal; as sleep progresses, it deepens and there is slower brain wave activity until REM sleep, when brain suddenly becomes much more active; in adults, first REM cycle triggered 90 min after going to sleep and lasts 5–10 min; EEG patterns return to non-REM for another 90 min sleep cycle.

- Each night most adults experience 5+ sleep cycles; REM periods grow progressively longer as sleep continues; last sleep cycle may produce REM period lasting an hour; non-REM sleep lasts 50% of 90-min sleep cycle in infants and 80% in adults; with aging, in addition to less REM sleep, people tend to awaken at transition from non-REM to REM sleep.

Importance of adequate sleep

Increased secretion of growth hormone (GH) and scavenging of free radicals in brain.

- GH is the anabolic "anti-aging" hormone; stimulates tissue regeneration, liver regeneration, muscle building, breakdown of fat stores, normalization of blood sugar regulation; helps convert fat to muscle; small amounts secreted during the day, but most secretion occurs during sleep.

- Sleep is the antioxidant for brain – free radicals are removed during this time; required to minimize neuronal damage due to free radical accumulation during waking; chronic sleep deprivation accelerates aging of brain; animal research: prolonged sleep deprivation causes neuronal damage.

THERAPEUTIC CONSIDERATIONS

Uncover causative psychological and physiological factors; counseling and/or stress reduction techniques (biofeedback, hypnosis) are indicated in many cases.

- **Exercise:** regular physical exercise improves sleep quality; perform in the morning or early evening, not before bedtime, and at moderate intensity; 20 min of aerobic exercise at heart rate between 60 and 75% of maximum (220 minus age in years).

- **Progressive relaxation:** based on simple procedure of comparing tension with relaxation; patient is taught what it feels like to relax by comparing relaxation with muscle tension; muscle first asked to contract forcefully for 1–2 s and then give way to feeling of relaxation; procedure goes progressively through all muscles of body and eventually deep state of relaxation results; begin contracting facial and neck muscles, then upper arms and chest, then lower arms and hands, abdomen, buttocks, thighs, calves, and feet; repeat two or three times, or until asleep.

- **Nocturnal glucose levels:** low nocturnal blood glucose is the cause of maintenance insomnia; drop in blood glucose promotes awakening via release of glucose regulatory hormones (epinephrine, glucagon, cortisol, and GH); rule out hypoglycemia in maintenance insomnia (see chapter on Hypoglycemia).

Serotonin precursor and cofactor therapy

Serotonin is the initiator of sleep; synthesis of CNS serotonin is dependent on tryptophan (*Textbook*, Ch. 126).

- **L-tryptophan** has modest effect on insomnia with dramatic relief in some patients; more effective in sleep onset and less effective in sleep maintenance; advantage of L-tryptophan over OTCs and Rx pills = no significant distortions of normal sleep processes whether given one time, for prolonged period, or upon withdrawal; dosages < 2,000 mg ineffective; L-tryptophan enhances melatonin synthesis; L-tryptophan reduces sleep latency, but in normal subjects the effects are at odds with serotonin, reducing REM and increasing non-REM sleep; some of L-tryptophan's sleep effects do not involve serotonin or melatonin; effects of L-tryptophan can be negated via kynurenine pathway – partially inhibited by niacin (30 mg), enhancing effects of L-tryptophan; sleep actions of L-tryptophan are cumulative – often takes a few nights to start working; L-tryptophan should be used for 1+ week to gauge effectiveness in chronic insomnia; L-tryptophan does exert good sleep-promoting effects with single administration (insomnia sleeping in "strange place"); high-dose L-tryptophan (4 g) during the day can promote sleep; high tryptophan-containing foods during the day may contribute to daytime sleepiness; evening meal high in tryptophan relative to competing amino acids may promote sleep.

- **5-HTP:** 5-hydroxytryptophan is one step closer to serotonin than L-tryptophan; not dependent on transport system for entry into brain; produces dramatically better results than L-tryptophan in promoting and maintaining sleep; increases REM sleep (by 25%) and increases deep sleep stages 3 and 4 without increasing total sleep time; sleep stages reduced to compensate for increases are non-REM stages 1 and 2, the least important stages; 5-HTP dosage for sleep promotion = 100–300 mg 30–45 min before retiring; start with lower dose for at least 3 days before moving up.

● **Cofactors for serotonin synthesis:** vitamin B_6, niacin, and magnesium are given with tryptophan to ensure conversion to serotonin; other amino acids compete for transport into CNS across blood–brain barrier, and insulin increases tryptophan uptake by CNS – avoid protein consumption near administration, and carbohydrate source (fruit or fruit juice) should accompany tryptophan; niacin has sedative effect, probably due to peripheral dilating action and shunting tryptophan towards serotonin synthesis.

Melatonin

Very effective in inducing and maintaining sleep in children and adults, in those with normal sleep patterns and those with insomnia; sleep effects of melatonin apparent only if melatonin levels are low – melatonin not like sleeping pill or 5-HTP; only produces sedative effect when melatonin levels are low; normally, just prior to retiring, melatonin secretion rises; melatonin supplement is only effective as sedative when pineal gland's own production of melatonin is very low; most effective for insomnia in elderly in whom low melatonin is common; dosage = 3 mg at bedtime; no serious side-effects at this dosage, but melatonin supplementation could disrupt normal circadian rhythm.

Restless legs syndrome and nocturnal myoclonus

These are significant causes of insomnia.

● *Restless legs syndrome* (RLS) characterized during waking by irresistible urge to move legs; almost all these patients have nocturnal myoclonus.

● *Nocturnal myoclonus* (NM) is a neuromuscular disorder with repeated contractions of one or more muscle groups, typically of leg, during sleep; each jerk lasts < 10 s; patient is unaware of myoclonus and complains only of frequent nocturnal awakenings or excessive daytime sleepiness; questioning sleep partner reveals myoclonus.

● If family history of RLS (1/3 of patients), high-dose folic acid (35–60 mg q.d.) helpful – require prescription – FDA limits amount per capsule to 800 µg; familial RLS is linked to higher need for folate; RLS is common in patients with malabsorption syndromes.

● If no family history, measure serum ferritin – best measure of iron stores; low Fe linked to RLS; serum ferritin is reduced in RLS patients compared with controls; serum Fe, B_{12}, folate, and hemoglobin do not differ; treatment with iron (ferrous sulfate) at dosage of 200 mg t.i.d. for 2 months reduced symptoms; Fe deficiency, with or without anemia, is a contributor to RLS in elderly and Fe supplements can produce significant improvement.

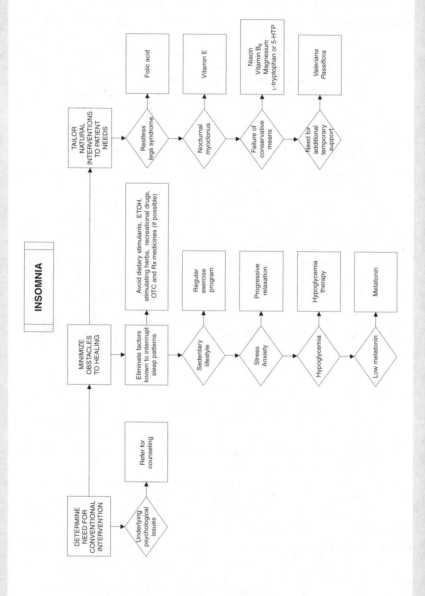

- Low serum ferritin found in psychiatric patients experiencing "akathisia" (from Greek word meaning "can't sit down"); akathisia is a drug-induced agitation caused by antidepressants (Prozac, Zoloft, Paxil); level of Fe depletion correlates with severity of akathisia; if serum ferritin < 35 μg/L, try 30 mg Fe bound to succinate or fumarate b.i.d. between meals; if this therapy causes abdominal discomfort, try 30 mg with meals t.i.d.

- For NM and muscle cramps at night, magnesium (250 mg at bedtime) and/or vitamin E (400–800 IU q.d.) may help; if patient > 50 years, *Ginkgo biloba* extract (80 mg t.i.d.) may also be used.

Botanicals with sedative properties

- ***Passiflora incarnata* (passion flower):** widely used by Aztecs as diaphoretic, sedative, and analgesic; constituents are harmol, harman, harmine, harmalol, harmaline, and passicol; harmine (called "telepathine" because of ability to induce contemplation and mild euphoria) used by Germans in World War II as "truth serum"; harma alkaloids are monoamine oxidase inhibitors – use with tryptophan or 5-HTP has additive effect.

- ***Valeriana officinalis* (valerian):** widely used in folk medicine as sedative and antihypertensive; aqueous extract of valerian root significantly improves sleep quality; criteria = sleep latency, night awakenings, subjective sleep quality, and sleepiness the next morning: has most significant effect among poor or irregular sleepers (particularly women), smokers, and people with long sleep latencies; exerts mild sedative effect; significantly reduces sleep latency, improves sleep quality, and reduces night-time awakenings in insomniacs; as effective in reducing sleep latency as small doses of barbiturates or benzodiazepines, but these drugs increase morning sleepiness, while valerian reduces morning sleepiness; compared with placebo, valerian shows significant effect, with 44% of subjects reporting perfect sleep and 89% reporting improved sleep; combination of valerian root extract (160 mg) and *Melissa officinalis* extract (80 mg) compared with benzodiazepine (triazolam 0.125 mg), and placebo – among insomniacs, valerian preparation's effect comparable to benzodiazepine, while increasing deep sleep stages 3 and 4; valerian preparation did not cause daytime sedation, diminished concentration, or impairment of physical performance.

THERAPEUTIC APPROACH

Treatment should be as conservative as possible; treat psychological factors; eliminate factors known to disrupt normal sleep patterns: stimulants (coffee, tea, chocolate, coffee-flavored ice cream, etc.), alcohol, hypoglycemia, stimulant-containing herbs (e.g. ephedra, guarana), marijuana and other recreational drugs, numerous OTC medications, prescription drugs; if this approach fails, use more aggressive measures; once normal sleep pattern established, supplements and botanicals should be slowly decreased; if patient suffers from RLS, add 5–10 mg q.d. folic acid; for NM use 400 IU q.d. natural vitamin E.

- **Lifestyle:** regular exercise program that elevates heart rate 50–75% for 20 min q.d.
- **Supplements:** taken 45 min before bedtime:
  - — niacin: 100 mg (decrease dose if uncomfortable flushing interferes with sleep induction)
  - — vitamin B_6: 50 mg
  - — magnesium: 250 mg
  - — tryptophan: 3–5 g; or 5-HTP: 100–300 mg
  - — melatonin: 3 mg.
- **Botanical medicines:** taken 45 min before bedtime:
  - — *Valeriana officinalis*:
    dried root (or as tea): 2–3 g
    tincture (1:5): 4–6 ml (1–1.5 tsp)
    fluid extract (1:1): 1–2 ml (0.5–1 tsp)
    dry powdered extract (0.8% valerenic acid): 150–300 mg
  - — *Passiflora incarnata*:
    dried herb (or as tea): 4–8 g
    tincture (1:5): 6–8 ml (1.5–2 tsp)
    fluid extract (1:1): 2–4 ml (0.5–1 tsp)
    dry powdered extract (2.6% flavonoids): 300–450 mg.

Intestinal dysbiosis and dysfunction

Introduction: overgrowth of inappropriate bacteria in GI tract is a widespread but unrecognized cause of chronic disorders throughout the body; symptoms mimic other disorders (*Textbook*, Chs 7, 9, 19, 21, 23, 31, 57, 131, 163, 165).

SMALL INTESTINE

- **Bacterial overgrowth:** normally relatively free of bacteria; overgrowth causes carbohydrate fermentation and protein putrefaction; bacteria and yeast contain decarboxylases, which convert amino acids histidine to histamine, tyrosine to tyramine, ornithine to putrescine, lysine to cadaverine (vasoactive amines); all cause constriction and relaxation of blood vessel smooth muscle, increased gut permeability ("leaky gut" syndrome) (*Textbook*, Ch. 21).

- **Diagnosis:** comprehensive digestive stool analysis (*Textbook*, Ch. 9); breath tests: hydrogen and methane after ingesting lactulose and glucose (*Textbook*, Ch. 7).

- **Symptoms:** indigestion, bloating, nausea, diarrhea, arthritis (rheumatoid).

- **Protective preventive factors:** HCl, pancreatic enzymes, liver secretions, peristalsis, immunological factors.

- **Factors associated with small intestinal bacterial overgrowth:** decreased digestive secretions (achlorhydria, hypochlorhydria, drugs inhibiting HCl, pancreatic insufficiency, decreased bile output due to liver or gall bladder disease); decreased motility (systemic sclerosis, systemic lupus erythematosus, intestinal adhesions, sugar-induced hypomotility, radiation damage; low secretory IgA (low immune function, food allergies, stress); weak ileocecal valve (long-term constipation, low-fiber diet).

- ***Candida albicans*** (*Textbook*, Ch. 48)

- **Treatment:** address cause; improve and supplement digestive secretions (*Textbook*, Ch. 55); decrease sugar consumption; increase dietary fiber

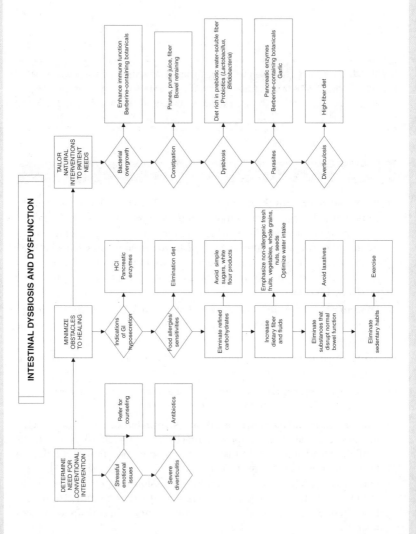

(*Textbook*, Ch. 57); restore secretory IgA: eliminate food allergens (*Textbook*, Ch. 51), enhance immune function (*Textbook*, Ch. 53), improve stress management; pancreatic enzymes and botanicals containing berberine inhibit bacteria: berberine is a broad-spectrum antibiotic, and it inhibits bacterial decarboxylase, which converts amino acids into vasoactive amines; pancreatic enzymes digest protein, inhibit pathogenic bacteria, yeast, protozoa, helminths.

COLON

Colon health is determined by dietary fiber, elimination of waste products (IBS – *Textbook*, Ch. 165; Crohn's and ulcerative colitis – *Textbook*, Ch. 163).

Constipation

- **Causes:** most common is a low-fiber refined diet; inadequate fluid intake; physical inactivity; pregnancy; advanced age; drugs; low potassium stores; diabetes; kidney disease; low thyroid; elevated calcium levels; pituitary disorders; structural anomalies; diverticulosis; IBS (alternating diarrhea and constipation); tumor; bowel nerve disorders; spinal cord disorders; disorders of splanchnic nerves; cerebral disorders; chronic use of enemas.

- **Treatment:** high-fiber diet, plentiful fluid consumption, and exercise: increase frequency and quantity of BM, decrease transit time, decrease absorption of toxins, and are preventive of other diseases; oat bran (1 cup bran cereal, increase to 1.5 cups over several weeks); whole prunes and prune juice (8 oz); 6–8 glasses liquids q.d.; fiber: 25–35 g of fiber; fiber formulas: psyllium seed, kelp, agar, pectin, plant gums (karaya, guar), purified semi-synthetic polysaccharides (methylcellulose, carboxymethylcellulose sodium); stimulant laxative abuse (even cascara or senna) requires bowel "retraining" 4–6 weeks.

- **Bowel retraining after laxative abuse:** eliminate causes of constipation; never repress urge to defecate; high-fiber diet (fruits, vegetables); 6–8 glasses fluid q.d.; sit on toilet same time q.d. (even without urge, after breakfast or exercise); exercise 20 min three times weekly; stop laxatives and enemas; week 1: every night before bed take stimulant laxative containing cascara or senna at lowest amount necessary to ensure BM every morning; weekly: decrease dosage by 50%; if constipation recurs, use previous week's dosage; decrease dosage if diarrhea occurs.

Diverticular disease

- Usually asymptomatic; if inflamed, perforated, or impacted, symptomatic diverticulitis results; 20% of people with diverticulosis develop diverticulitis: episodic lower abdominal pain and cramping, changed bowel habits (constipation or diarrhea), sense of abdominal fullness, fever, tenderness, rigidity over involved area.

- **Treatment:** high-fiber diet; severe diverticulitis: antibiotics.

Dysbiosis

- 500 different species of "normal" microflora; nine times as many bacteria in GI tract as cells in body.

- "Dysbiosis" is a state of altered gut microflora; first used by Russian scientist Elie Metchnikoff: theory – toxic compounds from bacterial breakdown of food cause degenerative disease.

- **Causes:** diet (high protein, sugar, fat; low fiber; food allergens); inadequate digestive secretions; stress; antibiotic/drug therapy; decreased immune function; malabsorption; intestinal infection; altered pH.

- **Treatment:** address major causes; re-seed GI tract with probiotics *Lactobacillus acidophilus* and *Bifidobacterium bifidum* (*Textbook*, Ch. 105); re-establish healthy symbiotic balance among microflora; parasites interfere with digestion, damage mucosa – increased mucous secretion, diarrhea.

- **Undigested unabsorbed carbohydrates** in small intestine or colon increase fermentation, overgrowth of toxic bacteria: gas, short-chain organic acids (e.g. lactic acid) are damaging to mucosa; aggravate problem by disaccharides (lactase, sucrase, isomaltase, maltase) in mucosa, increasing undigested disaccharides; damage enhances mucous secretion, separating carbohydrates from their digestive sites.

- **"Specific carbohydrate diet":** carbohydrates either predigested/easily digested and totally absorbed in duodenum; eliminate disaccharides, grain starches (e.g. wheat, rice, corn syrup), starchy vegetables (e.g. potatoes), legume starches; simple sugars (glucose, fructose in honey, fruits, some vegetables) and lactose-hydrolyzed milk products are allowed.

Parasites

- Diarrhea caused by parasites is the greatest single worldwide cause of illness and death.

- **Species:** Protozoa (*Giardia, Entamoeba coli, Endolimax nana, Blastocystis hominis, Entamoeba histolytica, Cryptosporidium*); nematodes (hookworm, *Trichuris trichiura, Ascaris lumbricoides, Clonorchis, Opisthorchis, Strongyloides stercoralis, Hymenolepis nana, Enterobius vermicularis, Taenia* species).

- **Signs and symptoms of parasitic infections:** abdominal pain and cramps, constipation, depressed secretory IgA, diarrhea, chronic fatigue, fever, flatulence, food allergy, foul-smelling stools, gastritis, HAs, hives, increased intestinal permeability, indigestion, irregular BMs, IBS, anorexia, low back pain, malabsorption, weight loss.

- **Treatment:** address underlying factors (e.g. achlorhydria, inadequate pancreatic enzyme output); monitor progress with multiple stool samples 2 weeks after therapy (*Textbook*, Ch. 131); pancreatic enzymes ($10 \times$ USP 750–1,000 mg 10–20 min before meals); berberine-containing plants (*Hydrastis canadensis, Berberis vulgaris, Berberis aquifolium, Coptis chinensis*) – dosage based on berberine content: solid (powdered dry) extract (4:1 or 8–12% alkaloid content): 250–500 mg t.i.d. (berberine dosage of 25–50 mg t.i.d. or up to 150 mg q.d.) (*Textbook*, Ch. 91); children – dosage based on body weight: 5–10 mg berberine/kg body weight.

Irritable bowel syndrome

DIAGNOSTIC SUMMARY

- Functional disorder of large intestine with no evidence of accompanying structural defect.

- Characterized by some combination of:
  — abdominal pain
  — altered bowel function, constipation, or diarrhea
  — hypersecretion of colonic mucus
  — dyspeptic symptoms (flatulence, nausea, anorexia)
  — varying degrees of anxiety or depression.

- Synonyms – nervous indigestion, spastic colitis, mucous colitis, and intestinal neurosis; splenic flexure syndrome is a variant of IBS in which gas in bowel leads to pain in lower chest or left shoulder.

GENERAL CONSIDERATIONS

Irritable bowel syndrome is the most common GI disorder in general practice; cause of 30–50% of all referrals to gastroenterologists; many sufferers never seek medical attention; 15% of population have IBS complaints; women predominate 2:1 (men do not report symptoms as often); etiology is attributed to physiological, psychological, and dietary factors; IBS is often diagnosis of exclusion – clinical judgment is needed to determine extent of diagnostic process; detailed history and physical exam can eliminate vagueness in diagnosing IBS; distension, relief of pain with BMs, and onset of loose or more frequent BMs with pain correlate best with diagnosis of IBS; comprehensive stool and digestive analysis (*Textbook*, Ch. 9), complete blood count, erythrocyte sedimentation rate, and serum protein concentration are necessary to determine diagnosis; if no discernible cause identified, sigmoidoscopy is indicated.

Conditions which may mimic IBS

- Gastrogenic dietary factors such as excessive tea, coffee, carbonated beverages, and simple sugars
- Infectious enteritis such as amebiasis and giardiasis
- Inflammatory bowel disease
- Lactose intolerance

Conditions which may mimic IBS

● Laxative abuse (an easy test to eliminate this possibility is to add a few drops of sodium hydroxide solution to a stool specimen; since most laxatives contain phenolphthalein, the stool will turn red)
● Intestinal candidiasis
● Disturbed bacterial microflora as a result of antibiotic or antacid usage
● Malabsorption diseases such as pancreatic insufficiency and celiac disease
● Metabolic disorders such as adrenal insufficiency, diabetes mellitus, and hyperthyroidism
● Mechanical causes such as fecal impaction
● Diverticular disease
● Neoplasm

THERAPEUTIC CONSIDERATIONS

Three major treatments to consider: (1) increasing dietary fiber; (2) eliminating allergic/intolerant foods; (3) controlling psychological components (*Textbook*, Chs 51, 55, 101).

● **Dietary fiber:** patients with constipation are more likely to respond to dietary fiber than those with diarrhea; food allergy has been ignored in studies of fiber; wheat bran is usually contraindicated since food allergy is a significant factor in IBS; fiber from fruit and vegetables rather than cereals is more beneficial in some patients; in certain cases, fiber may aggravate diarrhea (*Textbook*, Ch. 57).

● **Food allergy:** type of food sensitivity most significant in IBS is non-immunological – food intolerance rather than food allergy (*Textbook*, Ch. 51); 2/3 of patients with IBS have food intolerances; most common allergens are dairy (40–44%) and grains (40–60%); reaction appears related to prostaglandin synthesis or IgG rather than IgE mediation – skin tests and IgE-RAST are poor indicators of intolerances; ELISA ACT or ELISA IgE/IgG$_4$ may be better indicators (*Textbook*, Chs 10 and 15); many sensitivities are undetectable by current lab procedures; marked clinical improvement using elimination diets; many IBS patients have associated symptoms of vaso-motor instability (palpitation, hyperventilation, fatigue, excessive sweating, HAs) – consistent with food allergy/intolerance reactions.

● **Sugar:** meals high in refined sugar contribute to IBS and small intestinal bacterial overgrowth by decreasing intestinal motility; rapid rise in blood sugar slows GI tract peristalsis; glucose primarily absorbed in duodenum and jejunum, and hence the message affects this portion of GI tract the strongest – duodenum and jejunum become atonic.

● **Enteric-coated volatile oils:** peppermint oil and similar volatile oils inhibit GI smooth muscle action in lab animals and humans; reduce colonic spasm during endoscopy; enteric-coated peppermint oil is used to treat IBS.

— enteric coating may be necessary – menthol (major constituent of peppermint oil) and other monoterpenes in peppermint oil are rapidly absorbed; rapid absorption limits effects to upper intestine, causing relaxation of cardiac esophageal sphincter with esophageal reflux and heartburn; transient hot burning sensation in rectum on defecation (unabsorbed menthol) is noted in some patients

— dosage = 0.2 ml b.i.d. between meals

— improves rhythmic contractions of intestinal tract and relieves intestinal spasm

— effective against *Candida albicans* – overgrowth of *C. albicans* may be underlying factor in cases unresponsive to dietary advice and in patients consuming large amounts of sugar; nystatin (600,000 IU q.d. × 10 days) given to patients unresponsive to elimination diet produced dramatic improvement.

● **Psychological factors:** mental/emotional problems (anxiety, fatigue, hostile feelings, depression, sleep disturbances) reported by almost all patients with IBS; symptom severity and frequency correlate with psychological factors; poor sleep quality increases symptom severity.

— theories linking psychological factors to IBS: (1) "learning model" – when exposed to stressful situations some children learn to develop GI symptoms to cope with stress; (2) IBS is a manifestation of depression or chronic anxiety, or both; IBS sufferers have higher anxiety and greater feeling of depression; (3) IBS is either secondary to bowel disturbances (malabsorption) or the result of common etiological factor (stress, food allergy, or candidiasis)

— increased colonic motility during stress occurs in normal subjects and IBD sufferers; accounts for increased abdominal pain and irregular bowel functions seen in IBS and normal subjects during emotional stress; IBS sufferers may have difficulty adapting to life events; psychotherapy (relaxation therapy, biofeedback, hypnosis, counseling, or stress management training) reduces symptom frequency and severity, and enhances results of conventional treatment of IBS; anxiolytic drugs (tranquilizers, antispasmodics, antidepressants) have not yielded effective results.

● **Miscellaneous considerations:**

— Role of altered microbial flora in IBS has not been investigated; benefits of dietary fiber may be mediated by alterations in colon bacteria; *Lactobacillus acidophilus* supplementation is indicated in IBS (*Textbook*, Ch. 105).

— Old naturopathic remedy, Robert's (Bastyr's) formula, has long history of use in IBS (see Inflammatory bowel disease chapter).

IRRITABLE BOWEL SYNDROME

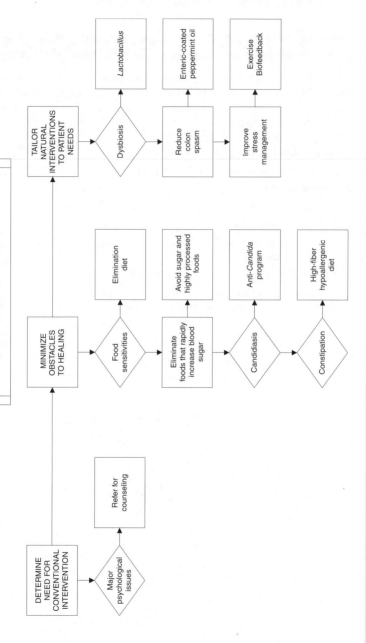

DETERMINE NEED FOR CONVENTIONAL INTERVENTION

Major psychological issues → Refer for counseling

MINIMIZE OBSTACLES TO HEALING

Food sensitivities → Elimination diet

Eliminate foods that rapidly increase blood sugar → Avoid sugar and highly processed foods

Candidiasis → Anti-*Candida* program

Constipation → High-fiber hypoallergenic diet

TAILOR NATURAL INTERVENTIONS TO PATIENT NEEDS

Dysbiosis → *Lactobacillus*

Reduce colon spasm → Enteric-coated peppermint oil

Improve stress management → Exercise / Biofeedback

— Increasing physical exercise is helpful – daily leisurely walks markedly reduce symptoms – stress reduction effects of exercise.

THERAPEUTIC APPROACH

Multifactorial disease requires consideration and integration of many factors: dietary fiber, determination and elimination of food allergies/intolerances, stress reduction, exercise; peppermint oil and Robert's formula as needed to ameliorate symptoms temporarily; since diagnosis is made by exclusion, careful diagnostic work-up is always indicated.

● **Diet:** increase fiber-rich foods (*Textbook*, Ch. 57); eliminate allergenic foods, refined sugar, and highly processed foods.

● **Supplements:**

— *Lactobacillus acidophilus*: 1–2 billion live organisms q.d.

● **Botanical medicine:**

— enteric-coated volatile oil preparations (peppermint oil): 0.2–0.4 ml b.i.d. between meals.

● **Physical therapy:** take daily, leisurely 20-min walks.

● **Counseling:** aid patient in developing effective stress reduction program; biofeedback particularly useful for these patients.

Kidney stones

DIAGNOSTIC SUMMARY

- Usually asymptomatic.
- Diagnosed adventitiously or by acute symptoms of urinary tract obstruction.
- Excruciating intermittent radiating pain originating in flank or kidney.
- Nausea, vomiting, abdominal distension.
- Chills, fever, and urinary frequency if infection.

GENERAL CONSIDERATIONS

- In the past, stone formation was almost exclusively in the bladder; today most stones form in upper urinary tract; 10% of all males experience renal stone during their lifetime; annual incidence = 0.1–6.0% of general population; incidence steadily increasing, paralleling rise in other diseases linked to "Western diet" (ischemic heart disease, cholelithiasis, hypertension, diabetes).
- In western hemisphere, kidney stones usually composed of calcium salts (75–85%), uric acid (5–8%), or struvite (10–15%); incidence varies geographically, reflecting environmental factors, diet, and components of drinking water.
- Males affected more than females; most patients over age 30.
- Human urine supersaturated with calcium oxalate, uric acid, and phosphates; remain in solution due to pH control and secretion of inhibitors of crystal growth.
- Primary and secondary metabolic diseases cause kidney stones – must be ruled out early in clinical process: hyperparathyroidism, cystinuria, vitamin D excess, milk-alkali syndrome, destructive bone disease, primary oxaluria, Cushing's syndrome, sarcoidosis.

DIAGNOSTIC CONSIDERATIONS

Stone formation: Conditions favoring stone formation:

- Factors increasing concentration of stone crystalloids – reduced urine volume (dehydration) and increased excretion of stone constituents.
- Factors favoring stone formation at normal urinary concentrations – urinary stasis, pH changes, foreign bodies, reduction of normal substances which solubilize stone constituents.

Causes of excessive excretion of relatively insoluble urinary constituents

Constituent	Cause of excess excretion	Laboratory findings
Calcium	(> 250 mg/day excreted) Absorptive hypercalciuria	Low serum PO_4 30–40% of all stone formers
	Renal hypercalciuria (renal tubular acidosis)	High serum PTH High urinary cAMP
	Primary hyperparathyroidism	High serum calcium High $1,25(OH)_2D_3$
	Hyperthyroidism High vitamin D intake Excess intake of milk and alkali	High serum calcium
	Aluminum salt intake	Low serum phosphate High $1,25(OH)_2D_3$
	Destructive bone disease Sarcoidosis Prolonged immobility	
Oxalate	Familial oxaluria	Rare
	Ileal disease, resection, or bypass Steatorrhea High oxalate intake Ethylene glycon poisoning Vitamin C excess (extremely unlikely)	Vitamin B_6 deficiency or abnormal oxalate metabolism
	Methoxyflurane anesthesia	
Uric acid	(> 750 mg/day excreted) Gout Idiopathic hyperuricosuria Excess purine intake Anti-cancer drugs	Rapid cell destruction
	Myeloproliferative disease	
Cystine	Hereditary cystinuria	

Physical changes in the urine and kidney

Condition	Possible cause
Increased concentration	Dehydration
	Stasis
	Obstruction
	Foreign body concretions
Urinary pH	Low – uric acid, cystine
	High – calcium oxalate and PO_4
Infection	Proteus – struvite
Uricosuria	Crystals of uric acid initiate precipitation of calcium oxalate from solution
Nuclei for stone formation	Cells, bacteria, blood clots, etc. initiate precipitation
Sponge kidney	Horseshoe kidney
Deformities of kidney	Caliceal obstruction or defect

THERAPEUTIC CONSIDERATIONS

- **Stone composition:** diagnosing type of stone critical to therapy; evaluate following criteria to determine stone composition, if one not available for analysis: diet; underlying metabolic or disease factors; serum and urinary calcium, uric acid, creatinine, and electrolyte levels; urinalysis; urine culture.

- **Dietary factors:** Calcium-containing stones are calcium oxalate, calcium oxalate mixed with calcium phosphate, or (very rarely) calcium phosphate alone; high incidence of Ca stones in affluent societies is linked to: low fiber, refined carbohydrates, high ETOH intake, high animal protein, high fat, high Ca food, vitamin D-enriched food.

  — dietary factors induce hyperuricemia, hypercalciuria, and stone formation – cumulative effect

  — vegetarians have decreased risk of developing stones; among meat eaters, those eating more fresh fruits and vegetables have lower incidence of stones; bran supplements and changing to wholewheat bread lower urinary calcium.

- **Weight and carbohydrate metabolism:** excess weight and insulin insensitivity induce hypercalciuria and higher risk; following glucose ingestion, urinary calcium rises along with decreased phosphate reabsorption; low plasma phosphate stimulates 1,25-dihydroxycholecalciferol production, increased intestinal absorption of Ca and hypercalciuria; sucrose and other simple sugars cause exaggerated increase in urinary calcium oxalate in 70% of recurrent kidney stone formers.

- **Magnesium and vitamin B₆:** Mg-deficient diet accelerates renal tubular Ca deposition in rats; Mg increases solubility of calcium oxalate and inhibits precipitation of calcium phosphate and calcium oxalate; low urinary Mg:Ca

Chemical and physical characteristics of urinary stones

Composition	Crystal name	Frequency	X-ray appearance	Urine characteristics	Crystal characteristics
Calcium oxalate	Whewellite	30–35%	Opaque	Non-specific	Small, hempseed or mulberry-shaped, brown or black color
Calcium oxalate + calcium phosphate		30–35	Opaque	pH > 5.5	Small, hempseed or mulberry-shaped, brown or black color
Calcium phosphate	Apatite	6–8	Opaque	pH > 5.5	Staghorn configuration, light color
Magnesium ammonium phosphate	Struvite Triple phosphate	15–20	Opaque	pH > 6.2 Infection	Staghorn configuration, light color
Uric acid		6–10	Translucent	pH < 6.0	Ellipsoid, tan or red-brown
Cystine		2–3	Opaque	pH < 7.2	Multiple, faceted, maple sugar color

ratio is an independent risk factor in stone formation; supplemental Mg alone prevents recurrences; Mg plus vitamin B_6 have even greater effect; pyridoxine reduces endogenous production and urinary excretion of oxalates; patients with recurrent oxalate stones show abnormal EGPT, EGOT, UGPT, and UGOT activation levels, indicating clinical insufficiency of B_6 and impaired glutamic acid synthesis; levels normalize after 3 months of treatment.

- **Glutamic acid:** decreased glutamic acid (due to B_6 deficiency or other reasons) linked to kidney stones – increased glutamic acid in urine reduces calcium oxalate precipitation; supplemental glutamic acid may be superfluous with adequate vitamin B_6.

- **Calcium:** Ca restriction enhances oxalate absorption and stone formation absorption; Ca supplements actually reduce oxalate excretion; Ca supplementation (300–1,000 mg q.d.) may be preventive.

- **Citrate:** citrate reduces urinary saturation of calcium oxalate and calcium phosphate; retards nucleation and crystal growth of Ca salts; potassium and sodium citrate for recurrent calcium oxalate are quite effective – ceasing stone formation in 90% of subjects; magnesium citrate may offer greatest benefit.

- **Vitamin K:** urinary glycoprotein inhibitor of calcium oxalate monohydrate growth requires post-transcription carboxylation of glutamic acid to form gamma-carboxyglutamic acid; vitamin K is an essential for this carboxylation; impairment of glutamic acid formation or vitamin K deficiency reduces this glycoprotein; vitamin K in green leafy vegetables may be one reason vegetarians have lower incidence of kidney stones.

- **Uric acid metabolism:** dietary purine intake linearly related to rate of urinary uric acid excretion; hyperuricosuria is a causative factor in recurrent Ca oxalate stones; high supplemental folic acid promotes purine scavenging and xanthine oxidase inhibition, decreasing excretion of uric acid (see chapter on gout).

- **Botanicals:**
  — Anthraquinones isolated from *Rubia*, *Cassia*, and *Aloe* species bind Ca and reduce growth of urinary crystals when used in oral doses lower than laxative dose; *Rubia tinctura*, *Rumex*, *Rheum*, *Polygonum aviculare*, *Aloe*, *Senna*, *Rhamnus alnus*, and *Mitchella repens* are sources of anthraquinones – used to prevent formation and reduce size of stone.

  — Furanocoumarin-containing herb, *Ammi visnaga*, is unusually effective at relaxing ureter, allowing stone to pass; calcium-channel-blocking capabilities act primarily upon ureters; atropine and papaverine have similar, but less active, smooth muscle-relaxing effects; *Peucedanum*, *Leptotania*, *Ruta graveolens*, and *Hydrangea* contain similar furanocoumarins promoting smooth muscle relaxation – historical uses in kidney stones.

- **Miscellaneous:**
  — *Hair mineral analysis*: heavy metals (mercury, gold, uranium, and cadmium) nephrotoxic; cadmium increases incidence of kidney stones.

— *Vitamin C*: in persons not on hemodialysis or suffering from recurrent kidney stones, severe kidney disease, or gout, high-dosage vitamin C will not cause kidney stones; vitamin C up to 10 g q.d. has no effect on urinary oxalate levels.

— *Decrease sodium chloride intake*: urinary Ca excretion increases 1 mmol (40 mg) for each 100 mmol (2,300 mg) increase in dietary Na^+ in normal adults; renal Ca stone formers with hypercalcemia have greater increase in urinary Ca per 100 mmol increase in salt intake.

THERAPEUTIC APPROACH

Accurately differentiate between stone types; recognize and control underlying metabolic diseases or structural abnormalities of urinary tract; goal = to prevent recurrence; dietary management effective, inexpensive, and free of side-effects; specific treatment determined by type of stone:

● reducing urinary calcium
● reducing purine intake
● avoiding high oxalate-containing foods
● increasing foods with a high magnesium:calcium ratio
● increasing vitamin K-rich foods.

Increase urine flow to dilute urine; maintain specific gravity < 1.015 and urinary volume of 2,000+ ml.

Acute obstruction: surgical removal or lithotripsy may be necessary.

● *Ammi visnaga* extract (12% khellin content): 250 mg t.i.d.
● *Rubia tinctura*, *Rumex crispus*, or *Aloe vera* at below laxative doses.

Calcium stones:

● **Diet:** increase fiber, complex carbohydrates, and green leafy vegetables; decrease simple carbohydrates and purines (meat, fish, poultry, yeast); increase high Mg:Ca ratio foods (barley, bran, corn, buckwheat, rye, soy, oats, brown rice, avocado, banana, cashew, coconut, peanut, sesame seed, lima beans, potato); if oxalate stones, reduce oxalate foods (black tea, cocoa, spinach, beet leaves, rhubarb, parsley, cranberry, nuts); limit dairy products.

● **Supplements:**
— vitamin B_6: 25 mg q.d.
— vitamin K: 2 mg q.d.
— magnesium: 600 mg q.d.
— calcium: 300–1,000 mg q.d.

● **Botanicals:** use any of the following in a dose below the laxative effect:
— *Rubia tinctura*

KIDNEY STONES

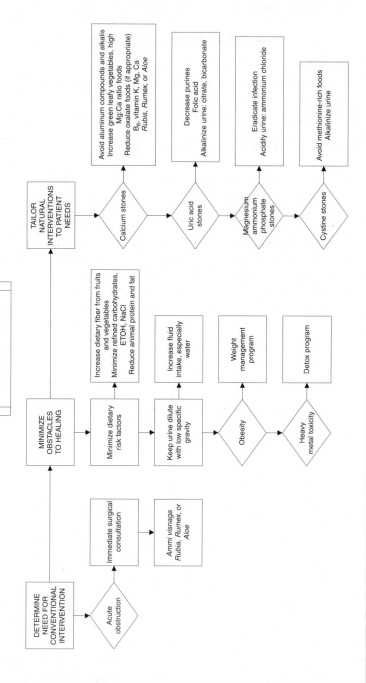

    — *Rumex crispus*

    — *Aloe vera.*

● **Miscellaneous:** avoid aluminum compounds and alkalis.

Uric acid stones:

● **Diet:** decrease purines (list above).

● **Supplements:** folic acid: 5 mg q.d.

● **Miscellaneous:** alkalinize urine – citrate, bicarbonate.

Magnesium ammonium phosphate stones:

● **Miscellaneous:**

    — eradicate infection (*Textbook*, Ch. 53)

    — acidify urine: ammonium chloride (100–200 mg t.i.d.).

Cystine stones:

● **Diet:** avoid methionine-rich foods (soy, wheat, dairy products [except whole milk], fish, meat, lima beans, garbanzo beans, mushrooms, and all nuts except coconut, hazelnut, and sunflower seeds).

● **Miscellaneous:** alkalinize urine – optimal pH is 7.5–8.0.

Leukoplakia

DIAGNOSTIC SUMMARY

- Adherent white patch or plaque appearing anywhere on oral mucosa.
- Asymptomatic until ulceration, fissuring, or malignant transformation.
- Diagnosis confirmed by biopsy.

GENERAL CONSIDERATIONS

Leukoplakia is the clinical term for a white plaque-like lesion anywhere on oral mucosa; generally reaction to irritation (cigarette smoking, tobacco, betel nut chewing) and early sign in HIV infection; most frequently in men aged 50–70; 90% of cases – represents epithelial hyperkeratosis and hyperplasia; 10% of cases – also epithelial dysplasia; lesions considered precancerous.

- **Oral cancer** is a common malignant neoplasm – 50,000 new cases and 12,000 deaths in the US alone each year; survival rates with chemotherapy, radiation, and surgery unchanged in the past few decades; prevent mortality by preventing occurrence – abstinence from tobacco and increased intake of antioxidants.

THERAPEUTIC CONSIDERATIONS

Removal of all irritants; electrodesiccation, cryosurgery, and proteolytic enzymes have not given predictably favorable results.

- **Vitamin A and beta-carotene:** clinically effective for leukoplakia; micronucleus test is a useful indicator of cancerous tendency of epithelial cells – immediate information on genotoxic damage; micronuclei formed during chromatid or chromosomal breakage; rate of formation linked to carcinogenesis in oral cavity; vitamin A and especially beta-carotene are quite effective in decreasing mean proportion of cells with micronuclei on buccal mucosa in Asian betel nut and tobacco chewers (*Textbook*, Chs 67 and 121); inverse relationship between serum retinol and carotene levels and cancer incidence holds true for oral carcinomas; clinical studies on leukoplakia used very high but effective retinol dosages

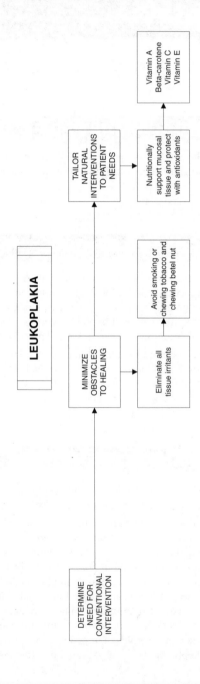

(150,000–900,000 IU q.d.); beta-carotene as effective as retinol in decreasing micronuclei with much higher therapeutic index; *note*: vulvar leukoplakia is responsive to retinol, and may be beta-carotene.

● **Other antioxidants:** vitamin E (400 mg q.d.) produces 65% response rate; utilize combination of antioxidants to accommodate their interactions and limitations; combination of vitamin C (1,000 mg q.d.), beta-carotene (30 mg q.d.), and vitamin E (400 mg q.d.) gives encouraging results.

THERAPEUTIC APPROACH

Leukoplakia is due to combination of excessive carcinogenic irritation and marginal or low levels of vitamin A; eliminate all sources of irritation; establish optimal vitamin A, beta-carotene, and antioxidant levels; main irritants are tobacco smoking and chewing, betel nut chewing, and ultraviolet exposure.

● **Supplements:**

— vitamin A: 5,000 IU q.d.

— beta-carotene: 30–90 mg q.d.

— vitamin C: 1,000–3,000 mg q.d.

— vitamin E: 400 IU q.d.

Macular degeneration

DIAGNOSTIC SUMMARY

- Progressive visual loss due to degeneration of macula.
- Ophthalmological exam may reveal spots of pigment near macula and blurring of macular borders.

GENERAL CONSIDERATIONS

The macula is the area of retina where most images focus and the portion of retina responsible for fine vision; macular degeneration (MD) is the leading cause of severe visual loss in US and Europe in persons aged 55 and older; second to cataracts as leading cause of decreased vision in persons over age 65; over 150,000 Americans are legally blind from age-related macular degeneration; 20,000 new cases each year.

- **Major risk factors:** smoking, aging, atherosclerosis, and hypertension; degeneration results from free radical damage; decreased blood and oxygen supply to retina are a harbinger of MD.

Types of age-related macular degeneration (ARMD)

In either form, patients experience blurred vision; straight objects appear distorted or bent; presence of dark spot near or around center of visual field; while reading, parts of words missing:

— atrophic ("dry") form: more frequent

— neovascular ("wet") form.

- **Dry ARMD:** 80–95% of people with ARMD have dry form; primary lesions = atrophic changes in retinal pigmented epithelium (RPE) (innermost layer of retina); cells of RPE gradually accumulate throughout life sacs of cellular debris (lipofuscin) – remnants of degraded molecules from damaged RPE or phagocytized rod and cone membranes; progressive lipofuscin engorgement of RPE cells extrude tissue components (hyaline, sialomuccin, cerebroside); hallmark excrescences beneath RPE seen on ophthalmoscopic exam called "drusen"; disease progresses slowly and only central vision lost; peripheral vision remains intact; total blindness from dry ARMD is rare; no standard medical treatment.

● **Wet ARMD:** neovascular form affects 5–20% of those with ARMD; involves growth of abnormal blood vessels; can be treated effectively in early stages with laser photocoagulation; disease rapidly progresses to point where surgery is ineffective – perform surgery ASAP.

THERAPEUTIC CONSIDERATIONS

Treatment for wet form is laser photocoagulation; treating dry form and preventing wet form involve antioxidants and natural substances which correct underlying pathophysiology (free radical damage and poor oxygenation of macula); reduce risk factors for atherosclerosis; increase dietary fresh fruits and vegetables; use nutritional and botanical antioxidants.

● **Reducing and preventing atherosclerosis:** risk factor for MD; in subjects younger than 85, plaques in carotid bifurcation indicated 4.7-fold increased prevalence of MD; lower extremity atherosclerosis linked to 2.5 times greater risk (see chapter on atherosclerosis).

● **Dietary fruits and vegetables:** diet rich in fruits and vegetables offers lowered risk for ARMD – increased intake of antioxidant vitamins and minerals; non-provitamin A carotenes lutein, zeaxanthin, and lycopene and flavonoids more protective against ARMD than traditional nutritional antioxidants; macula (and central portion, the fovea) owes its yellow color to high concentration of lutein and zeaxanthin – prevent oxidative damage to retina and protect against MD; individuals with lycopene in lowest quintile are twice as likely to have ARMD.

● **Nutritional supplements:** antioxidants (vitamin C, selenium, beta-carotene, vitamin E) are important for treatment and prevention; combination better than any single nutrient alone – none alone accounts for impaired antioxidant status in ARMD; decreased antioxidant status reflects decreases in combination of nutrients; progression of dry ARMD halted (but not reversed) with commercial antioxidant combination; another combination containing beta-carotene, vitamins C and E, zinc, copper, manganese, selenium, and riboflavin was able to maintain or improve visual acuity in these patients.

● **Zinc:** essential in metabolism of retina, and elderly have high risk for Zn deficiency.

● **Flavonoid-rich extracts:** bilberry (*Vaccinium myrtillus*), *Ginkgo biloba*, and grape seed (*Vitis vinifera*) are very beneficial in preventing and treating ARMD: excellent antioxidants; improve retinal blood flow and function; capable of halting progressive visual loss of dry ARMD and may even improve visual function; bilberry extracts standardized to 25%

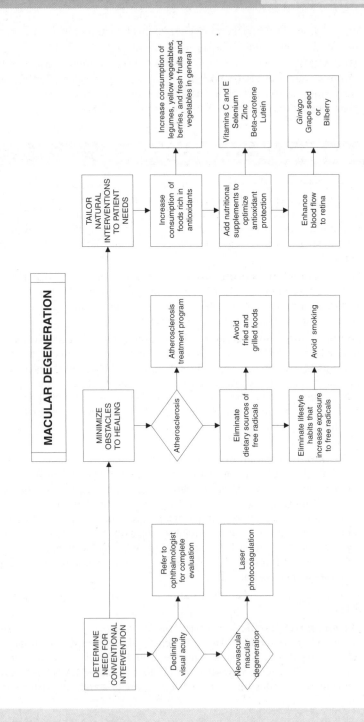

anthocyanidins most useful; *Vaccinium* anthocyanosides have very strong affinity for retinal pigmented epithelium (RPE), the functional portion of retina affect by ARMD – reinforcing collagen structures of retina and preventing free radical damage; *Ginkgo biloba* extract (24% ginkgo flavonglycoside and 6% terpenoids) is a better choice if patient also has signs of cerebrovascular insufficiency; grape seed extract most useful with photophobia or poor night vision.

- **Lifestyle:** oxidant exposure is the major factor in MD; smoking increases risk in men and women.

THERAPEUTIC APPROACH

Prevention or treatment at early stage most effective; treatment for wet form of ARMD is laser photocoagulation ASAP; dry form – use antioxidants and promote retinal blood flow; refer any patient 55 years or older complaining of visual loss to ophthalmologist for complete evaluation, especially if visual loss progressing rapidly.

- **Diet:** avoid fried and grilled foods, and other sources of free radicals; increase legumes (high in sulfur-containing amino acids), yellow vegetables (carotenes), flavonoid-rich berries (blueberries, blackberries, cherries, etc.) and vitamin E- and vitamin C-rich foods (fresh fruits and vegetables).

- **Supplements:**
    — vitamin C: 1 g t.i.d.
    — vitamin E: 600–800 IU q.d.
    — selenium: 400 µg q.d.
    — zinc: 30 mg q.d.
    — beta-carotene (mixed carotenoids recommended): 50,000 IU q.d.
    — lutein: 5 mg q.d.

- **Botanical medicines** (choose one):
    — *Ginkgo biloba* extract (24% ginkgo heterosides): 40–80 mg t.i.d.
    — *Vaccinium myrtillus* (bilberry) extract (25% anthocyanidin content): 40–80 mg t.i.d.
    — grape seed extract (95% procyanidolic content): 150–300 mg q.d.

Male infertility

DIAGNOSTIC SUMMARY

- Inability to conceive child after 6 months of unprotected sex in absence of female causes
- Total sperm count < 5 million/ml
- Presence of > 50% abnormal sperm
- Inability of sperm to impregnate egg as determined by postcoital or hamster egg penetration tests.

GENERAL CONSIDERATIONS

- In US, 15% of couples have difficulty conceiving a child; in 1/3 of cases, the man is responsible; in another 1/3, both responsible; another 1/3, female responsible; 6% of men aged 15–50 are infertile.
- Most male infertility reflects abnormal sperm count (oligospermia) or quality; natural barriers in female reproductive tract allow only 40 of 20 million ejaculated sperm to reach vicinity of egg; strong correlation between number of sperm in ejaculate and fertility; in 90% of oligospermia cases, the reason is deficient sperm production; in 90% of these cases, the cause for decreased sperm formation is unidentified – labeled "idiopathic oligospermia or azoospermia"; azoospermia is the complete absence of living sperm in semen.

Causes of male infertility

- Deficient sperm production
- Ductal obstruction
  - congenital defects
  - post-infectious obstruction
  - cystic fibrosis
  - vasectomy
- Ejaculatory dysfunction
  - premature ejaculation
  - retrograde ejaculation
- Disorders of accessory glands
  - infection
  - inflammation
  - antisperm antibodies

Causes of male infertility

● Coital disorders
  — defects in technique
  — premature withdrawal
  — erectile dysfunction

DIAGNOSTIC CONSIDERATIONS

Semen analysis is the most widely used test of male fertility potential; semen analyzed for concentration of sperm and sperm quality; sperm count and quality in male population deteriorating over last few decades; men now supply 40% of number of sperm per ejaculate compared with 1940 levels.

Possible causes of falling sperm counts

● Increased scrotal temperature
  — tight-fitting clothing and briefs
  — varicoceles are more common
● Environmental
  — increased pollution
  — heavy metals (lead, mercury, arsenic, etc.)
  — organic solvents
  — pesticides (DDT, PCBs, DBCP, etc.)
● Dietary
  — increased saturated fats
  — reduced intake of fruits, vegetables, and whole grains
  — reduced intake of dietary fiber
  — increased exposure to synthetic estrogens

As sperm counts have declined, line differentiating infertile and fertile men has been reduced progressively from 40 million/ml to 5 million/ml; quality more important than quantity – high sperm count meaningless if percentage of healthy sperm not also high.

"Normal" spermatogenesis

Criteria	Value
Volume	1.5–5.0 ml
Density	> 20 million sperm/ml
Motility	> 30% motile
Normal forms	> 60%

If most sperm abnormally shaped or non-motile, the man is infertile despite normal sperm concentration; low sperm count does not always mean a man is infertile.

Causes of temporary low sperm count

- Increased scrotal temperature
- Infections, the common cold, the flu, etc.
- Increased stress
- Lack of sleep
- Overuse of alcohol, tobacco, or marijuana
- Many prescription drugs
- Exposure to radiation
- Exposure to solvents, pesticides, and other toxins

Conventional semen analysis must be interpreted with caution; functional tests indicated when screening couples for in vitro fertilization.

Male fertility tests

Test	Fertility prediction accuracy
Semen analysis	30%
Hamster egg penetration test	66%

- **Postcoital test:** measures ability of sperm to penetrate cervical mucus after intercourse; in vitro variant of this test based on the fact that human sperm can, under appropriate conditions, penetrate hamster eggs; fertile males exhibit range of penetration of 10–100%; penetration < 10% is indicative of infertility.
- **Antisperm antibodies** produced by men attack tail of sperm, impeding motility and penetration of cervical mucus; antibodies produced by women attack head; antibodies in semen are a sign of past or current infection in male reproductive tract.

THERAPEUTIC CONSIDERATIONS

- Standard medical treatment of oligospermia is effective when cause is known (increased scrotal temperature, chronic infection of male sex glands, pharmaceuticals, endocrine disturbances – hypogonadism and hypothyroidism); 90% of cases are idiopathic oligospermia; azoospermia caused by ductal obstruction is surgically correctable.
- Rational approach is to enhance factors promoting spermogenesis; sperm formation is linked to scrotal temperature and nutritional status – healthful diet plus nutritional factors; avoid dietary sources of estrogens; botanicals that increase sperm counts; glandular therapy.

Controlling sperm-damaging factors

Scrotal temperature: normal temperature between 94 and 96°F; above 96°F.

- Sperm production inhibited or halted; mean scrotal temperature higher in infertile than in fertile men; reducing scrotal temperature may be enough make them fertile.

- Best methods: avoid tight-fitting underwear, tight jeans, and hot tubs; avoid exercises that raise scrotal temperature while wearing synthetic fabrics, tight shorts, or tight bikini underwear, e.g. rowing machines, simulated cross-country ski machines, treadmills, and jogging.

- Allow testicles to hang free to recover from heat build-up; wear boxer-type underwear; apply cold shower or ice to scrotum; use "testicular hypothermia device" or "testicle cooler" – must be worn daily during waking hours, fairly comfortable and easy to conceal.

- Rule out varicocele that can increase temperatures high enough to inhibit sperm production and motility – surgical repair may be necessary, but try scrotal cooling first.

Genitourinary infections: major role in many cases; many infections asymptomatic; antisperm antibodies are good indicators of chronic infection; wide range of microbes can infect male GU system.

- ***Chlamydia*** is the most common and serious; major cause of acute non-bacterial prostatitis and urethritis – symptoms are pain/burning upon urination or ejaculation; more serious is *Chlamydia* infection of epididymis and vas deferens – scarring and blockage can occur; antibiotics essential – tetracyclines and erythromycin; because *Chlamydia* lives within host cells, total eradication difficult; chronic infections can be asymptomatic; 28–71% of infertile men have evidence of chlamydial infection; only limited improvements in sperm count and quality; isolated cases of tremendous improvement after antibiotics; both partners should take antibiotic, but should be used only if evidence of chronic infection and recommendations in chapter on chlamydial infections employed for 3+ months; antisperm antibodies may indicate chronic *Chlamydia*; in absence of positive culture, rectal ultrasonography and anti-*Chlamydia* antibodies confirm diagnosis.

Avoiding estrogens: increased exposure to environmental estrogens during fetal development and reproductive years is a major cause of increased disorders of development and function of male sexual system; avoiding hormone-fed animal and milk products is important for male sexual vitality, especially in oligospermia and hypotestosteronemia.

- Estrogens have been detected in drinking water and are harmful to male sexual vitality; presumably recycled synthetic estrogens (birth control pills), which are more potent: do not bind to sex-hormone-binding globulin (SHBG); use purified or bottled water; weakly estrogenic xenobiotics (PCBs, dioxin, DDT) resist biodegradation and are recycled in environment, and interfere with spermatogenesis.

- Greatest impact during fetal development – inhibit multiplication of Sertoli cells: number of Sertoli cells is directly proportional to number of sperm produced; Sertoli cell multiplication occurs during fetal life and before puberty under control of FSH; estrogens inhibit FSH secretion, causing reduced number of Sertoli cells and reduced sperm counts.

● Low-fiber, high-fat diet is linked to higher levels of estrogens because estrogens excreted in bile are reabsorbed.

● If testosterone is low or marginal, or if estrogen elevated, legumes (beans), especially soy foods, may benefit; soy is a good source of isoflavonoids = "phytoestrogens"; soy isoflavonoids have 0.2% of estrogen activity of estradiol; isoflavones bind to estrogen receptors; weak estrogenic action = anti-estrogenic, preventing binding of endogenous estrogen to receptors; phytoestrogens may reduce effects of estrogens by stimulating production of SHBG that binds estrogen; soy, other legumes, nuts and seeds are good sources of phytosterols that aid steroid hormone synthesis, including testosterone.

Heavy metals: sperm susceptible to damage by heavy metals (lead, cadmium, arsenic, mercury); hair mineral analysis indicated on all men with oligospermia.

Nutritional considerations

● **Vitamin C and other antioxidants:** free radical/oxidative damage to sperm is the major cause of idiopathic oligospermia; free radicals are abundant in semen of 40% of infertile men.

— Three factors combine to render sperm susceptible to free radical damage: (1) high membrane concentration of polyunsaturated fatty acids (PUFAs), (2) active generation of free radicals, (3) lack of defensive enzymes.

— Health of sperm is dependent upon antioxidants; men exposed to increased levels of free radicals are more likely to have abnormal sperm and sperm counts; sperm is sensitive to free radicals – dependent upon integrity and fluidity of cell membrane for proper function; improper membrane fluidity activates enzymes that impair motility, structure, and viability of sperm; major determinant of membrane fluidity is concentration of omega-3 PUFAs (DHA), which are very susceptible to free radical damage.

— Sperm have low superoxide dismutase and catalase and generate free radicals to break barriers to fertilization.

— Source of oxidants: smoking and pollutants, linked to decreased sperm counts and motility plus increased abnormal sperm.

— Antioxidants (vitamin C, beta-carotene, selenium, vitamin E) protect sperm; vitamin C protects sperm DNA; ascorbate is much higher in seminal fluid compared with other body fluids, including blood; low dietary vitamin C is likely to lead to infertility; smoking reduces vitamin C throughout the body; non-smokers benefit from vitamin C as much as smokers.

- — Sperm become agglutinated when antibodies bind to them; antibodies to sperm are linked to chronic GU tract or prostatic infection; when > 25% of sperm is agglutinated, fertility is unlikely; vitamin C reduces percentage of agglutinated sperm; vitamin C is very effective in treating male infertility due to antibodies against sperm.
- — Vitamin E is the main antioxidant in sperm membranes – inhibits free radical damage to PUFAs, enhances ability of sperm to fertilize egg in vitro, decreases malondialdehyde in sperm pellet suspensions; dosage = 600–800 IU q.d.

- **Fats and oils:** saturated fats, hydrogenated oils, *trans* fatty acids, and cotton, coconut and palm oil should be avoided; coconut and palm oils are saturated; cotton seed contains toxic pesticide residues plus gossypol, a substance that inhibits sperm function and may be used as male antifertility agent; saturated fats decrease membrane fluidity and interfere with sperm motility; increase omega-3 PUFAs.

- **Zinc:** most critical trace mineral for male sexual function – hormone metabolism plus sperm formation and motility; Zn deficiency decreases testosterone and sperm counts; levels much lower in infertile men with oligospermia; study – supplements increased testosterone and sperm counts in men with infertility > 5 years and resulted in impregnation of wives; RDA = 15 mg; sources: whole grains, legumes, nuts, and seeds; supplement dosage = 45–60 mg q.d.

- **Vitamin B_{12}:** involved in cellular replication; deficiency reduces sperm counts and motility; supplementation without deficiency improves sperm counts in men with < 20 million/ml or motility rate < 50%.

- **Arginine:** required for replication of cells – essential in sperm formation; may be effective treatment of male infertility; critical determinant is the level of oligospermia: if counts < 20 million/ml, arginine is less beneficial; dosage of L-arginine = 4+ g q.d. for 3 months; reserve for use after other nutritional measures have been tried.

- **Carnitine:** transports fatty acids into mitochondria; deficiency reduces energy production from fats; carnitine levels very high in epididymis and sperm – epididymis derives energy requirements from fatty acids, and sperm do so traversing epididymis; motility of ejaculated sperm correlates with carnitine – the higher the carnitine content, the more motile; carnitine deficit reduces sperm development, function and motility; increases sperm count and mobility in idiopathic asthenospermia; dosage = 300–1,000 mg L-carnitine t.i.d.; try other measures first due to high cost.

Botanical medicines

- **Ginseng:** Panax ginseng (Chinese or Korean ginseng) and *Eleutherococcus senticosus* (Siberian ginseng) are effective in male infertility; long history as male "tonics"; Panax promotes growth of testes, increases sperm formation and testosterone levels, and increases sexual activity and mating behavior in studies with animals; Siberian ginseng increases reproductive capacity and sperm counts in bulls; Panax has more potent effects (stimulant) than *Eleutherococcus*; Siberian contains no ginsenosides – not a true ginseng; has many of the same effects but milder than Panax.

● **Pygeum africanum:** improves fertility if diminished prostatic secretion plays significant role; increases prostatic secretions; improves composition of seminal fluid – increases total seminal fluid, alkaline phosphatase and protein; most effective if alkaline phosphatase activity reduced (< 400 IU/cm³) and no evidence of inflammation or infection (no WBCs or IgA); lack of IgA in semen is a good indicator of clinical success; improves capacity to achieve erection in patients with BPH or prostatitis as determined by nocturnal penile tumescence – BPH and prostatitis are often linked to erectile dysfunction and other sexual disturbances.

Glandular therapy

Basic concept underlying using glandular substances from animals = "like heals like"; in hypotestosteronemia or oligospermia, extracts of bovine testicular tissues effective orally because of active hormones; dosage and efficacy vary from one manufacturer to another.

THERAPEUTIC APPROACH

Refer to urologist or fertility specialist for complete evaluation; scrotal cooling – loose cotton underwear, avoid activities that elevate testicular temperature, apply cold water to testes; optimize nutrition (antioxidants and zinc); identify and eliminate environmental pollutants; use fertility-enhancing botanicals.

● **General measures:**
  — maintain scrotal temperatures between 94 and 96°F
  — avoid exposure to free radicals
  — identify and eliminate environmental pollutants
  — stop/reduce all drugs (antihypertensives, anti-neoplastics [cyclophosphamide] and anti-inflammatories [sulfasalazine]).

● **Diet:**
  — avoid dietary free radicals, saturated fats, hydrogenated oils, *trans* fatty acids, and cottonseed oil
  — increase legumes (soy – phytoestrogens and phytosterols), dietary antioxidant vitamins, carotenes, and flavonoids (dark-colored vegetables and fruits), essential fatty acids, and zinc (nuts and seeds)
  — 8 to 10 servings of vegetables, 2–4 servings of fresh fruits, and half a cup of raw nuts or seeds.

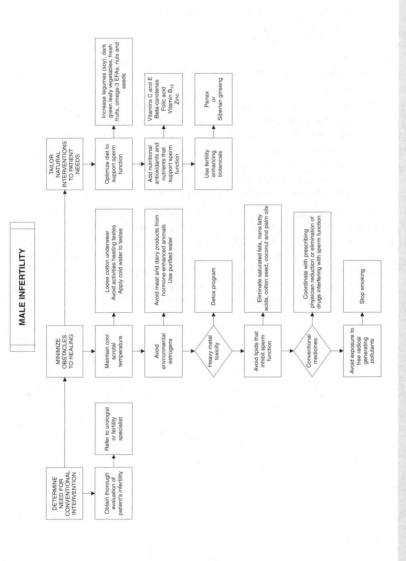

● **Nutritional supplements:**

— multiple vitamin-mineral
— vitamin C: 1,000–3,000 q.d. in divided doses
— vitamin E: 600–800 IU q.d.
— beta-carotene: 100,000–200,000 IU q.d.
— folic acid: 400 µg q.d.
— vitamin B_{12}: 1,000 µg q.d.
— zinc: 30–60 mg q.d.

● **Botanical medicines:**

— Panax ginseng (t.i.d.)
   high-quality crude ginseng root: 1.5–2 g q.d.
   standardized extract (5% ginsenosides): 500 mg
— *Eleutherococcus senticosus* (t.i.d.)
   dried root: 2–4 g
   tincture (1:5): 10–20 ml
   fluid extract (1:1): 2.0–4.0 ml
   solid (dry powdered) extract (20:1): 100–200 mg.

Dosage of ginseng based on ginsenoside content; typical dose (taken t.i.d.) = saponin content of at least 25 mg ginsenosides with ratio Rb1 to Rg1 of 2:1 (for high-quality ginseng root extract containing 5% ginsenosides, dose = 500 mg); response to ginseng is individually unique – observe possible ginseng toxicity (*Textbook*, Ch. 100); begin at lower doses and increase gradually; Russian approach for long-term Panax or Siberian ginseng is to use ginseng cyclically – 15–20 days on, followed by 2 weeks off.

Menopause

DIAGNOSTIC SUMMARY

- Cessation of menstruation in older women for 6–12 months.
- Average age of onset is 51 years.
- Hot flashes in 65–80%.
- Atrophic vaginitis.
- Frequent bladder infections in 15%.

GENERAL CONSIDERATIONS

Causes of menopause: thought to occur when there are no eggs left in the ovaries; at birth, there are about 1 million eggs (ova), which drops to 300,000–400,000 at puberty; only 400 actually mature during reproductive years; absence of active follicles reduces estrogen and progesterone – pituitary increases FSH in large and continuous quantities; LH and FSH cause ovaries and adrenals to secrete androgens which can be converted to estrogens by fat cells of hips and thighs; converted androgens are the source of most circulating estrogen in postmenopausal women; total estrogen is still far below reproductive levels.

Menopause as social construct: social and cultural factors contribute greatly to how women react to menopause; modern society values allure of everlasting youth – cultural devaluing of older women; cultural view of menopause is directly related to symptoms of menopause; if the cultural view is negative, symptoms are common; if menopause is viewed in a positive light, symptoms are less frequent; study of rural Mayan Indians – no woman experienced hot flashes or any other symptom and no woman showed evidence of osteoporosis, despite hormonal patterns identical to postmenopausal women in US; Mayan women saw menopause as a positive event, providing acceptance as a respected elder as well as relief from child-bearing.

Estrogen replacement therapy

Benefits of HRT: relief from hot flashes and other symptoms; reduction in osteoporosis; but dietary, exercise, and lifestyle factors offer identical benefits without risks; short-term (< 6 months) HRT for symptoms only provides temporary relief – not permanent cure and only delays the inevitable; long-term HRT not justified in most women – risks outweigh benefits; exception are women at high risk for osteoporosis; estrogen-progesterone combinations are preferred to estrogen alone; exception are women with or at high risk for disease aggravated by estrogen – breast cancer, active liver diseases, and certain cardiovascular diseases – in which case progesterone alone indicated.

HRT and cancer: most likely form of cancer adversely affected by HRT is breast cancer; estrogen replacement therapy is associated with 1–30% increase in risk of breast cancer; association increases with age and length of use; avoid HRT, except in specific cases (serious osteoporosis).

Types of HRT:

● Estrogen is given alone without progestin = "unopposed estrogen therapy" – high risk for endometrial and other cancers (breast); unopposed estrogen given q.d. or during 25-day cycles separated by 3–6 days without.

● To reduce endometrial cancer, estrogen given in combination with progestin-like progesterone, either cyclically or continuously; cyclical method = estrogen for 25 days and progestin for last 10–12 days of cycle, with 3–6 day hormone-free interval during which bleeding occurs – menstruation continues in 90% of women.

● To prevent monthly bleeding, estrogen and progesterone given q.d. without hormone-free interval = "combined continuous HRT".

● "Natural-type" estrogens preferred to synthetic, e.g.:

— conjugated estrogens (Premarin, Genisis)
— esterified estrogens (Evex, Menest)
— micronized 17-beta-estradiol (Estrace)
— transdermal 17-beta-estradiol (Estraderm, Systen).

● Conjugated estrogens are metabolized in body to active forms (17-beta-estradiol; liver catabolizes active estrogens before they produce effects – large amounts given, since 17-beta-estradiol is not absorbed well orally; absorbed well through skin – estrogen patches and vaginal creams; patches are preferable to conjugated estrogens – approximate body's secretions by delivering 17-beta-estradiol in slow, sustained manner.

● Best form of progesterone is the natural derivative, medroxyprogesterone acetate – preferred to synthetic versions (megesterol, norethindrone, norgestrel); examples of medroxyprogesterone are Provera, Cycrin, and Amen.

Major symptoms

● **Hot flashes:** most common symptoms; can be accompanied by increased heart rate, HAs, dizziness, weight gain, fatigue, and insomnia; 65–80% of menopausal women in US experience hot flashes; often first sign menopause approaching – may begin prior to cessation of menses; in most cases, most uncomfortable in first and second years after menopause; as body adapts to decreased estrogen, hot flashes subside.

- **Atrophic vaginitis:** vaginal lining may become thin and dry from lack of estrogen, causing dyspareunia, increased susceptibility to infection, and vaginal itching or burning; avoid substances which dry mucous membranes (antihistamines, ETOH, caffeine); stay well hydrated; prefer clothes made from natural fibers (cotton); regular intercourse is beneficial – increases blood flow to vaginal tissues, improving tone and lubrication; exogenous lubricant (oil or K-Y Jelly) essential.

- **Bladder infections:** 15% of menopausal women experience frequent cystitis from breakdown in natural defenses which protect against UTIs; primary goal is to enhance normal host protective measures—increasing flow of urine via proper hydration, promoting pH inhibiting microbial growth, and preventing bacterial adherence to bladder endothelium.

- **Cold hands and feet:** common to women in general; three major causes: hypothyroidism, low iron, and poor circulation; use basal body temperature test (*Textbook*, App. 8) to evaluate functional thyroid activity; serum ferritin is the best indicator of body Fe stores; also CBC and chemistry panel, with LDL/HDL cholesterol; complete physical exam attending to any other signs of vascular insufficiency; treat identified cause directly.

- **Forgetfulness with inability to concentrate:** common symptoms of menopause; may result from decreased oxygen and nutrient supply to brain.

Role of hypothalamus and endorphins

Many symptoms result from altered function of hypothalamus, the bridge between CNS and endocrine system; hypothalamus is responsible for control of body temperature, metabolic rate, sleep patterns, reactions to stress, libido, mood, and release of pituitary hormones; endorphins critical to proper functioning of hypothalamus; exercise and acupuncture enhance endorphin output.

THERAPEUTIC CONSIDERATIONS

Natural approach is to improve physiology via diet, exercise, nutritional supplements, and botanical medicines.

Baseline evaluation of menopausal woman (to be repeated annually):

- detailed personal and family medical history
- breast exam and instructions on self-exam
- pelvic exam
- lab tests

- complete blood count
- blood chemistry panel
- cholesterol evaluation: HDL, LDL, and VLDL
- thyroid function panel, including T_3, T_4, and TSH
- baseline mammography (if indicated)
- baseline bone densitometry.

Bone density studies can be used as a gauge as to whether HRT is necessary.

Diet

Increase plant foods, especially phytoestrogens; reduce animal foods; consume fruit and vegetables.

- **Phytoestrogen-containing foods:** fennel, celery, and parsley (Umbelliferae) contain phytoestrogens; fennel has confirmed estrogenic action; soy, nuts, whole grains, apples, and alfalfa also have phytoestrogens; lignins and isoflavonoids are converted by intestinal bacteria to diphenolic estrogenic compounds which decrease hot flashes, increase maturation of vaginal cells and may inhibit osteoporosis; decrease breast, colon, and prostate cancer.

- **Soy:** isoflavones (genistein) and phytosterols of soybeans have mild estrogenic effect; 1 cup soybeans has 300 mg isoflavone = 0.45 mg conjugated estrogens = one tablet Premarin; associated with reduced risk of cancer; increase number of superficial cells lining the vagina. This increase offsets the vaginal drying and irritation that are common in postmenopausal women; the lower the protein content, the higher the level of isoflavonoids; products from whole soybeans are higher in isoflavonoids than those from soy protein concentrates; protects LDL from oxidation – preventing cardiovascular disease.

- **Dietary fat:** positive correlation between breast cancer risk and saturated fat intake in postmenopausal women; total caloric intake not linked to increased risk to breast cancer.

Nutritional supplements

- **Vitamin E:** relieves hot flashes and menopausal vaginal complaints compared with placebo; improves not only symptoms, but also blood supply to vaginal wall when taken for 4+ weeks; 400 IU q.d. is effective in 50% of postmenopausal women with atrophic vaginitis; vitamin E oil, creams, ointments, or suppositories are used topically to provide symptomatic relief of atrophic vaginitis; effective in relieving dryness and irritation of atrophic vaginitis.

- **Hesperidin and vitamin C:** hesperidin improves vascular integrity and relieves capillary permeability; combined with vitamin C, citrus flavonoids

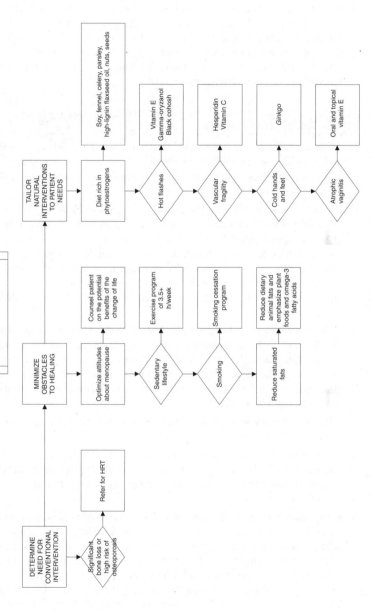

MENOPAUSE

DETERMINE NEED FOR CONVENTIONAL INTERVENTION

Significant bone loss or high risk of osteoporosis → Refer for HRT

MINIMIZE OBSTACLES TO HEALING

Optimize attitudes about menopause → Counsel patient on the potential benefits of the change of life

Sedentary lifestyle → Exercise program of 3.5+ h/week

Smoking → Smoking cessation program

Reduce saturated fats → Reduce dietary animal fats and emphasize plant foods and omega-3 fatty acids

TAILOR NATURAL INTERVENTIONS TO PATIENT NEEDS

Diet rich in phytoestrogens → Soy, fennel, celery, parsley, high-lignin flaxseed oil, nuts, seeds

Hot flashes → Vitamin E Gamma-oryzanol Black cohosh

Vascular fragility → Hesperidin Vitamin C

Cold hands and feet → Ginkgo

Atrophic vaginitis → Oral and topical vitamin E

may relieve hot flashes, nocturnal leg cramps, nose bleeds, and easy bruising.

● **Gamma-oryzanol (ferulic acid):** a growth-promoting substance in grains and isolated from rice bran oil, it enhances pituitary function and promotes endorphin release by the hypothalamus; helpful in women with post-oophorectomy menopause; extremely safe natural substance; no significant side-effects produced in experimental and clinical studies; lowers blood cholesterol and triglyceride levels.

Botanical medicines

● **"Uterine tonics"** are beneficial; effects are from phytoestrogens and the ability to improve blood flow to female organs; nourish and tone female glandular and organ system = non-specific mode of action making many botanicals useful.

● **Phytoestrogens:** not associated with adverse side-effects; very effective in inhibiting mammary tumors – by occupying estrogen receptors and by other unrelated anticancer mechanisms; estrogenic effects only 2% as strong as estrogens; low activity has balancing action – if estrogen is low, phytoestrogen effect will counterbalance this; if high, phytoestrogen binding to estrogen receptors competes with estrogen, decreasing estrogen effects; this balancing action allows the same plants to be used for PMS and menopause.

● *Angelica sinensis* **(Dong Quai):** historical use in Asia for hot flashes (*Textbook*, Ch. 65); good uterine tonic, causing initial increase in uterine contraction followed by relaxation; increases uterine weight and glucose utilization by liver and uterus in lab animals – reflect estrogenic activities; efficacy may be based on mild estrogenic effects and other components acting to stabilize blood vessels.

● *Glycyrrhiza glabra* **(licorice):** estrogen-like activity responsible for many of its beneficial effects (*Textbook*, Ch. 90).

● *Vitex agnus-castus* **(chaste tree):** native to Mediterranean; berries historically used for female complaints; profound effects on pituitary function; beneficial effects in menopause may be due to altering LH and FSH secretion (*Textbook*, Ch. 123).

● *Cimicifuga racemosa* **(black cohosh):** widely used by American Indians and later by American colonists for menstrual cramps and menopause; relieves hot flashes, depression and vaginal atrophy; noticeable benefits within 4 weeks after beginning cimicifuga therapy; after 6–8 weeks complete resolution of symptoms achieved in most patients; very well tolerated; only 7–10% of patients report mild transitory stomach complaints or other mild side-effects; no contraindications or limitations of use – suitable natural alternative to HRT for menopause, especially when HRT is contraindicated (e.g. in history of cancer, unexplained uterine bleeding, liver and gall bladder disease, pancreatitis, endometriosis, uterine fibroids, or fibro-cystic breast disease (*Textbook*, Ch. 75).

- ***Ginkgo biloba***: indicated for its effects on vascular system; useful in improving cold hands and feet, and forgetfulness accompanying menopause; improves blood flow to hands and feet in human clinical trials; effective in treating peripheral vascular disease of extremities; improves mental health in patients with cerebral vascular insufficiency and may exert similar effects in menopause; increases blood flow to brain; enhances energy production within brain, increasing uptake of glucose by neurons, and improving transmission of nerve signals – transmission rate of nerve signals is critically important to memory, which is directly related to speed at which nerve impulse can be transmitted; improves memory in elderly and college-aged women: should be taken consistently for at least 12 weeks to determine effectiveness.

Lifestyle factors

- **Exercise:** clinical studies indicate that regular physical exercise decreases frequency and severity of hot flashes: women exercising can pass through a natural menopause without HRT; physically active women who have no hot flashes whatsoever spend 3.5 h/week exercising; women who exercise less are more likely to have hot flashes; regular exercise also beneficial to mood, bone health, and cardiovascular wellness.
- **Cigarette smoking:** greatly increases risk of early menopause – double the risk of menopause between ages 44 and 55; former smokers have lower risk, showing partial reversal of effect.

THERAPEUTIC APPROACH

In most cases, HRT is unnecessary; for women at high risk for osteoporosis or with already documented significant bone loss, HRT may be indicated; for atrophic vaginitis, use topical vitamin E; if the woman is smoking, facilitate smoking cessation program.

- **Diet:** increase phytoestrogens – soyfoods; fennel, celery, parsley; high-lignin flaxseed oil; nuts and seeds.
- **Supplements:**
    - vitamin E: 800 IU q.d. until symptoms improve, then 400 IU q.d.
    - hesperidin: 900 mg q.d.
    - vitamin C: 1,200 mg q.d.
    - gamma-oryzanol: 300 mg q.d.
- **Botanical medicines (t.i.d.):**
    - *Angelica sinensis*:

powdered root or as tea: 1–2 g
tincture (1:5): 4 ml (1 tsp)
fluid extract: 1 ml (1/4 tsp)

— *Glycyrrhiza glabra*:
powdered root or as tea: 1–2 g
fluid extract (1:1): 4 ml (1 tsp)
solid (dry powdered) extract (4:1): 250–500 mg

— *Vitex agnus-castus*:
powdered berries or as tea: 1–2 g
fluid extract (1:1): 4 ml (1 tsp)
solid (dry powdered) extract (4:1): 250–500 mg

— *Cimicifuga racemosa*:
powdered rhizome: 1–2 g
tincture (1:5): 4–6 ml
fluid extract (1:1): 3–4 ml (1 tsp)
solid (dry powdered) extract (4:1): 250–500 mg

— Standardized extract:
dosage should provide 1–2 µg of 2% deoxyacteine b.d.

— *Ginkgo biloba* extract:
24% ginkgo flavonglycoside content: 40 mg.

● **Lifestyle:** regular exercise program – at least 30 min three times a week.

Menorrhagia

DIAGNOSTIC SUMMARY

● Excessive menstrual bleeding, i.e. blood loss > 80 ml, occurring at regular cyclical intervals (cycles are usually, but not necessarily, of normal length).
● Often caused by local lesions, e.g. uterine myomas (fibroids), endometrial polyps, endometrial hyperplasia, adenomyosis, and endometritis.

GENERAL CONSIDERATIONS

Menorrhagia is largely subjective – objective measure of blood loss rarely done; poor correlation between measured blood loss and patient assessment of bleeding; patients with menorrhagia have increased menstrual blood flow during first 3 days (up to 92% of total menses lost at this time) – mechanisms responsible for ceasing menses as effective in women with menorrhagia as in normal women, despite very high blood loss.

● **Etiology:** consult gynecology textbook to rule out pathological causes.

Pathological causes of menorrhagia

Cause	Possible etiology
Anovulation	Excessive estrogen
	Failure of midcycle surge of LH
	Hypothyroidism
	Hyperprolactinemia
	Polycystic ovarian disease
Intrauterine structural defects	Fibroids
	Polyps
	Cancer
	Ectopic pregnancy
	Intrauterine devices
Bleeding disorders	See table on hemorrhagic disorders (below)

● **Abnormalities of prostaglandin metabolism:** menorrhagic endometrium incorporates arachidonic acid (AA) into neutral lipids to much greater extent than normal, while incorporation into phospholipids is decreased; increased AA release during menses increases production of series 2 prostaglandins, a major factor in excess bleeding and dysmenorrhea; excess bleeding during first 3 days due to vasodilatory properties of PGE_2 and PGI_2 and anti-aggregating activity of PGI_2; pain of dysmenorrhea due to overproducing $PGF_{2\alpha}$.

● **Other contributing factors:** iron deficiency, hypothyroidism, vitamin A deficiency, intrauterine devices, local factors (uterine myomas, endometrial polyps, adenomyosis, endometrial hyperplasia, salpingitis, endometritis).

● **Estimating menstrual blood loss:** no correlation between measured blood loss and number of pads used during each period and duration of period; a woman's assessment of her blood loss is very subjective (40% of women with loss > 80 ml felt periods were only moderately heavy/scanty, while 14% of those with loss < 20 ml felt periods were heavy); serum ferritin may be best indicator of excessive menstrual blood loss.

THERAPEUTIC CONSIDERATIONS

● **Psychological:** subjective nature of complaint – psychological component may be etiological; but women complaining of menorrhagia more likely to receive antidepressant and more likely to have hysterectomy; iron deficiency and thyroid insufficiency can disturb mood (see chapter on affective disorders); many women have had needless hysterectomy, uterine curettage, and/or antidepressant medication; rule out organic factors first.

● **Iron deficiency:** blood loss > 60 ml/period causes negative Fe balance; chronic Fe deficiency can cause menorrhagia:
   — many patients without organic pathosis respond well to Fe supplements alone
   — high rate of organic pathosis (fibroids, polyps, adenomyosis) in patients unresponsive to Fe supplements
   — serum iron levels rise in many patients given Fe supplements
   — less response to Fe therapy when initial serum Fe is high
   — menorrhagia correlates with depleted tissue Fe stores (bone marrow) irrespective of serum Fe level
   — 75% of patients on Fe supplements improve, compared with 32.5% on placebo.

Hematological screening and serum ferritin (first to indicator of decreased Fe levels) are essential; iron supplementation: dose = 100 mg elemental Fe q.d. = prophylactic therapy to prevent menorrhagia and depletion of Fe-containing enzymes before hematological changes observed; decreased serum ferritin is a good indicator of need for Fe supplementation.

● **Vitamin A:** serum retinol is significantly lower in women with menorrhagia than healthy controls; 25,000 IU vitamin A b.i.d. × 15 days can reduce or normalize blood loss in such patients.

● **Vitamin C and bioflavonoids:** capillary fragility is believed to play a role in many cases of menorrhagia; vitamin C (200 mg t.i.d.) and bioflavonoids can reduce menorrhagia; vitamin C increases Fe absorption – therapeutic effect may be also due to enhanced Fe absorption.

● **Vitamin E:** free radicals may play a causative role in endometrial bleeding, particularly with intrauterine device; vitamin E (100 IU every 2 days) has improved patients within 10 weeks; vitamin E may work via antioxidant activity or prostaglandin metabolism.

● **Vitamin K and chlorophyll:** although bleeding time and prothrombin levels are usually normal in menorrhagia, vitamin K (crude preparations of chlorophyll) has clinical and limited research support; also, some women may have inherited or acquired bleeding disorder.

Acquired generalized hemorrhagic disorders

Factor	Possible cause
Deficiency of vitamin K	Low intake, impaired absorption, antimicrobial inhibition of gut flora that synthesize vitamin K
Drug-induced hemorrhage	Heparin, warfarin
Dysproteinemias	Myeloma, macroglobinemia
Disseminated intravascular coagulation	
Severe hepatic disease	
Circulating inhibitors of coagulation	
Primary fibrinolysis	

● **Thyroid abnormalities:** overt hypothyroidism or hyperthyroidism is linked to menstrual disturbances; minimal thyroid dysfunction (minimal subclinical insufficiency, determined by thyroid stimulation [TRH] test) may cause menorrhagia; such patients may respond dramatically to thyroxine; patients with long-standing menstrual dysfunction (and no obvious uterine pathosis) may need TRH testing.

● **Essential fatty acids:** majority of tissue arachidonic acid derived from diet; reducing dietary animal products and increasing linoleic, linolenic and dihomo-gamma-linolenic acid may curtail blood loss by decreasing AA.

● **Botanicals:**
   — *Geranium maculatum*
   — *Trillium pendulum*
   — *Areca catechu*
   — *Caulophyllum thalictroides*
   — *Hamamelis virginiana*
   — *Capsella bursa pastoris* (shepherd's purse)

Shepherd's purse historically used to manage obstetric/gynecologic hemorrhage; effective in menorrhagia due to functional abnormalities and fibroids; hemostatic action may be due to high oxalic and dicarboxylic acids.

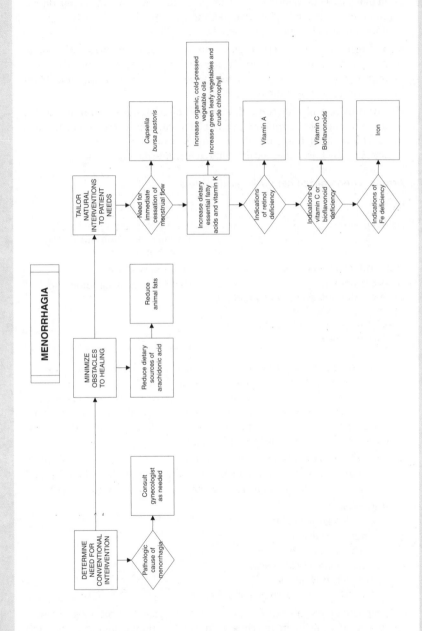

Reserve botanicals for intractable cases, situations requiring immediate cessation of blood loss, and/or as a short-term adjunct to above-mentioned therapies.

THERAPEUTIC APPROACH

Rule out serious pathological causes; if functional – test prothrombin time, hematological status, and thyroid function; correct abnormalities as indicated; quantitative measuring of blood loss should be worked out with patient; serum ferritin can help monitor progress.

● **Diet:** low in sources of arachidonic acid (animal fats); high in linolenic and linoleic acids (vegetable oil sources); green leafy vegetables and other sources of vitamin K.

● **Supplements (q.d.):**
  — vitamin C: 1,000 mg
  — bioflavonoids: 250 mg
  — vitamin A: 25,000 IU
  — vitamin E: 200 IU
  — chlorophyll: 25 mg (use a crude form)
  — iron: 25 mg.

● **Botanical medicine:**
  — *Capsella bursa pastoris*: 1 tsp/cup t.i.d. if needed to control very heavy bleeding.

Migraine headache

DIAGNOSTIC SUMMARY

- Recurrent, paroxysmal attacks of headache.
- Headache is typically pounding and unilateral, but may become generalized.
- Attacks often preceded by psychological or visual disturbances; accompanied by anorexia, nausea, and gastrointestinal upset; and followed by drowsiness.

GENERAL CONSIDERATIONS

Migraine HAs are caused by excessive dilation of blood vessel in the head; affect 15–20% of men and 25–30% of women; more than half of patients have family history of migraine; can occur without warning or with warning symptoms (auras); auras last a few minutes and include: blurring or bright spots in vision, anxiety, fatigue, disturbed thinking, and numbness or tingling on one side of body.

- Vascular HA pain – throbbing or pounding sharp pain; non-vascular HA (tension HA) pain – steady, constant, dull pain starting at back of head or in forehead and spreading over entire head, giving sensation of pressure or vise grip applied to skull.
- Pain of HA comes from outside brain because brain tissue does not have sensory nerves; pain arises from meninges and scalp plus blood vessels and muscles when these are stretched or tensed.
- Most common non-vascular HA is the tension HA, caused by tightened muscles of face, neck, or scalp, resulting from stress or poor posture; tightened muscles pinch nerve or its blood supply, causing pain and pressure; relaxation of muscle usually brings immediate relief.

Classification and diagnosis

Migraine classification

	Common	Classic	Complicated
Incidence	80%	10%	10%

(continued over)

(continued)

	Common	Classic	Complicated
Pain	Frontal, uni/bilateral	Unilateral	Unpredictable, may be absent
Aura	Unusual	0.5 h, striking	Neurological aura, vertigo, syncope, diplopia, hemiparesis
Duration of headache	1–3 days	2–6 h	Unpredictable
Physical examination	Unhappiness	Pallor, vomiting	Mild neurological signs, speech disorder, hemi-paresis, unsteadiness, cranial nerve III palsy

- **Cluster HA** once considered migraine-type since vasodilation is a key component; now separately classified; also called histamine cephalgia, Horton's HA, or atypical facial neuralgia; much less common than migraine.
- **Chronic daily HA (CDH):** 40% of patients in HA clinics; also called chronic tension HA, migraine with interparoxysmal HA, transformed migraine, evolutive migraine, mixed HA syndrome, tension-vascular HA.

Types of chronic daily headache

- Transformed migraine
  — drug-induced
  — non-drug-induced
- Chronic tension-type headache
- New daily persistent headache
- Post-traumatic headache

Pathophysiology

Migraine linked to vasomotor instability; mechanisms unknown.

- **Vasomotor instability:** superficial temporal vessels visibly dilated; local compression of these vessels or carotid artery temporarily relieves pain; other types of extracranial vasodilation (heat- or exercise-induced) not problematic; patients pale during HA despite extracranial vasodilation and lower skin temperature of affected side suggests constriction of small vessels = intracranial vasoconstriction; greatly reduced blood flow during prodromal stage, followed by stage of increased blood flow persisting for > 48 h; decreased regional cerebral blood flow in classic, but not common, migraine; abnormal blood flow confined to cerebral cortex, while deeper structures perfused normally; may involve inherited abnormality of vasomotor control: patients have orthostatic symptoms more often than normal, and are abnormally sensitive to vasodilatory physical and chemical agents.

- **Platelet disorder:** migraine platelet shows increased spontaneous aggregation, different manner of serotonin release, and different platelet composition; Hanington theory: most common precipitant of migraine is stressor causing increased plasma catecholamine, triggering serotonin release, platelet aggregation and vasoconstriction; migraine platelets aggregate more readily than normal, spontaneously and when exposed to serotonin, adenosine diphosphate and catecholamines (similar to transient cerebral ischemic attacks – TIAs); attack onset accompanied by elevated plasma serotonin, followed by increased urinary 5-hydroxyindoleacetic acid (5-HIAA – breakdown product of serotonin metabolism); blood serotonin is normally stored in platelets and released by aggregation and in response to stimuli (catecholamines); total serotonin content in normal and migraine platelets is identical; quantity of serotonin released by migraine platelets, in response to serotonin stimulation, is normal (or subnormal) after attack, but progressively higher as next attack approaches; classic migraine patients have twofold increase in incidence of mitral valve prolapse; prolapsing mitral valve damages platelets and increases aggregation.

- **Neuronal disorder:** theory – trigeminovascular neurons, which innervate pial arteries, release peptide substance P either in direct response to initiators or secondarily to changes in CNS; substance P is a mediator of pain, released into arteries, linked to vasodilation, mast cell degranulation, and increased vascular permeability; arterial endothelial cells may respond to substance P by releasing vasoactive substances; functional changes within noradrenergic system may be threshold for migraine activation; potentiators may exert effects by modulating sympathetic activity; chronic stress is a potentiator in this model.

- **Migraine as a "serotonin deficiency" syndrome:** increased 5-HIAA in urine during migraine; cause is increased breakdown of serotonin due to increased activity of monoamine oxidase (MAO); migraine sufferers have low tissue serotonin: migraine is a "low serotonin syndrome"; low serotonin may cause decreased pain threshold; positive clinical results with serotonin precursor 5-hydroxytryptophan (5-HTP) (*Textbook*, Ch.92); link between low serotonin and HA is the basis of many migraine prescription drugs; monoamine oxidase inhibitors (which increase serotonin) prevent HAs; increasing serotonin relieves chronic migraines; 5-HTP in preventing migraine – increased serotonin produced over time decreases sensitivity of migraine-triggering $5-HT_{1c}$ serotonin receptors and increases sensitivity for migraine-inhibiting $5-HT_{1d}$ receptors – lowered tendency to experience HA; 5-HTP is more effective over time (better results after 60 days of use than after 30).

- **Unified hypothesis:** three-stage process of migraine – initiation, prodrome, and headache; initiation dependent on accumulation over time of several stressors that ultimately affect serotonin metabolism; at critical point of susceptibility (or threshold), cascade event initiated; susceptibility is a combination of decreased tissue serotonin, platelet changes, altered responsiveness of key cerebrovascular end-organs, increased sensitivity of intrinsic noradrenergic system of brain, and build-up of histamine, arachidonic acid metabolites, or other mediators of inflammation; platelet changes – increased adhesiveness, enhanced tendency to release serotonin, and increased membrane arachidonic acid; when platelets are stimulated to secrete serotonin, platelet aggregation, vasospasm, and inflammatory processes cause local cerebral ischemia; this is followed by rebound vasodilation and release of peptide substance P and other mediators of pain.

THERAPEUTIC CONSIDERATIONS

Identify precipitating factor; food intolerance/allergy is the most important; many other factors are primary causes or contributors; assess role HA medicines play, especially in chronic HAs.

Drug reaction

Seventy per cent of patients with CDH suffer from drug-induced HAs; there are two main forms of drug-induced CDH: analgesic rebound HA and ergotamine rebound HA; withdrawal of medicine induces prompt improvement in most cases.

Analgesic-rebound headache (A-RHA):   should be suspected in any patient with chronic headaches who is taking large quantities of analgesics and experiencing daily predictable HA; critical dosage leading to A-RHA = 1,000 mg acetaminophen or aspirin; analgesic medicines typically contain additional substances (caffeine or sedative like butabarbital) – further contribute to problem and may lead to withdrawal HA, nausea, abdominal cramps, diarrhea, restlessness, sleeplessness, and anxiety; withdrawal symptoms start at 24–48 h and subside in 5–7 days.

Ergotamine-rebound headache (E-RHA):   ergotamine is the most widely used drug for severe acute migraine and cluster HAs; works by constricting blood vessels of head, preventing or relieving excessive dilation responsible for HA pain; administered i.m., by inhalation, or by suppository – poorly absorbed if given orally; quite effective, but associated with side-effects.

● Symptoms of acute poisoning include: vomiting, diarrhea, dizziness, rise or fall of blood pressure, slow/weak pulse, dyspnea, convulsions, and loss of consciousness.

● Symptoms of chronic poisoning are those resulting from blood vessel contraction and reduced circulation (numbness and coldness of extremities, tingling, chest pain, heart valve lesions, hair loss, decreased urination, and gangrene of fingers and toes) and those resulting from nervous system disturbances (vomiting, diarrhea, HA, tremors, contractions of facial muscles, and convulsions).

● Regular ergotamine use in migraine is linked to dependency syndrome – severe chronic HA with increased HA intensity – upon ceasing medicine; most migraines rarely occur more than once or twice a week – presence of daily migraine-type HA in persons taking ergotamine is a good clue for E-RHA; dosage can be a clue – weekly dosages > 10 mg (some patients take 10–15 mg q.d.).

● Stopping ergotamine causes predictable, protracted, debilitating HA with nausea and vomiting within 72 h and may last another 72 h; improvement after cessation is common; ginger may lessen ergotamine withdrawal symptoms.

Diet

Food allergy/intolerance: plays role in many cases; detection and removal of allergens/intolerant foods will eliminate or greatly reduce symptoms in majority of patients (success ranges from 30 to 93%); incidence of food allergy similar for the three major types of migraine; mechanism unknown; several theories:

● idiopathic response to a pharmacologically active substance, such as tyramine

● monoamine oxidase deficiency

● platelet phenolsulfotransferase deficiency; immunologically mediated food allergy

● platelet abnormalities, etc.

Egger theory – chronic alteration of non-specific responsiveness of cerebral vascular end-organ via long-term antigenic stimulation (analogous to asthmatic response of bronchioles to exercise or cold after antigen contact); food allergies cause platelet degranulation and serotonin release; lab detection of food allergies is most convenient for patient; challenge testing is most reliable, but there is delayed response, requiring several days of repeated challenge; ingestion of large amounts of several foods is needed to detect the marginally reactive.

Dietary amines: chocolate, cheese, beer, and wine precipitate migraines – contain histamine and/or other vasoactive compounds triggering migraines in sensitive individuals by causing blood vessels to expand.

● Red wine is more problematic than white wine due to 20–200 times the amount of histamine, and stimulates release of vasoactive compounds by platelets; much higher in flavonoids – inhibits enzyme (phenolsulfotransferase) which breaks down serotonin and other vasoactive amines in platelets; migraine sufferers have much lower levels of this enzyme; high vasoactive amine foods (cheese, chocolate) worsen problem.

- Standard treatment of histamine-induced HA is histamine-free diet plus vitamin B_6.

- Enzyme diamine oxidase, which breaks down histamine in small intestine mucosa before absorption into circulation, influences whether a person reacts to dietary histamine; persons sensitive to dietary histamine have less of this enzyme than controls; diamine oxidase is vitamin B_6-dependent – compounds inhibiting B_6 also inhibit diamine oxidase = food coloring agents (hydrazine dyes: FD&C yellow #5), drugs (isoniazid, hydralazine, dopamine, penicillamine), birth control pills, ETOH, and excessive protein intake – yellow dye #5 (tartrazine) is consumed in greater quantities (15 g q.d.) than RDA for vitamin B_6 (2.0 mg for males and 1.6 mg for females).

- Vitamin B_6 (1 mg/kg body weight) improves histamine tolerance, presumably by increasing diamine oxidase activity; women have lower diamine oxidase – may explain higher incidence of histamine-induced HAs; women are more frequently intolerant of red wine; level of diamine oxidase in women increases by over 500 times during pregnancy – common for women with histamine-induced HAs to experience complete remission during pregnancy.

Nutritional supplements

- **5-HTTP:** increases endorphins; at least as effective as other pharmacological agents used to prevent migraine; much safer and better tolerated; dosage = 200–600 mg q.d. (*Textbook*, Ch. 92).

- **EFAs and arachidonic acid:** little research attention; platelet aggregation and arachidonic acid metabolites play major role mediating events causing prodromal cerebral ischemia; manipulating dietary EFAs may be very useful; reducing animal fats and increasing fish significantly change platelet and membrane EFA ratios and decrease platelet aggregation.

- **Riboflavin:** another hypothesis – migraines caused by reduced energy production within mitochondria of cerebral blood vessels; riboflavin can increase mitochondrial energy efficiency; dosage = 400 mg q.d. for 3+ months; improved patients 68.2% as determined by migraine severity score used by researchers; no side-effects reported.

- **Magnesium:** low Mg is linked to migraine and tension HAs; low brain and tissue Mg found in patients with migraines; key Mg functions are to maintain tone of blood vessels and prevent overexcitability of nerve cells; Mg supplements may only be effective in patients with low tissue or low ionized levels of Mg; low tissue Mg is common in migraine patients – unnoticed because serum Mg is normal, but is unreliable indicator because most body Mg stores are intracellular; low serum Mg is an end-stage deficiency; use red blood cell (erythrocyte) Mg and ionized Mg^{2+} (most biologically active form) in serum; Mg improves mitral valve prolapse that can damage platelets, causing release of histamine, platelet-activating factor, and serotonin; 85% of patients with mitral valve prolapse have chronic Mg deficiency; oral Mg improves mitral valve prolapse; Mg bound to citrate, malate, aspartate, or other Krebs cycle compound is better absorbed and tolerated than inorganic forms with laxative effect; use 50 mg vitamin B_6 q.d. to increase intracellular Mg.

● **Intravenous magnesium for acute migraine:** extremely effective in some cases of acute migraine, tension, and cluster HAs; dosage = 1–3 g i.v. Mg (over 10-min period); 90% success rate in patients with low ionized Mg^{2+}.

Physical medicine

Effective in shortening duration and decreasing intensity of an attack, but relatively ineffective in actually curing this disorder.

● **Cervical manipulation:** no influence on frequency of recurrence, duration, or disability; greater reduction in pain associated with attacks.

● **Temporomandibular joint dysfunction syndrome (TMJ):** incidence of migraine in patients with TMJ is similar to that in general population; incidence of HA due to muscle tension is much higher; correction of TMJ dysfunction may be useful in treating migraine, but it is far more important in muscle tension HAs.

● **Transcutaneous electrical stimulation (TENS):** TENS is effective in migraine and muscle tension HAs (55% responded to treatment vs. 18% placebo response); inappropriately applied TENS (TENS applied below perception threshold) is ineffective.

● **Acupuncture:** relieves migraine pain; mechanism of relief is not endorphin-mediated; acupuncture increases endorphins in controls, but low levels of serum endorphins in migraine patients do not increase with treatment; mechanism may be via normalization of serotonin levels; effective in relieving pain when it normalizes serotonin levels, but ineffective in relieving pain and raising serotonin in patients with very low serotonin; some success reducing frequency of migraine attacks – 40% of subjects experienced 50–100% reduction in severity and frequency in one study; five treatments (over period of 1 month) decreased recurrence in 45% of patients over period of 6 months.

● **Biofeedback and relaxation therapy:** most widely used non-drug therapy for migraine headaches is thermal biofeedback and relaxation response training; as effective as drug approach, but was without side-effects.

Botanical medicines

● *Tanacetum parthenium* **(feverfew):** 70% of surveyed migraine sufferers eating feverfew q.d. for prolonged periods claimed decreased

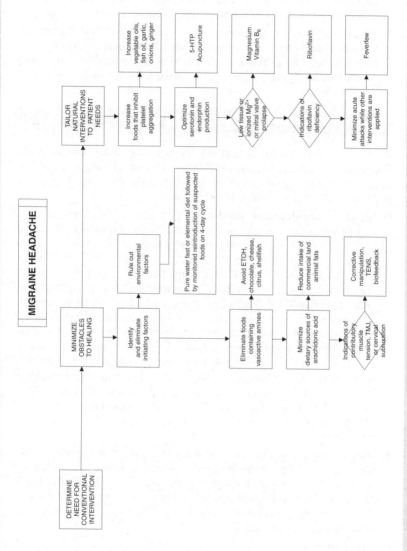

MIGRAINE HEADACHE

DETERMINE NEED FOR CONVENTIONAL INTERVENTION

MINIMIZE OBSTACLES TO HEALING

Identify and eliminate initiating factors

Rule out environmental factors

Pure water fast or elemental diet followed by monitored reintroduction of suspected foods on 4-day cycle

Eliminate foods containing vasoactive amines

Avoid ETOH, chocolate, cheese, citrus, shellfish

Minimize dietary sources of arachidonic acid

Reduce intake of commercial land animal fats

Indications of contributory muscle tension, TMJ, or cervical subluxation

Corrective manipulation, TENS, biofeedback

TAILOR NATURAL INTERVENTIONS TO PATIENT NEEDS

Increase foods that inhibit platelet aggregation

Increase vegetable oils, fish oil, garlic, onions, ginger

Optimize serotonin and endorphin production

5-HTP
Acupuncture

Low tissue or ionized Mg^{2+} or mitral valve prolapse

Magnesium
Vitamin B_6

Indications of riboflavin deficiency

Riboflavin

Minimize acute attacks while other interventions are applied

Feverfew

frequency and/or intensity of attacks (many of these patients unresponsive to orthodox medicines); studies indicate feverfew treats and prevents migraine by inhibiting release of blood vessel-dilating substances from platelets, inhibiting production of inflammatory substances, and re-establishing proper blood vessel tone; efficacy of - feverfew is dependent upon adequate parthenolide, its active principle.

- **Zingiber officinalis (ginger):** root has significant effects against inflammation and platelet aggregation; much anecdotal information on migraine, but little clinical evidence; most active anti-inflammatory components are found in fresh preparations and ginger oil.

THERAPEUTIC APPROACH

Migraine is a multifaceted disease; may be symptom rather than a disease; determine which factors are responsible for each patient's migraine process; identification of precipitating factors and avoidance thereof reduce frequency; avoidance reduces cumulative effect of initiators.

- **Identify problematic foods:** high incidence (80–90%) of food allergy/intolerance in migraine warrants 1 week of careful avoidance of all foods to which patient may be allergic/intolerant – pure water fast or elemental diet (oligoantigenic diet may be used but is less desirable, since allergens may be inadvertently included); avoid all other possible allergens (vitamin preparations, unnecessary drugs, herbs); food-sensitive patients will exhibit strong exacerbation of symptoms early in the week, followed by almost total relief by the end of fast/modified diet – this sequence is due to addictive characteristic of reactive foods; when patient symptom-free, one new food reintroduced (and eaten several times) q.d. with symptoms carefully recorded; some recommend reintroduction on 4–day cycle; suspected foods (symptom onset ranges from 20 min to 2 weeks) eliminated, and apparently safe foods rotated through 4–day cycle (*Textbook*, Ch. 58); when symptom-free period of at least 6 months is established, 4-day rotation diet is no longer necessary.

- **Diet:** eliminate food allergens; use 4-day rotation diet until patient symptom-free for 6 months; eliminate foods containing vasoactive amines and reintroduce carefully after symptoms controlled; eliminate ETOH, cheese, chocolate, citrus fruits, and shellfish; reduce sources of arachidonic acid (land animal fats); increase foods inhibiting platelet aggregation (vegetable oils, fish oils, garlic, onion).

- **Supplements:**
  - magnesium: 250–400 mg t.i.d.
  - vitamin B_6: 25 mg t.i.d.
  - 5-HTP: 100–200 mg t.i.d.

● **Botanical medicines:**

— *Tanacetum parthenium*: 0.25–0.5 mg parthenolide b.i.d.

— ginger (*Zingiber officinalis*):
fresh ginger: approximately 10 g q.d. (6 mm slice)
dried ginger: 500 mg q.i.d.
extract standardized to contain 20% of gingerol and shogaol 100–200 mg t.i.d. for prevention and 200 mg every 2 h (up to six times daily) in the treatment of an acute migraine.

● **Physical medicine:**

— TENS to control secondary muscle spasm
— Acupuncture to balance meridians
— Biofeedback

Primary classifications of headache

Vascular headache

● Migraine headache
— classic migraine
— common migraine
— complicated migraine
— variant migraine

● Cluster headache
— episodic cluster
— chronic cluster
— chronic paroxysmal hemicrania

● Miscellaneous vascular headaches
— carotidynia
— hypertension
— exertional
— hangover
— toxins and drugs
— occlusive vascular disease

Non-vascular

● Tension headache
— common tension headache
— temporomandibular joint (TMJ) dysfunction

● Increased or decreased intracranial pressure

● Brain tumors

● Sinus infections

● Dental infections

● Inner or middle ear infections

Factors that trigger migraine headaches

- Low serotonin levels
  — genetics
  — shunting of tryptophan into other pathways
- Foods
  — food allergies
  — histamine-releasing foods
  — histamine-containing foods
- Alcohol, especially red wine
- Chemicals
  — nitrates
  — MSG (monosodium glutamate)
  — nitroglycerin
- Withdrawal from caffeine or other drugs which constrict blood vessels
- Stress
- Emotional changes, especially let-down after stress, and intense emotions, such as anger
- Hormonal changes, e.g. menstruation, ovulation, birth control pills
- Too little or too much sleep
- Exhaustion
- Poor posture
- Muscle tension
- Weather changes, e.g. barometric pressure changes, exposure to sun
- Glare or eyestrain

Foods which most commonly induce migraine headaches

Food	Egger et al	Hughes et al	Monro et al
Cow's milk	67%	57%	65%
Wheat	52	43	57
Chocolate	55	57	26
Egg	60	24	22
Orange	52	–	13
Benzoic acid	35	–	–
Cheese	32	–	–
Tomato	32	14	–
Tartrazine	30	–	–
Rye	30	–	–
Rice	–	–	30
Fish	22	29 (shell)	17
Grapes	12	33	–
Onion	–	24	–
Soy	17	24	–
Pork	22	–	17
Peanuts	12	29	–
Alcohol	–	29	9

Food	Egger et al	Hughes et al	Monro et al
MSG	–	19	–
Walnuts	–	19	–
Beef	20	14	–
Tea	17	–	17
Coffee	15	19	17
Nuts	12	19 (cashew)	17
Goat's milk	15	14	–
Corn	20	9	–
Oats	15	–	–
Cane sugar	7	19	–
Yeast	12	14	–
Apple	12	–	–
Peach	12	–	–
Potato	12	–	–
Chicken	7	14	–
Banana	7	–	–
Strawberry	7	–	–
Melon	7	–	–
Carrot	7	–	–

Factors involved with histamine-induced headaches

Histamine levels increased by:
- Histamine in alcoholic beverages (particularly red wine)
- Histamine in food
- Histamine-releasing foods
- Food allergy
- Vitamin B_6 deficiency

Histamine breakdown inhibited by:
- Vitamin B_6 antagonists
  — alcohol
  — drugs
  — food additives (e.g. yellow dye #5, monosodium glutamate)
- Vitamin C deficiency

Histamine release prevented by:
- Di-sodium chromoglycate
- Quercetin
- Antioxidants (e.g. vitamin C, vitamin E, selenium, etc.)

Histamine breakdown promoted by:
- Vitamin B_6
- Vitamin C

Multiple sclerosis

DIAGNOSTIC SUMMARY

- Sudden, transient motor and sensory disturbances including impaired vision.
- Diffuse neurologic signs, with remissions and exacerbations.
- Diagnosis is made almost entirely on characteristic clinical presentation.

GENERAL CONSIDERATIONS

No coherent theory accounts for all evidence about epidemiology, etiology, and pathogenesis; pathologic hallmark = zones of demyelination (plaques) varying in size and location; symptoms correspond generally to distribution of plaques.

- **Epidemiology:** in two-thirds of cases, onset between ages 20 and 40 (rarely after 50); 60% female: 40% male; areas with highest prevalence located in higher latitudes, in northern and southern hemispheres (50–100 cases/100,000 vs. 5–10/100,000 in tropics) – northern US, Canada, Great Britain, Scandinavia, northern Europe, New Zealand, Tasmania; exception – uncommon in Japan.

  — initial event occurs in early life – people who move from low-risk to high-risk area before age 15 acquire high risk of MS; those who move after adolescence retain low risk; incidence increasing

  — possible reasons for geographic distribution are solar exposure, genetics, diet, other environmental factors.

Etiology

MS may be the epitome of a multifactorial disease.

- **Virus infection:** demyelination can be induced by viral infection; demyelination may be direct viral lysis of myelin-producing cells, or viral infection leading to autoimmunity; viral infection can alter balance of suppressor to helper T-cells, allowing immune-mediated demyelination; viruses isolated from cultures of material from MS patients may represent contamination or were adventitious, rather than causal; high percentage of MS patients have elevated CSF antibody titers to two or more viruses; measles-specific antibody in MS patients accounts for small percentage of total IgG;

CSF of most MS patients contains elevated IgG, electrophoretic pattern of which characterizes infectious process; "sense antibody" hypothesis is that antibody exists as consequence of unrecognized virus; "non-sense antibody" hypothesis is that IgG in CNS is non-specific; no current evidence of common infectious agent as antigen for increased IgG; hyperactivity of circulating B-cells during acute attacks may cause excess IgG within CNS.

● **Autoimmune reaction:** in MS, sensitivity to myelin basic protein is not demonstrated; if MS is autoimmune, it is due to some other antigen; no antigen exclusive to MS patients has ever been found; many immune abnormalities identified in MS patients – support autoimmune etiology; suppressor T-cell numbers fall just prior to acute attack and rise when attack ends; suppressor cell decline should permit many latent autoimmune conditions to manifest; alternative explanation – changes in T-suppressor activity during acute attacks may be secondary to viral suppression.

● **Diet:** diets high in gluten and milk much more common in areas where there is high prevalence of MS; strong association between diet rich in animal and dairy products and incidence of MS; saturated fatty acids, animal fat, animal minus fish fat, and latitude correlate independently and positively with MS mortality; ratio of polyunsaturated fatty acids (PUFAs) to saturated fatty acids (P/S ratio) and ratio of unsaturated fatty acids to saturated fatty acids are correlated independently and negatively with MS mortality; incidence of MS is low in Japan, where intake of marine foods, seeds, and fruit oil is high; deficiencies of omega-3 oils may interfere with lipid elongation and permanently impair normal myelin formation; MS patients may have defect in EFA absorption and/or transport, causing functional deficiency; dietary saturated fats increase need for EFAs.

● **Excessive lipid peroxidation:** there is reduced glutathione peroxidase (GSH-Px) activity in RBCs and WBCs of MS patients; GSH-Px protects cells from free radical damage – decreased activity leaves myelinated sheath sensitive to lipid peroxidation; GSH-Px has two forms: selenium-dependent and non-selenium-dependent; GSH-Px activity in MS patients is independent of Se concentration and probably due to genetic factors; increased occurrence of MS in individuals with inherent low RBC GSH-Px (GSH-PxL), compared with persons with high RBC GSH-Px (GSH-PxH); decreased GSH-Px activity in myelin-producing cells would render them very susceptible to lipid peroxidation.

DIAGNOSTIC CONSIDERATIONS

Early symptoms of multiple sclerosis

Type	Frequency	Symptoms
Motor	42%	Feeling of heaviness, weakness, leg dragging, stiffness, tendency to drop things, clumsiness

Type	Frequency	Symptoms
Sensory	18%	Tingling, "pins and needles" sensation, numbness, dead feeling, band-like tightness, electrical sensations
Visual	34%	Blurring, fogginess, haziness, eyeball pain, blindness, double vision
Vestibular	7%	Light-headedness, feeling of spinning, sensation of drunkenness, nausea, vomiting
Genitourinary	4%	Incontinence, loss of bladder sensation, loss of sexual function

Difficult disease to diagnose early, when most are effectively treated; symptoms develop over a few days, remain stable for a few weeks, and then recede; recurrences are common; course of disease is extremely variable; diagnosed primarily on clinical grounds; helpful lab procedures are:

● CSF: IgG elevated in 80–90% of MS patients.

● Agarose electrophoresis: oligoclonal bands in 90%.

● Nerve fiber conduction in visual, auditory, and somatosensory pathways shows abnormalities in 94% with established disease, and 67% of patients with suspected disease.

● Magnetic resonance imaging assesses level of lesions in nervous system.

● EFA analysis (*Textbook*, Ch. 13) for early signs of lipid abnormalities and to monitor efficacy of EFA supplements.

THERAPEUTIC CONSIDERATIONS

Three approaches: dietary therapy, nutritional supplements, physical therapy.

Diet

Swank diet: low saturated fats, maintained over long period, retard disease process and reduce number of attacks:

● saturated fat < 10 g q.d. (reduces animal protein)

● polyunsaturated oils: 40–50 g q.d. (margarine, shortening, hydrogenated oils not allowed)

● cod liver oil: 1+ tsp q.d.

● protein: normal allowance

● fish: 3+ times/week.

Protein sources: legumes, grains, vegetables; fish is a source of omega-3 fatty acids to maintain neural function and myelin production – incorporated into myelin sheath, optimizing fluidity and neural transmission;

Benefits of Swank diet:

- decreased platelet aggregation observed in MS
- decreased autoimmune response
- normalized EFAs in the serum, RBCs, and CSF in MS patients.

Excess platelet aggregation and microemboli may damage blood–brain barrier, alter microcirculation of CNS, induce subcutaneous hemorrhage, cause cerebral ischemia; damaged blood–brain barrier may allow influx into CSF of plasma constituents (microbes, antibodies, toxic chemicals, etc.) toxic to myelin; ischemia may contribute to demyelination by promoting release of lysosomal enzymes and cellular death; FAs have modulatory effect on immune system.

Food allergy: MS patients may have increased frequency of villous atrophy similar to celiac disease and food allergies; no convincing evidence that gluten-free or allergy elimination diets are universally beneficial in MS; may be warranted to eliminate food allergens (as long as other dietary measures are also included, e.g. Swank diet); there is anecdotal evidence that specific individuals have been helped.

Nutritional supplements

Linoleic acid: patients supplementing with linoleic acid had smaller increase in disability and reduced severity and duration of relapses compared with controls; better results if dietary saturated fatty acids restricted, effective amounts of linoleic acid used (20+ g q.d.), and regimen maintained for long period (normalization of RBC fatty acid levels may require at least 2 years of supplementation).

- Linoleic acid may be useful in MS due to immunosuppression; individuals with minimal disability respond better than those with severe disability; PUFAs influence cell-mediated immunity.
- Beneficial effects of EFAs are mediated by prostaglandins (PGs) and a splenic factor; inhibitors of PG synthesis (aspirin and NSAIDs) and splenectomy prevent protective effect of linoleic acid in experimental allergic encephalomyelitis (EAE); spleen synthesizes immunologically active prostaglandins; avoid NSAIDs and splenectomy in MS.
- EFA supplements may correct lipid composition of oligodendrocytes, Schwann cells, and other myelin-producing cells; several years of supplementation may be required for complete therapeutic benefit.

Flax and marine oils: flaxseed oil contains linoleic and alpha-linolenic acid (ALA) (omega-3); linolenic acid has greater effect on platelets and is required for normal CNS composition; strong rationale for supplementing EPA and DHA ("marine lipids" of fish and cod liver oil) in MS, although no direct clinical investigation has been reported; EPA greatly inhibits platelet aggregation and DHA present in large quantities in lipids of brain.

Selenium and vitamin E: Se supplements will not increase activity of glutathione peroxidase in most MS patients, but may benefit some; vitamin E is indicated due to increased lipid peroxidation and increased intake of PUFAs; combination of Se, ascorbate, and E have increased GSH-Px activity in MS patients fivefold.

Vitamin B$_{12}$: acquired B$_{12}$ deficiency and inborn errors of metabolism involving B$_{12}$ cause demyelination of CNS nerve fibers; B$_{12}$ levels in serum, RBCs, and CNS are low in MS; B$_{12}$ deficiency in MS may aggravate disease or promote another cause of progressive demyelination; there is a significant decrease in unsaturated B$_{12}$ binding capacities in MS patients, indicating defect in transport of B$_{12}$ into cells; 60 mg q.d. methylcobalamin improved visual and brain stem auditory evoked potentials by nearly 30% in severe chronic progressive MS; motor function did not improve, indicating afferent pathways benefit from B$_{12}$ while efferent pathways do not; no side-effects attributed to high-dose B$_{12}$; methylcobalamin is the main form in body and directly related to methylation reactions; CSF and blood B$_{12}$ in MS patients may be lower and homocysteine (indication of impaired B$_{12}$ nutriture) higher than healthy subjects.

Pancreatic enzymes: MS associated with increased circulating immune complexes; protease enzymes reduce these in autoimmune diseases; clinical improvements correspond with decreases in immune complexes; pancreatic enzymes reduce severity and frequency of MS flare-ups; especially good in visual disturbance, urinary bladder and intestinal malfunction, and sensory disturbances; little effect on spasticity, dizziness, or tremor.

Other considerations

- **Malabsorption:** study of MS patients – 42% had fat malabsorption, 42% had high levels of undigested meat fibers in feces, 27% had an abnormal D-xylose absorption, and 12% had malabsorption of B$_{12}$; multiple subclinical deficiencies possible.

- **Physical therapy:** patient should lead as normal and active a life as possible; exercise is beneficial; avoid overwork and fatigue; passive movement and massage for weakened spastic limbs.

- **Natural alpha-interferon:** recombinant beta-interferon is a popular medical treatment; naturally derived alpha-interferon from leukocytes is advantageous; 5–30 million IU per week for 3–12 months and observed for 2 years after first injection – no major toxicity, with some initially reporting fatigue, flu-like symptoms, or myalgias that abated after 1 month of treatment; first year, 80% of patients improved or stabilized in first year, 76% remained improved or stabilized in second year; better results at higher dosages for longer periods; 83% remission rate in relapsing/remitting patients – better than the 30% rate for beta-interferon.

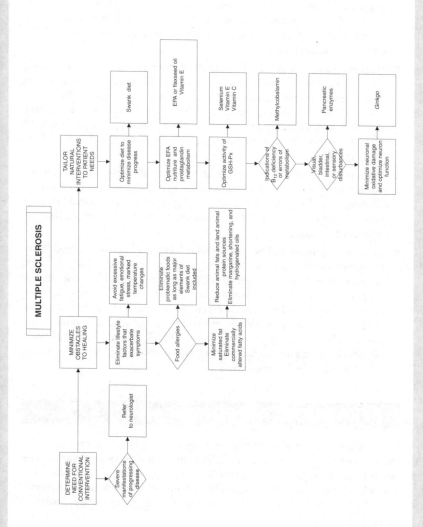

MULTIPLE SCLEROSIS

DETERMINE NEED FOR CONVENTIONAL INTERVENTION

Severe manifestations of progressing disease → Refer to neurologist

MINIMIZE OBSTACLES TO HEALING

Eliminate lifestyle factors that exacerbate symptoms → Avoid excessive fatigue, emotional stress, marked temperature changes

Food allergies → Eliminate problematic foods as long as major elements of Swank diet included

Minimize saturated fat Eliminate commercially altered fatty acids → Reduce animal fats and land animal protein sources Eliminate margarine, shortening, and hydrogenated oils

TAILOR NATURAL INTERVENTIONS TO PATIENT NEEDS

Optimize diet to minimize disease progress → Swank diet

Optimize EFA nurture and prostaglandin metabolism → EPA or flaxseed oil Vitamin E

Optimize activity of GSH-Px → Selenium Vitamin E Vitamin C

Indications of B$_{12}$ deficiency or errors of metabolism → Methylcobalamin

Visual, bladder, intestinal, or sensory disturbances → Pancreatic enzymes

Minimize neuronal oxidative damage and optimize neuron function → Ginkgo

- *Ginkgo biloba* **extract:** free radical damage in CNS in MS patients indicates need for antioxidants; ginkgo acts as antioxidant, improves platelet function, and enhances nerve cell functions (*Textbook*, Ch. 88).

- **Hyperbaric oxygen (HBO):** of eight well-designed trials with HBO, only one showed favorable results; patients had chronic progressive or chronic stable MS; HBO supplied at pressures of 1.75–2 ATA during 20 sessions of 90 min over a period of 4 weeks; side-effects generally minor but included ear and visual problems.

- **Oral antigen therapy:** oral myelin basic protein (MBP) exerts profoundly suppressive effect on EAE induced in rats; MBP-induced oral tolerance characterized by inhibition of EAE clinical neurologic signs, reduced CNS histopathosis, significant decreased T-lymphocyte proliferative response specific for fed antigen, and decreased serum antibody specific for MBP; preliminary results in humans are equally impressive; still in investigational phase.

- **Exercise:** improves fitness and quality of life in MS; aerobic training (three 40-min sessions per week of combined arm and leg ergometry) improved all measures of physical function, social interaction, emotional behavior, home management, total sickness impact profile score and recreation, but no benefit on fatigue.

- **Electromagnetic fields:** extracerebral applications of picotesla low-frequency electromagnetic fields may rapidly reverse conduction blocks in demyelinating fibers; reversal of conduction block believed to change axonal Na^+ and K^+ channels and synaptic nerve transmitter release – may account for immediate improvement in vision and other neurologic deficits; has value – immediate improvement of fine and large muscle control, speech, balance, fatigue, body image, cataplexy, and mood; evaluation impossible – small number of patients, uncontrolled, authored by one clinician, and published in one journal.

THERAPEUTIC APPROACH

Begin ASAP – the earlier therapy is initiated, the better the results; non-specific measures – avoid excessive fatigue, emotional stress, and marked temperature changes; natural therapy of MS not proven to be highly effective, but will help, and poses no threat to patient's health; once MS progressed to significant disability, unlikely to be affected to any great degree by these measures.

- **Diet:** Swank diet:
  - — saturated fat < 10 g q.d.
  - — PUFAs: 40–50 g q.d. (margarine, shortening, and hydrogenated oils not allowed)
  - — normal amounts of protein
  - — fish 3+ times per week.

Fresh whole foods emphasized; animal foods (except cold-water fish) reduced or completely eliminated.

● **Supplements:**

— EPA: 1.8 g q.d. (or flaxseed oil: 1 tbsp q.d.)
— selenium: 200 μg q.d.
— vitamin E: 800 IU q.d.
— vitamin B_{12} (methylcobalamin): 60 mg q.d.
— pancreatin (10×): 350–700 mg t.i.d. (on empty stomach).

● **Botanical medicines:**

— *Ginkgo biloba* extract (24% ginkgo flavonglycosides): 40–80 mg t.i.d.

Nausea and vomiting of pregnancy

DIAGNOSTIC SUMMARY

● Morning or evening nausea and vomiting occurring during first trimester of pregnancy.

GENERAL CONSIDERATIONS

Fifty per cent of women complain of morning sickness at some time during pregnancy; hormonal and metabolic changes of pregnancy contribute and emotional factors affect perception and severity of experience; psychological support is paramount to effective metabolic therapy.

THERAPEUTIC CONSIDERATIONS

● **Pyridoxine:** deficiency, plus estrogen-mediated alterations in tryptophan metabolism, may cause many cases (see chapter on PMS); recent studies have prompted researchers to recommend B_6 as first-line treatment; yet > 1/3 of patients still had N&V with B_6 supplementation; perhaps larger dosage more effective or perhaps ginger is a better choice (alone or with B_6).

● **Vitamins K and C:** together these have considerable clinical efficacy – 91% of patients showing complete remission within 72 h; mechanism unknown; little effect *given alone*.

● ***Zingiber officinale*** **(ginger):** alleviates symptoms of GI distress, including N&V typical of pregnancy; mechanism uncertain – may be due more to aromatic and carminative effects on GI tract than CNS effects; in hyperemesis gravidum, ginger root powder (250 mg q.i.d.) reduces severity of nausea and number of attacks of vomiting in early pregnancy (< 20 weeks); high safety and relatively small doses required; antiemetic drugs problematic in pregnancy due to teratogenicity; becoming well-accepted in orthodox obstetrics.

● **Psychological aspects:** 50% of normal women experience no N&V during pregnancy and some women suffer beyond first trimester; mild first

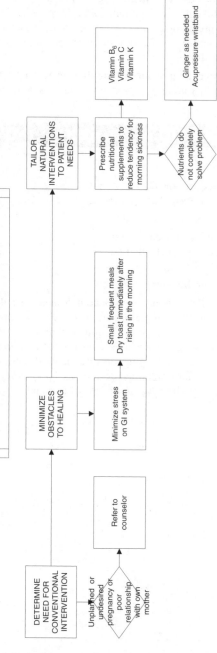

NAUSEA AND VOMITING OF PREGNANCY

DETERMINE NEED FOR CONVENTIONAL INTERVENTION

Unplanned or undesired pregnancy or poor relationship with own mother

Refer to counselor

MINIMIZE OBSTACLES TO HEALING

Minimize stress on GI system

Small, frequent meals
Dry toast immediately after rising in the morning

TAILOR NATURAL INTERVENTIONS TO PATIENT NEEDS

Prescribe nutritional supplements to reduce tendency for morning sickness

Vitamin B$_6$
Vitamin C
Vitamin K

Nutrients do not completely solve problem

Ginger as needed
Acupressure wristband

trimester N&V has strong physiological basis (hormone changes) and is predictive of positive outcome; serious or longer-lasting symptoms may have psychological component; N&V is more common in unplanned, undesired pregnancies and in women with negative relationships with their own mothers; third trimester problems are also linked to such negative relationships.

- **Acupressure**: acupressure wristbands relieve morning sickness in many subjects; reduce anxiety, depression, behavioral dysfunction, and nausea.

THERAPEUTIC APPROACH

- **Diet:**
    — small, frequent meals
    — dry toast immediately after rising.
- **Supplements:**
    —vitamin B_6: 25 mg b.i.d.–t.i.d.
    —vitamin C: 250 mg b.i.d.–t.i.d.
    —vitamin K: 5 mg q.d.
- **Botanical medicines:**
    — *Zingiber officinale* (ginger): research dosage = 1 g dry powdered ginger root (small dose); prefer fresh (or freeze-dried) ginger root or extracts concentrated for gingerol at equivalent dosage; for N&V of pregnancy, dosage = 1–2 g dry powdered ginger or as decoction; for ginger extracts standardized to 20% gingerol and shogaol, dosage = 100–200 mg.
    — counseling: for unplanned or undesired pregnancy or when poor relationship with their own mother; refer to qualified counselor.

Obesity

DIAGNOSTIC SUMMARY

Obesity is defined as:
- Weight > 10% above "normal".
- Body fat > 30% for women and 25% for men.

GENERAL CONSIDERATIONS

Frequency of obesity in US adults > 1/3; number of obese children doubled from 1960 to 1991; odds = 4:1 against children ever achieving normal weight as adult if they enter adolescence obese, and 28:1 if they end teen years obese.

Visual observation

- *Endomorph* – relatively large body with short arms and legs.
- *Mesomorph* – large muscular chest that dominates over abdomen with prominent bony joints.
- *Ectomorph* – relatively small frame (slender and delicate bone structure) with long arms and legs.

Endomorph at greatest risk for obesity, mesomorph at moderate risk, and ectomorph at extremely low risk; patterns of body fat distribution = gynecoid (female) and android (male).

Anthropometric measurements

Height, weight, body circumferences or diameters (waist, chest, or hip circumferences and distances between ileac crests, greater trochanters or acromioclavicular joints), and skinfold thickness.

- **Height and weight indices:** most widely used are tables of desirable weights for height from Metropolitan Life Insurance Company – merely reflect weights of those with lowest mortality of insured persons, but may not reflect US population; weight ranges for lowest mortality do not reflect optimal healthy weight for height; difficult to assess degree of obesity (body fat %); weight alone is a poor reflector of body fat composition.

- **Body mass indices (BMIs):** Quetelet index is the most widely accepted method and correlates well with skinfold thickness measurements of body fat; Quetelet's index = W/H^2 (W = weight [kg]; H = height [m]); least correlation with body height and highest correlation with independent measures of body fatness; value of 27 or greater for either sex indicates obesity; score between 24 (for females) or 25 (for males) and 27 = overweight; measures of relative weight cannot distinguish adiposity, muscularity, and edema; Quetelet index correlates well with hydrostatic and skinfold measurements.

- **Skinfold thickness:** amount of total body fat can be estimated by measuring thickness of subcutaneous fat (skinfold or fatfold thickness); measured with skinfold calipers at several sites on body to improve accuracy – triceps, biceps, subscapular, and suprailiac skinfolds; limitations: inability to control inter- and intra-subject variation in skinfold compressibility, inability to palpate fat–muscle interface, impossibility of obtaining interpretable measurements on very obese persons, interobserver variability, and use of different types of skinfold calipers; nevertheless, it is the easiest and least expensive method for estimating body fat percentage; more precise methods: bioelectrical impedance, ultrasound, total body electrical conductivity (TOBEC), and hydrostatic weighing.

- **Body density:** provides quantitative technique for measuring body fat; determined from specific gravity, calculated by measuring weight of body in and out of water; patient weighed under water and out of water, accounting for lung residual volume; information is used to fractionate body into fat and non-fat components – fat is lighter than water, and lean tissue is heavier than water; relatively easy if facilities available; "gold standard" method, but fallen out of favor due to body composition analyzers; requires considerable patient cooperation; impossible for use with elderly, ill, or hospitalized patients.

- **Bioelectric impedance:** based on measuring conduction of applied electrical current through tissues; constant low-level AC results in impedance to current flow that is frequency-dependent, according to type of tissue; intra- and extracellular fluids are electrical conductors; cell membranes are electrical condensers; low-frequency (1 kHz) current mainly traverses extracellular fluids; higher frequencies (500–800 kHz) penetrate intra- and extracellular fluids; fat-free mass has much greater conductivity than fat; safe non-invasive procedure providing rapid measurement.

Types of obesity

Categories based on size and number of fat cells and fat distribution in body.

- **Hyperplastic obesity:** increased number of adipocytes throughout body; number of fat cells in body is dependent on the diet of mother while person in utero and early infant nutrition; excess calories during early life can increase number of fat cells for life; harder to develop new fat cells in adulthood; hyperplastic obesity begins in childhood; hyperplastic obesity is linked to fewer health effects than other types of obesity.

- **Hypertrophic obesity:** increased size of each fat cell; linked to diabetes, heart disease, hypertension; fat distribution around waist = "male-pattern"/"android" – typical of obese male; waist > hips = android obesity; hips > waist = "female-pattern"/"gynecoid" obesity.

- **Hyperplastic–hypertrophic obesity:** increased number and size of fat cells.

CAUSES OF OBESITY

Psychological factors

TV watching is linked to onset of obesity with dose-related effect – leads to childhood obesity and overweight in adults; physiological effects of watching TV that promote obesity are: reduced physical activity, lowered resting (basal) metabolic rate to that of trance-like states.

Physiological factors

Obese persons may be very sensitive to specific internal cues; physiological theories support the concept that obesity is not just due to overeating and explain variable correlation between caloric intake and weight.

Low serotonin theory: brain serotonin influences eating behavior; diets deficient in tryptophan increase appetite significantly, causing binge eating of carbohydrates; low tryptophan leads to low brain serotonin, a condition the brain interprets as starvation, stimulating appetite control centers; carbohydrate meal increases tryptophan delivery to brain, elevating serotonin synthesis; low serotonin leads to "carbohydrate craving"; blood tryptophan and subsequent brain serotonin plummet with dieting, the reason most diets fail; upper end of spectrum of carbohydrate addiction is bulimia (binge eating plus purging via forced vomiting or laxatives), causing stomach rupture, erosion of dental enamel, and heart disturbances due to loss of potassium.

Set point theory: "set point" is the weight the body tries to maintain by regulating amount of food/calories consumed; each person has a programmed "set point" weight.

- Individual fat cells may control set point – when fat cell gets smaller, it sends powerful message to the brain to eat; obese person has more and larger fat cells, giving an overpowering urge to eat; explains why most diets fail – obese person diets until signal is too strong to ignore, then rebound overeats, exceeds previous weight, and the set point is now set at a higher level = "ratchet effect" and "yo-yo dieting".

- Set point tied to fat cell insulin sensitivity – if cells insensitive to insulin, glucose transport into cells is impaired and burning fat for energy is impaired; obesity and diabetes are strongly linked to diet of saturated fats and refined carbohydrates, disrupting internal mechanisms that control glucose levels (see chapter on diabetes); overcome fat cell's set point by increasing sensitivity of fat cells to insulin – through exercise, diet, and specific nutriceuticals; diet that does not improve insulin sensitivity will fail long-term; increasing insulin sensitivity reduces insulin secretion; elevated insulin increases fatty acid transport into fat cells; when fat cells replete with fat, the body manufactures more fat cells; impossible to reduce number of existing fat cells via natural means.

- Loss of muscle mass (prime burner of fat) caused by dieting is an additional factor.

Diet-induced thermogenesis: some of excess consumed calories are converted immediately to heat; determines patient's susceptibility to weight gain; in lean individuals, meal stimulates up to 40% increase in heat production.

- Overweight persons show only 10% increase – excess energy stored rather than converted to heat; major factor is insulin insensitivity; another cause is impaired sympathetic nervous system (SNS) activity.

- Natural plant stimulants can activate SNS; even after weight loss, persons predisposed to obesity have decreased diet-induced thermogenesis – support insulin sensitivity and proper metabolism indefinitely.

- Another factor is the amount of brown fat – cells contain multiple fat storage compartments with triglycerides localized in smaller droplets surrounding numerous mitochondria; extensive vascular network and mitochondrial density give increased capacity to metabolize fatty acids – does not metabolize fatty acids to ATP as efficiently as other tissues – increases heat production; lean people have higher ratio of brown to white fat than overweight people; amount of brown fat in modern humans is extremely small (0.5–5% of total body weight), but has profound effect on diet-induced thermogenesis – 1 oz of brown fat (0.1% of body weight) can make a difference between maintaining body weight or adding 10 lb/year.

- Lean people respond differently to excess calories – must increase caloric intake by 50% to increase and maintain higher weight; to maintain reduced weight, formerly obese persons must restrict food intake to 25% less than lean person of similar weight and body size; persons predisposed to obesity are more sensitive to weight gain-promoting effects of high-fat diet, tend to consume more fat than lean persons and tend to exercise less.

THERAPEUTIC CONSIDERATIONS

Only 5% of markedly obese persons are able to attain and maintain "normal" weight; 66% of those just a few pounds overweight are able to do so.

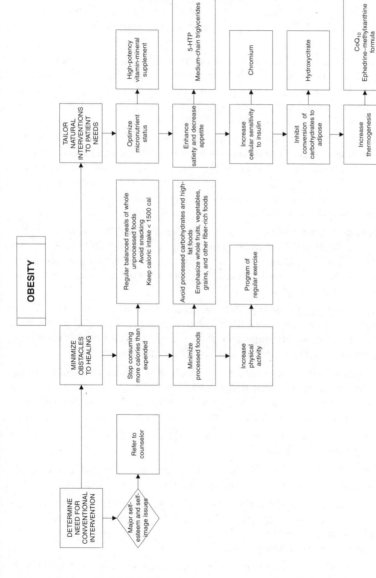

- In order to lose weight, energy intake must be < energy expenditure – decrease caloric intake or increase rate at metabolism; to lose 1 lb, a person must consume 3,500 fewer calories than expended; loss of 1lb/week requires negative caloric balance of 500 cal q.d. – decrease amount of calories ingested or exercise; weight reduction by reduced intake alone or exercise alone (45-min jog, tennis × 1 h, or brisk walk × 1.25 h) is difficult; most sensible approach is diet plus exercise.

- Most people begin to lose if they decrease caloric intake < 1,500 cal q.d. and do aerobic exercise 15–20 min three to four times/week; starvation and crash diets give rapid weight loss (muscle and water), but cause rebound weight gain; prefer gradual reduction (0.5–1 lb/week) via long-standing healthy dietary/lifestyle habits.

5-HTTP: able to reduce calorie intake and promote weight loss despite fact that female subjects made no conscious effort to lose weight; helps overweight people adhere to dietary recommendations; promotes weight loss by promoting satiety, reducing calories consumed at meals; mild nausea during first 6 weeks but never severe enough for any women to drop out of study groups; no other side-effects reported.

Thermogenic formulas: combination plant stimulants (ephedrine, caffeine) can activate SNS, increasing metabolic rate and diet-induced thermogenesis; weight loss induced by normalizing possible underlying defect in metabolism; must be used rationally and not abused – not panaceas, not for everyone, and may induce side-effects.

- Ephedrine suppresses appetite, but main mechanism for weight loss is increasing metabolic rate of adipose tissue; greatest effects in person with low basal metabolic rate and/or decreased diet-induced thermogenesis; thermogenic effects are enhanced by methylxanthines.

- Good methylxanthine sources are coffee (*Coffea arabica*), tea (*Camellia sinensis*), cola nut (*Cola nitida*), and guarana (*Paullinea cupana*); optimum dosage of crude plant preparation/extract depends on content of active constituents; prefer standardized preparations.

- Promote fat loss and preserve lean muscle mass; patients experience improved energy levels.

- Formulas containing ephedrine and caffeine can produce increased BP, increased heart rate, insomnia, and anxiety.

- FDA recommends that ephedrine not be taken by patients with heart disease, hypertension, thyroid disease, diabetes, or difficulty in urination due to prostate enlargement; ephedrine should not be used by patients on antihypertensives or antidepressants.

- Tremendous variation in response to ephedrine and caffeine; patients with slow liver phase I detox (*Textbook*, Ch. 16) are extremely sensitive to CNS stimulatory effects.

- Side-effects at daily dosage of 60 mg ephedrine and 600 mg caffeine decrease with time – tolerance or induction of liver phase I detox; 60% of subjects on ephedrine–caffeine combination have long-term reports of dizziness, HA, insomnia, and heart palpitations.

- Systolic and diastolic BP actually decrease, indicating that the effect of weight loss more than compensates for any increase in BP caused by ephedrine and caffeine; blood glucose, triglycerides, and cholesterol also decrease with weight loss and are not affected by ephedrine and caffeine.

Fiber supplements: increasing dietary fiber promotes weight loss; best sources are psyllium, chitin, guar gum, glucomannan, gum karaya, and pectin – water-soluble fibers; taken with water before meals, these fibers bind to water in stomach to form a gelatinous mass that induces satiety; enhance blood sugar control, decrease insulin levels, reduce number of calories absorbed by body by 30–180 cal q.d. = 3–18 lb weight loss in 1 year.

- avoid products that contain a lot of sugar or other sweeteners to camouflage taste

- drink adequate amounts of water with any fiber supplement, especially in pill form.

Guar gum, from Indian cluster bean (*Cyamopsis tetragonoloba*), gives best results; water-soluble fibers are fermented by intestinal bacteria, producing a great deal of gas – increased flatulence and abdominal discomfort; start with dosage between 1 and 2 g before meals and at bedtime, gradually increasing dosage to 5 g.

Chromium: plays key role in cellular sensitivity to insulin; essential to proper blood sugar control; no RDA exists, health requirement = 200 µg q.d.; Cr levels are depleted by refined carbohydrates, and lack of exercise.

- Decreases fasting glucose, improves glucose tolerance, lowers insulin levels, and decreases total cholesterol and triglycerides, and increases HDL; important in hypoglycemia – increases number of insulin receptors on RBCs.

- Lowers body weight yet increases lean body mass by increasing insulin sensitivity; results are most striking in elderly and in men; promotes increase in lean body weight percentage – fat loss plus muscle gain; greater muscle mass gives greater fat burning potential.

- All effects of Cr are due to increased insulin sensitivity; marginal Cr deficiency is quite common; Cr supplements improve blood sugar control and lower cholesterol and triglycerides.

Medium-chain triglycerides (MCTs):   these are saturated fats (extracted from coconut oil) in 6 to 12 carbon chains.

- Used by body differently from long-chain triglycerides (LCTs), which are the most abundant fats in nature; LCTs are storage fats for humans and plants in 18 to 24 carbon chains.

- MCTs promote weight loss rather than weight gain; may promote weight loss by increasing thermogenesis; LCTs are usually stored in fat deposits – energy is conserved and so a high-fat diet decreases metabolic rate; the thermogenic effect of high-calorie diets with 40% fat as MCTs was compared with 40% fat as LCTs – thermogenic effect (calories wasted 6 h after meal) of MCTs was twice as high as LCTs; excess energy in the form of MCTs is not efficiently stored as fat, but wasted as heat; MCTs can increase diet-induced thermogenesis by 50%; thermic effect of MCTs over 6 h is three times that of LCTs.

- LCTs elevate the blood fat level by 68%, while MCTs have no effect; substituting MCTs for LCTs can produce weight loss as long as calorie level remains the same; to get full benefit from MCTs, LCTs should be low; use as oil for salad dressing, bread spread, or as supplement; dosage = 1–2 tbsp q.d.; closely monitor diabetics and persons with liver disease for ketoacidosis.

Hydroxycitrate: natural substance isolated from fruit of Malabar tamarind (*Garcinia cambogia*), a yellowish fruit the size of an orange, with thin skin, and deep furrows similar to acorn squash, native to southern India; dried fruit contains 30% hydroxycitric acid; powerful lipogenic inhibitor in animals; not yet proven in humans; reduces food intake and body weight gain in rats; may also suppress appetite; low-fat diet must be maintained, as it only inhibits conversion of carbohydrates to fat; may be safe, natural aid for weight loss; dosage = 500 mg t.i.d.; combined with Cr and thermogenic formula may produce greater effect, inhibiting fat production and increasing fat catabolism.

Coenzyme Q$_{10}$: essential compound for converting fatty acids into energy; may help promote weight loss; CoQ$_{10}$ is low in 52% of overweight subjects tested; enhances weight loss in obese subjects compared with placebo.

THERAPEUTIC APPROACH

Proper diet; adequate exercise; positive mental attitude; right supportive natural measures.

- **Diet** (*Textbook*, Ch. 44).
- **Psychological support:** consider referral for counseling to heal assaults on self-esteem and self-image.
- **Lifestyle:** exercise is absolutely critical to effective weight loss program (*Textbook*, Ch. 38).
- **Supplements** (*Textbook*, Ch. 44):
  — 5-HTP: begin at 50–100 mg 20 min before meals for 2 weeks and then double dosage (to maximum of 300 mg) if weight loss < 1 lb/week; higher dosages of 5-HTP (e.g. 300 mg) are associated with nausea, but this symptom disappears after 6 weeks of use.

— chromium: 200–400 µg q.d.

— medium-chain triglycerides: incorporate 1–2 tbsp into diet

— hydroxycitrate: 500 mg t.i.d.

— coenzyme Q_{10}: 100–300 mg q.d.

- **Botanical medicines:** combinations of ephedrine source (*Ephedra sinica*) with methylxanthine source – coffee (*Coffea arabica*), tea (*Camellia sinensis*), cola nut (*Cola nitida*), or guarana (*Paullinea cupana*) – at dosage to provide 20–30 mg q.d. of ephedrine and 80–100 mg q.d. of methylxanthines.

Osteoarthritis

DIAGNOSTIC SUMMARY

- **Symptoms:** mild early morning stiffness, stiffness following periods of rest, pain that worsens on joint use, and loss of joint function.
- **Signs:** local tenderness, soft tissue swelling, joint crepitus, bony swelling, restricted mobility, Heberden's (proximal interphalangeal joints) and/or less common Bouchard's (distal interphalangeal joints) nodes, and other signs of degenerative loss of articular cartilage.
- **X-ray findings:** narrowed joint space, osteophytes, increased density of subchondral bone, subchondral sclerosis, bony cysts, soft tissue swelling, and periarticular swelling.

GENERAL CONSIDERATIONS

Osteoarthritis (OA) characteristics = joint degeneration, loss of cartilage, and alterations of subchondral bone; most common form of arthritis – highest morbidity rate of any illness; primarily in elderly; 35% incidence in knee as early as age 30 (often diagnosed as chondromalacia patellae); incidence increases dramatically with age; > 40 million Americans have OA, including 80% of persons over age 50; under age 45, much more common in men; after age 45, much more common in women.

- **Diseases thought to be OA of specific joints:** hands (Heberden's and Bouchard's nodes); hip (Malum coxae sinilis); temporomandibular (Costen's syndrome); knee (Chondromalacia patellae); spine (ankylosing hyperostosis – interstitial skeletal hyperostosis).
- Weight-bearing joints and peripheral and axial articulations are principally affected; hyaline cartilage destruction followed by hardening and formation of large bone spurs (calcified osteophytes) in joint margins – pain, deformity, and limited joint motion; inflammation usually minimal.
- **Two categories:** *primary OA* – "wear-and-tear" after fifth and sixth decades, with no predisposing abnormalities; cumulative effects of decades of use stress collagen matrix; damage releases enzymes that destroy collagen components; with aging, ability to synthesize restorative collagen decreases; *secondary OA* – predisposing factor for degeneration; factors include: congenital abnormalities in joint structure or function (e.g. hyper-

mobility and abnormally shaped joint surfaces), trauma (obesity, fractures along joint surfaces, surgery, etc.), crystal deposition, presence of abnormal cartilage, previous inflammatory disease of joint (RA, gout, septic arthritis, etc.).

DIAGNOSIS

Onset subtle – morning joint stiffness first symptom; then pain on joint motion worsened by prolonged activity and relieved by rest; no signs of inflammation; clinical picture varies with joint involved: disease of hands – pain and limitation of use; knee involvement – pain, swelling, and instability; hip – local pain and limp; spinal OA (very common) – compression of nerves and blood vessels – pain and vascular insufficiency; RA associated with much more inflammation of surrounding soft tissues; best diagnostic tool is X-ray of suspected joint – joint space narrowing, loss of cartilage, and presence of bone spurs (osteophytes).

- **Pain:** lack of correlation between severity of OA (X-ray) and degree of pain; 40% of patients with worst X-ray classification for OA are pain-free; cause of pain in OA is still not well-defined; depression and anxiety increase experience of OA pain.

THERAPEUTIC CONSIDERATIONS

Cellular and tissue response is purposeful and aimed at repair of anatomic defects; process is arrestable and sometimes reversible; therapeutic goal is to enhance collagen matrix repair and regeneration by chondrocytes; studies to determine "natural course" of OA show marked clinical improvement and radiologic recovery of joint space in almost 50% of cases with no therapy – medical intervention may promote disease progression.

- **Aspirin and NSAIDs:** ASA is effective in relieving pain and inflammation, and is inexpensive; therapeutic dose high (2–4 g q.d.) and toxicity frequent – tinnitus, gastric irritation; side-effects of other NSAIDs are GI upset, HAs, and dizziness – only recommended for short periods of time; unexpected side-effects may increase rate of cartilage degeneration – inhibit collagen matrix synthesis and accelerate cartilage destruction; NSAID use is associated with acceleration of OA; NSAIDs suppress symptoms but accelerate OA progression.

Hormonal considerations

Endocrine forces may initiate or accelerate OA by altering chondrocyte's microenvironment; all hormones act on connective tissue cells: fibroblasts, osteoblasts and chondrocytes.

- **Estrogen:** higher prevalence of OA in women suggests estrogen involvement; estradiol worsens OA; anti-estrogen drug tamoxifen improves experimental OA by decreasing erosive lesions – therapeutic role for estrogen blockade; botanicals (e.g. *Glycyrrhiza glabra* and *Medicago sativa*) used for OA contain "phytoestrogens" that bind to estrogen receptors, acting as estrogen antagonists; food sources of phytoestrogens are soy, fennel, celery, parsley, nuts, whole grains, and apples.

- **Insulin, growth hormone (GH) and somatomedin (SMM):** diabetics have greater incidence and more severe OA than non-diabetics; insulin insensitivity or deficiency, increased GH, and decreased SMMs (insulin-like growth factors secreted by liver in response to GH); insulin stimulates chondrocytes to increase synthesis and assembly of proteoglycans; most prominent early change in articular cartilage is decreased proteoglycans and state of aggregation – insulin insensitivity or deficiency predisposes to OA; excessive GH is detrimental to bone and joint structures – increased incidence of OA in acromegaly; women with primary osteoporosis have higher basal GH than controls; GH detrimental to chondrocytes; SMMs mediate normal chondrocyte activity; impaired hepatic function, diabetes, and malnutrition suppress liver secretion – increased risk of OA.

- **Thyroid:** hypothyroidism increases risk of OA compared with age- and sex-matched population samples.

Dietary considerations

Achieve normal body weight – minimize stress on weight-bearing joints affected with OA; healthy diet, rich in complex carbohydrates and dietary fiber (*Textbook*, Ch. 175).

- **Nightshade vegetables:** Childers' theory – genetically susceptible individuals might develop arthritis from long-term, low-level consumption of the solanum alkaloids found in Solanaceae (nightshade) plants: tomatoes, potatoes, eggplant, peppers, and tobacco; alkaloids may inhibit normal collagen repair; theory as yet unproven, but diet beneficial to some patients.

- **Antioxidant nutrients:** Framingham Osteoarthritis Cohort Study: high intake of antioxidant nutrients, especially vitamin C, gave threefold reduced risk of cartilage loss and OA disease progression in middle and highest tertiles of vitamin C intake; advocate diet rich in plant-based antioxidants.

Nutritional supplements

- **Glucosamine sulfate:** stimulates manufacture of glycosaminoglycans (GAGs) and promotes incorporation of sulfur into cartilage; with age, there is reduced ability to synthesize sufficient glucosamine – cartilage loses gel-like nature and ability to absorb shock – may be the major factor leading to OA; significantly more effective than placebo in improving pain and movement after 4 weeks (1,500 mg q.d.) in double-blind crossover; longer GS use gives greater therapeutic benefit; rate and severity of GS side-effects not different from placebo; head-to-head studies: better long-term results than NSAIDs relieving OA pain and inflammation despite little anti-inflammatory or analgesic effect of GS; NSAIDs offer only symptomatic relief and may promote disease process; GS treats root cause (cartilage synthesis), improving symptoms and helping body to repair damage; higher dosages may be required for obese patients; patients with peptic ulcers should take GS with food; individuals taking diuretics may need increased dosage to compensate for reduced efficacy; improvement with GS lasts 6–12 weeks after end of treatment – taken for long periods of time or in repeated short-term courses; high safety and excellent tolerability – suitable for long-term use (*Textbook*, Ch. 89).

- **Chondroitin sulfate (CS):** contains mixture of intact or partially hydrolyzed GAGs of molecular weights 14,000 to > 30,000; composed of repeating units of derivatives of GS; absorption rate of GS = 90–98%; absorption of intact CS = 13% – CS 50–300 times larger than GS; key reason why GS is effective is small molecular size, allowing diffusion through joint cartilage to chondrocyte; CS levels are typically elevated in synovial tissues of OA patients; less effective than GS.

- **Niacinamide:** Kaufman and Hoffer – treatment of RA and OA with high-dose niacinamide (i.e. 900–4,000 mg q.d. in divided doses); improves joint function, range of motion, muscle strength and endurance, and sedimentation rate; benefits within 1–3 months of use; peak benefits between 1 and 3 years of continuous use; 29% improvement in global arthritis impact vs. 10% worsening with placebo; pain levels do not change, but niacinamide patients reduce NSAID use; reduces ESR by 22% and increases joint mobility by 4.5° over controls (8° vs. 3.5°); no other changes in blood chemistry; side-effects are mild GI complaints, managed by taking with food or fluids; high dose can result in significant side-effects (e.g. glucose intolerance and liver damage) – requires strict supervision.

- **Methionine:** *S*-adenosylmethionine (SAM) is formed in body by combining essential amino acid methionine to adenosyl-triphosphate (ATP); SAM deficiency in joint tissue causes loss of gel-like nature and shock-absorbing qualities of cartilage; very important in synthesis of cartilage components; supplemental SAM increases cartilage formation (determined by MRI) in osteoarthritis of hands; mild analgesic and anti-inflammatory effects in animal studies; similar reductions in pain scores and clinical symptoms to NSAIDs; SAM administered orally at dose of 1,200 mg q.d. is significantly more effective than NSAIDs (physicians' and patients' judgments); better tolerated than placebo; efficacy described as very good or good in 71% of cases, moderate in 21%, and poor in 9%; tolerance assessed as very good or good in 87%, moderate in 8%, and poor in 5% of cases; SAM offers significant advantages over NSAIDs.

● **Superoxide dismutase (SOD):** intra-articular injections of SOD have significant therapeutic effects; whether oral SOD is absorbed orally is yet to be determined; preliminary indications unfavorable.

● **Vitamin E:** 600 IU is significantly beneficial – antioxidant and membrane-stabilizing actions; in vitro, it inhibits activities of lysosomal enzymes and stimulates increased deposition of proteoglycan.

● **Vitamin C:** deficient intake is common in elderly – altered collagen synthesis and compromised connective tissue repair; in vitro vitamin C has anabolic effect on cartilage; excess of ascorbic acid needed in human chondrocyte protein synthesis; in vivo study of experimental OA in guinea pigs – cartilage erosion is much less, and overall histologic and biochemical changes in and around OA joint are much milder in animals on high doses of vitamin C; vitamins C and E have synergistic effects – enhance stability of sulfated proteoglycans.

● **Pantothenic acid:** acute deficiency in the rat causes pronounced failure of cartilage growth and lesions similar to OA; clinically improves OA symptoms at dosage of 12.5 mg; results often do not manifest until 7–14 days; larger, double-blind study of RA patients – no significant benefit at dosage at 500 mg.

● **Vitamins A and E, pyridoxine, zinc, copper, and boron:** required for synthesis of collagen and maintenance of normal cartilage; deficiency of any one of these allows accelerated joint degeneration; supplements at appropriate potencies may promote cartilage repair; boron used to treat OA in Germany since mid-1970s; 6 mg boron (sodium tetraborate decahydrate) – 71% of patients improved compared with 10% on placebo; open trial: boron at 6–9 mg q.d. gave effective relief in 90% of arthritis patients including OA, juvenile arthritis, and RA; boron is of value in arthritis – many OA patients experience complete resolution.

Physical therapy

Exercise, heat, cold, diathermy, and ultrasound often improve joint mobility and reduce pain in OA, especially when administered regularly; benefit of physical therapy – achieving proper hydration within joint capsule; short-wave diathermy may be of greatest benefit; combining short-wave diathermy with periodic ice massage, rest, and appropriate exercises may be most effective approach; ultrasound and laser therapy also helpful; best exercises are isometrics and swimming – increase circulation to joint and strengthen surrounding muscles without excess strain on joints; increasing quadriceps strength improves clinical features and reduces pain in knee OA; walking helps improve functional status and relieve pain in knee OA.

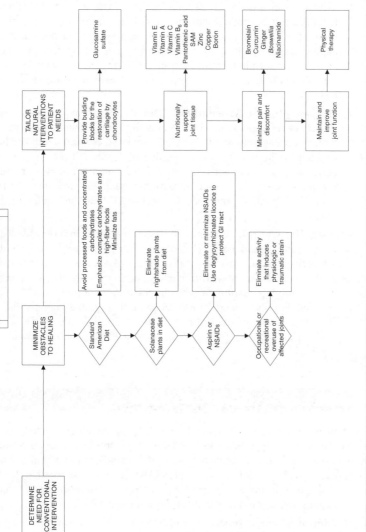

Botanical medicines

When inflammation is present, botanicals and nutritional factors possessing anti-inflammatory activity are indicated, e.g. bromelain, curcumin, and ginger.

● **Yucca:** double-blind trial – saponin extract of yucca has positive therapeutic effect; results gradual with no direct joint effects; improvement due to indirect effects on GI flora; bacterial lipopolysaccharides (endotoxins) depress the biosynthesis of proteoglycans; yucca may decrease bacterial endotoxin absorption, reducing inhibition of proteoglycan synthesis; other saponin-containing herbs and other ways of reducing endotoxin load may be useful.

● ***Harpagophytum procumbens* (Devil's claw):** experimental animal models of inflammation – Devil's claw has anti-inflammatory and analgesic effect comparable to phenylbutazone; other studies indicate little, if any, anti-inflammatory effect; equivocal research from mechanism of action is inconsistent with current anti-inflammatory models or failure to use quality-controlled (standardized) extracts; main components of Devil's claw are saponins – therapeutic effect in OA may be similar to that of yucca.

● ***Boswellia serrata:*** large branching tree native to India; exudative gum resin ("salai guggul") used for centuries; newer preparations concentrated for active components (boswellic acids) give better results; boswellic acid extracts have anti-arthritic effects in animal models; mechanisms of action – inhibit inflammatory mediators, prevent decrease in GAG synthesis, and improve blood supply to joint tissues; herbal formulas with *Boswellia* yield good clinical results in OA and RA; dosage for boswellic acids in arthritis = 400 mg t.i.d.; no side-effects due to boswellic acids reported.

THERAPEUTIC APPROACH

Clinical study of comprehensive, integrated program for OA yet to be conducted; therapeutic approach – reduce joint stress, promote collagen repair, and eliminate foods and other factors that inhibit collagen repair; control all diseases or predisposing factors; avoid NSAIDs as much as possible; if aspirin used, deglycyrrhizinated *Glycyrrhiza glabra* (licorice) may protect GI tract from damaging effects and ASA should be discontinued ASAP.

● **Diet:** avoid simple, processed, and concentrated carbohydrates; emphasize complex-carbohydrate, high-fiber foods; minimize fats; eliminate Solanaceae foods (tomatoes, potatoes, eggplant, peppers, and tobacco); liberally consume flavonoid-rich berries or extracts.

● **Supplements:**
— glucosamine sulfate: 1,500 mg q.d.

— niacinamide: 500 mg six times/day (under strict supervision – monitor liver enzymes)
— vitamin E: 600 IU q.d.
— vitamin A: 5,000 IU q.d.
— vitamin C: 1,000–3,000 mg q.d.
— vitamin B_6: 50 mg q.d.
— pantothenic acid: 12.5 mg q.d.
— SAM: 400 mg t.i.d.
— zinc: 45 mg q.d.
— copper: 1 mg q.d.
— boron: 6 mg q.d.

- **Botanical medicines:**

   — *Medicago sativa*: equivalent to 5–10 g q.d.
   — yucca leaves: 2–4 g t.i.d.
   — *Harpagophytum procumbens*:
      dried powdered root – 1–2 g t.i.d.
      tincture (1:5) – 4–5 ml t.i.d.
      dry solid extract (3:1) – 400 mg t.i.d.
   — *Boswellia serrata*: equivalent to 400 mg boswellic acids t.i.d.

- **Physical therapy and exercise:** avoid physical activity that induces physiologic or traumatic strain (occupational or recreational overuse); normalize posture; orthopedically correct structural abnormalities to limit joint strain; monitored daily non-traumatic exercise (isometrics and swimming); short-wave diathermy, hydrotherapy, and other PT modalities which improve joint perfusion.

Osteoporosis

DIAGNOSTIC SUMMARY

- Usually asymptomatic until severe backache.
- Most common in postmenopausal white women.
- Spontaneous fractures of the hip and vertebra.
- Decrease in height.
- Demineralization of spine and pelvis as confirmed by X-ray techniques.

GENERAL CONSIDERATIONS

Normal decline in bone mass after age 40 in both sexes (2% loss/year); women at much greater risk due to lower bone density prior to age 40; post-menopausal (PM) osteoporosis is the most common form; 1 in 4 PM women has osteoporosis (OP); 20 million people are affected in US.

Major risk factors for osteoporosis in women

- Postmenopausal
- White or Asian
- Premature menopause
- Positive family history
- Short stature and small bones
- Leanness
- Low calcium intake
- Inactivity
- Nulliparity
- Gastric or small-bowel resection
- Long-term glucocorticosteroid therapy
- Long-term use of anticonvulsants
- Hyperparathyroidism
- Hyperthyroidism
- Smoking
- Heavy alcohol use

Entire skeleton involved, but bone loss greatest in spine, hips, and ribs – weight-bearing causes susceptibility to pain, deformity or fracture; 1.5 million fractures yearly from osteoporosis, including 250,000 hip fractures – fatal in 12–20% of cases plus long-term care for half who survive; 1/3 of all women and 1/6 of all men fracture hips in their lifetime.

Etiology

Involves mineral (inorganic) and non-mineral (organic protein matrix) components of bone; lack of dietary calcium in adult causes osteomalacia ("softening of bone"); in osteomalacia, only Ca is deficient in bone; in osteoporosis, there is a lack of Ca, other minerals plus decreased non-mineral framework (organic matrix); Ca and vitamin D are the most important nutritional factors; hormones critical – incorporation of Ca into bone is dependent upon estrogen.

- **Gastric acid:** Ca absorption depends on being ionized/solubilized by stomach acid; 40% of postmenopausal women are hypochlorhydric; patients with insufficient stomach HCl absorb only 4% of Ca as calcium carbonate – a person with normal HCl absorbs 22%; hypochlorhydric patients need Ca in soluble/ionized state (citrate, lactate, gluconate); 45% of Ca is absorbed from calcium citrate in patients with hypochlorhydria.

- **Vitamin D:** stimulates Ca absorption; synthesized by action of sunlight on 7-dehydrocholesterol in skin – considered more a hormone than a vitamin; sunlight converts 7-dehydrocholesterol into vitamin D_3 (cholecalciferol); liver converts D_3 into 25-hydroxycholecalciferol ($25\text{-}(OH)D_3$) (five times more potent than D_3), which is converted by kidneys to 1,25-dihydroxycholecalciferol ($1,25\text{-}(OH)_2D_3$) (10 times more potent than D_3); liver or kidney disorders impair conversion of D_3; many patients with osteoporosis have high $25\text{-}OH\text{-}D_3$ but low $1,25\text{-}(OH)_2D_3$ – suggests impaired kidney conversion; boron theorized to help this conversion.

- **Hormonal factors:** blood Ca level strictly circumscribed; Ca decrease triggers parathyroid hormone (PTH) release and decreases secretion of calcitonin by thyroid and parathyroids; Ca increase decreases secretion of PTH and increases calcitonin; PTH increases serum Ca by activating osteoclast catabolism of bone, decreasing kidney Ca excretion, increasing kidney conversion of $25\text{-}(OH)D_3$ to $1,25\text{-}(OH)_2D_3$, and increasing intestinal Ca absorption; estrogen deficiency makes osteoclasts more sensitive to PTH, increasing bone breakdown.

DIAGNOSTIC CONSIDERATIONS

Best diagnosed by bone densitometry – prefer dual energy X-ray absorptiometry (DEXA) – measures hip and lumbar spine densities; for high-risk women, get baseline bone density and then monitor bone loss by urine tests for bone breakdown products (cross-linked N-telopeptide of type I collagen or deoxypyridium); urine tests give quicker feedback than DEXA (up to 2 years to detect therapeutic response); reducing urinary markers of bone breakdown over a 2-year period increases bone density measurements.

THERAPEUTIC CONSIDERATIONS

Primary goals: (1) preserve mineral mass, (2) prevent loss of protein matrix and other structural components, (3) assure optimal repair to remodel damaged bone.

Hormone replacement therapy: benefits of HRT outweigh risks in women susceptible to OP or already suffering major bone loss; prefer estrogen–progesterone combinations to estrogen alone; exceptions are women at high risk for breast cancer or suffering diseases aggravated by estrogen (breast cancer, active liver diseases, certain cardiovascular diseases) – use progesterone alone.

Lifestyle factors: coffee, alcohol, and smoking cause negative Ca balance and are linked to increased risk of OP; regular exercise reduces risk; exercise is most critical for maintaining healthy bones – physical fitness is the major determinant of bone density; 1 h of moderate activity three times/week prevents bone loss and increases bone mass in PM women.

General dietary factors

Vegetarian diet (lacto-ovo and vegan) is linked to lower risk of OP; bone mass in vegetarians and omnivores differs only after fifth decade – decreased OP in vegetarians is not due to increased initial bone mass, but decreased bone loss; high-protein or high-phosphate diet is linked to increased urinary Ca excretion; refined sugar increases urinary Ca excretion (average American consumes daily 125 g sucrose, 50 g corn syrup and other sugars, 15 oz carbonated beverage loaded with phosphates, and over-abundant protein).

● **Soft drinks:** major factor for OP – high phosphates and no Ca, leading to lower blood Ca and higher blood phosphate; consumption in children is a risk factor for impaired calcification of growing bones; strong correlation between maximum bone mineral density and risk of OP; significant inverse correlation between serum Ca and number of bottles of soft drink consumed per week.

● **Green leafy vegetables:** green leafy vegetables protect against OP – sources of Ca, vitamin K_1, and boron:

— vitamin K_1 converts inactive osteocalcin to active form; osteocalcin is a major non-collagen protein in bone that anchors Ca into protein matrix; vitamin K deficits impair bone mineralization due to inadequate osteocalcin; low blood K_1 found in patients with OP-linked fractures; severity of fracture is strongly correlated with circulating vitamin K;

the lower the level of circulating vitamin K, the lower the bone density; sources are dark green leafy vegetables, broccoli, lettuce, cabbage, spinach, green tea; minerals (Ca, boron) – protective effect

— supplemental boron (3 mg q.d.) in PM women reduces urinary Ca excretion and increases 17-beta-estradiol; boron activates certain hormones, including estrogen and vitamin D; boron required for converting vitamin D to $1,25\text{-}(OH)_2D_3$ within kidney; fruits and vegetables are main dietary sources of boron.

Nutritional supplements

- **Calcium:** supplements reduce bone loss in PM women; Ca alone does not completely halt Ca loss, but slows rate by 30–50%; protects against hip fractures; with exercise and dietary recommendations, Ca is part of effective treatment for most women; Ca supplements alone significantly prevent bone loss; greater benefit using more absorbable forms (citrate or bound to other Krebs cycle intermediates); continued Ca supplementation produces sustained reduction in rate of loss of total bone mineral density in healthy PM women and reduces incidence of bone fractures; improves bone density in perimenopausal women; beware of lead contamination in some Ca supplements; prefer products lab-tested for purity and potency; avoid natural oyster shell Ca, dolomite, and bone meal products unless manufacturer can document purity; calcium hydroxyapatite (purified bone meal) tested at 20% absorption compared with 30% for carbonate or citrate.

- **Vitamin D:** vitamin D_3 alone at 700 IU q.d. may reduce annual rate of hip fracture from 1.3 to 0.5% – nearly a 60% reduction; increases hip bone density; combined with Ca produces slightly better results; vitamin D can be helpful in elderly people living in nursing homes, people living further away from equator, and those who do not regularly get outside; dosage = 400 IU q.d. vitamin D_3; level of active vitamin D does not differ substantially from 400–800 IU; taking higher dosages offers no significant benefit and may adversely affect magnesium levels.

- **Magnesium:** may be as important as Ca in preventing and treating OP; women with osteoporosis have lower bone Mg content and other indicators of Mg deficiency than people without OP; enzyme responsible for conversion of $25\text{-}(OH)D_3$ to $1,25\text{-}(OH)_2D_3$ is Mg-dependent; Mg mediates PTH and calcitonin secretion; slightly improves bone density in PM women.

- **Vitamin B_6, folic acid, and vitamin B_{12}:** low levels of these nutrients are common in elderly; important in conversion of amino acid methionine to cysteine; deficiency or defect in enzymes responsible for conversion causes increase in homocysteine – implicated in atherosclerosis and osteoporosis (*Textbook*, Ch. 52); hyperhomocysteinemia demonstrated in PM women; may contribute to osteoporosis by interfering with collagen cross-linking, leading to defective bone matrix; folic acid reduces homocysteine

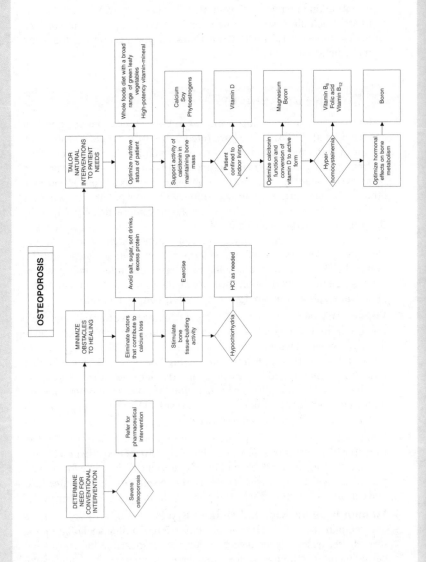

in PM women even though none were deficient in folic acid according to standard folic acid lab criteria; vitamins B_6 and B_{12} are also necessary in metabolism of homocysteine; combinations of these vitamins will produce better results than either one of them alone.

- **Silicon:** necessary for cross-linking collagen strands, contributing to strength and integrity of connective tissue matrix of bone; silicon concentrations increased at calcification sites in growing bone; recalcification in bone remodeling may depend on silicon.

- **Fluoride:** fluoride administration is a popular therapy, but validity still in question; fluoride's predominant effects: stimulating osteoblasts and positive Ca balance; incorporated into crystalline structure of bone as fluoroapatite, but bone matrix is poorly formed and weak; long-term excessive exposure causes bone fragility; therapeutic index for fluoride quite narrow; recommended daily dose of 60–75 mg sodium fluoride causes side-effects in 33–50% of patients – joint pain, stomach aches, nausea, vomiting; less troublesome if taken with meals; enteric-coated and timed-released show fewer side-effects and better clinical results; not recommended in treatment of osteoporosis.

- **Phytoestrogens:** may be suitable alternatives to estrogens to prevent OP in menopausal women; ipriflavone is a semi-synthetic isoflavonoid similar to soy isoflavonoids that increases bone density by 2 and 5.8% after 6 and 12 months, respectively, in women with OP; longer-term studies are documenting safety and efficacy of ipriflavone; naturally occurring isoflavonoids (genistein and daidzein in soy) may exert similar benefits; soy isoflavonoid protection against breast cancer alone warrants regular consumption of soyfoods; mechanism of action may be enhancement of calcitonin effects on Ca metabolism as ipriflavone exerts no estrogen-like effects.

THERAPEUTIC APPROACH

Osteoporosis preventable if appropriate dietary and lifestyle measures are followed; bone is dynamic, living tissue that requires constant supply of high-quality nutrition and regular stimulation (exercise); primary goal is prevention; in severe cases of OP, use natural measures in conjunction with appropriate medical care, including pharmaceuticals.

- **Diet** (*Textbook*, Ch. 44): avoid items promoting Ca excretion – salt, sugar, protein, soft drinks.
- **Supplements:**
    — high-potency multiple vitamin-mineral formula
    — calcium: 800–1,200 mg q.d.
    — vitamin D: 400 IU q.d.
    — magnesium: 400–800 mg q.d.
    — boron (as sodium tetrahydraborate): 3–5 mg q.d.

Otitis media

DIAGNOSTIC SUMMARY

Acute otitis media
- Earache or irritability.
- History of recent upper respiratory tract infection or allergy.
- Red, opaque, bulging ear drum with loss of the normal features.
- Fever and chills.

Chronic or serous otitis media
- Painless hearing loss.
- Dull, immobile tympanic membrane.

GENERAL CONSIDERATIONS

Otitis media (OM) is inflammation, swelling, or infection of middle ear; two types:

- **Acute OM:** usually preceded by URI or allergy; common microorganisms are *Streptococcus pneumoniae* (40%) and *Haemophilus influenzae* (25%).

- **Chronic OM** (also known as serous, secretory, or non-suppurative OM, chronic OM with effusion; and "glue ear"): constant swelling of middle ear.

Acute OM affects two-thirds of American children by age 2; chronic OM affects two-thirds of children under age 6; OM is the most common diagnosis in children – accounts for > 50% of all visits to pediatricians; $8 billion spent annually on medical and surgical treatment.

Standard medical treatment

Antibiotics, analgesics (e.g. acetaminophen), and/or antihistamines; if long-standing infection unresponsive to drugs, surgery performed – involves placing a tiny plastic myringotomy tube through ear drum to drain fluid into throat via Eustachian tube; children with tubes in their ears are more likely to have further problems with OM; surgery unnecessary for most children; only 42% of these surgeries are judged as being appropriate; no significant differences in clinical course of acute OM between conventional treatments and placebo – no differences between non-antibiotic treatment, ear tubes, ear tubes with antibiotics, and antibiotics alone; children not receiving antibiotics may have fewer recurrences than those receiving antibiotics; recent international review: antibiotics not recommended for OM in most children.

Causes

- **Primary risk factors for OM:** day-care attendance, wood-burning stoves, parental smoking or exposure to other second-hand smoke, food allergies, not being breast-fed.

- **Common mechanism** is abnormal Eustachian tube (ET) function, the underlying cause in virtually all cases of OM; ET regulates gas pressure in middle ear, protects middle ear from nose and throat secretions and bacteria, and clears fluids from middle ear; swallowing opens ET via action of surrounding muscles; infants and small children are susceptible to ET problems due to smaller diameter and more horizontal orientation; ET obstruction allows fluid build-up and bacterial infection if immunity is impaired and pathogenic microbes present; obstruction results from collapse of tube (weak tissues and/or abnormal opening mechanism), blockage by allergy-induced mucus, mucosal edema, or infection.

THERAPEUTIC CONSIDERATIONS

Treatment goals are to ensure ET patency by identifying and addressing causative factors, and to support immune system.

- **Bottle-feeding:** recurrent ear infection linked to early bottle-feeding; breast-feeding (minimum 4 months) is protective – may be due to cow's milk allergy and protective effect of human milk against infection; bottle-feeding while child lying on back (bottle-propping) leads to regurgitation of bottle contents into middle ear; human milk is protective due to high antibody content inhibiting microbes; breast-fed infants have thymus glands 20 times larger than formula-fed infants.

- **Food allergy:** 85–93% of OM children have allergies: 16% to inhalants only, 14% to food only, 70% to both; prolonged breast-feeding may prevent OM by avoiding food allergens, particularly if mother avoids sensitizing foods (those to which she is allergic) during pregnancy and lactation; excluding/limiting foods to which children are commonly allergic (wheat, egg, fowl, dairy), particularly during first 9 months, is also of value; child's digestive tract is permeable to antigens, especially during first 3 months – control eating patterns (infrequent repetition of any food, avoid common allergenic foods, and introduce foods in controlled manner – one food at a time, carefully watching for reaction);

  — allergic reaction causes blockage of ET – inflammatory edema of ET mucosa and nasal edema causing Toynbee phenomenon (swallowing with both mouth and nose closed, forcing air and secretions into middle

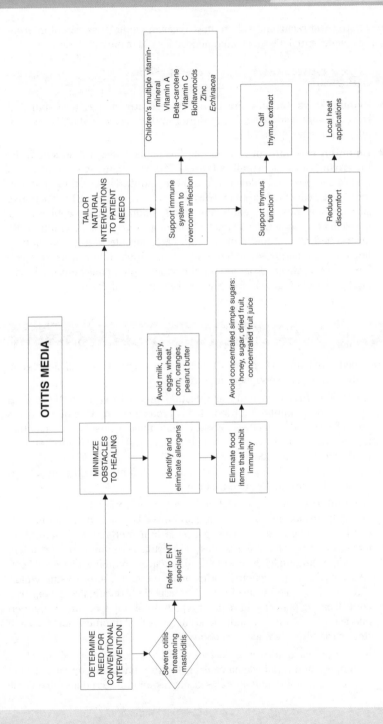

OTITIS MEDIA

DETERMINE NEED FOR CONVENTIONAL INTERVENTION

Severe otitis threatening mastoiditis → Refer to ENT specialist

MINIMIZE OBSTACLES TO HEALING

Identify and eliminate allergens → Avoid milk, dairy, eggs, wheat, corn, oranges, peanut butter

Eliminate food items that inhibit immunity → Avoid concentrated simple sugars: honey, sugar, dried fruit, concentrated fruit juice

TAILOR NATURAL INTERVENTIONS TO PATIENT NEEDS

Support immune system to overcome infection → Children's multiple vitamin-mineral / Vitamin A / Beta-carotene / Vitamin C / Bioflavonoids / Zinc / *Echinacea*

Support thymus function → Calf thymus extract

Reduce discomfort → Local heat applications

ear); chronic OM – always consider allergy; 93.3% of children tested were allergic to foods, inhalants, or both; 92% of OM children improve when treated with serial dilution titration therapy for inhalants and elimination diet for food allergens; statistically significant association between food allergy and recurrent OM in 78% of patients; elimination diet ameliorates chronic OM in 86% of patients; challenge diet with suspected offending food(s) provokes recurrence of serous OM in 94% of patients.

— *most common food allergens in order of frequency*: cow's milk, wheat, egg white, peanut, soy, corn, tomato, chicken, apple.

● **Thymus gland extract:** thymus secretes hormones acting on WBCs to ensure proper development and function; oral calf thymus extracts given to children improve immune function, decrease food allergies, and improve resistance to chronic respiratory infections; may be of particular benefit in chronic OM (*Textbook*, Ch. 53).

● **Humidifiers:** popular treatments for OM and URIs in children; significantly more effusions (fluid in ETs) observed in lab animals kept in low-humidity environments compared with those kept in more moderate environs; low humidity may induce nasal swelling and reduce ventilation of ET, or may dry ET lining causing inability to clear fluid and increased secretions; mast cells of ET mucosa may release histamine and produce edema; increasing humidity with humidifier may be important modality to treat OM with effusion.

THERAPEUTIC APPROACH

Recognize and eliminate allergies, particularly food allergies, and support immune system.

● **Diet:** usually not possible to determine exact allergen during acute attack; eliminate most common allergic foods: milk and dairy, eggs, wheat, corn, oranges, peanut butter; eliminate concentrated simple carbohydrates (sugar, honey, dried fruit, concentrated fruit juice) that inhibit immune system.

● **Nutritional supplements:**
— children's multiple vitamin-mineral formula
— vitamin A: 50,000 IU q.d. × 2 days in children under age 6 years, and × 4 days in children over 6
— beta-carotene (natural mixed carotenoids): age in years × 20,000 IU q.d. (up to 200,000 IU q.d.)
— vitamin C: age in years × 50 mg every 2 h
— bioflavonoids: age in years × 50 mg every 2 h
— zinc: age in years × 2.5 mg q.d. (up to 30 mg)

— thymus extract: equivalent of 120 mg pure polypeptides with molecular weights < 10,000 or 500 mg of crude polypeptide fractions q.d.

● **Botanical medicines:**

— *Echinacea* sp.: 1/2 adult dosage for children under age 6; full adult dosage (below) for children over age 6 (*Echinacea* very safe for children); all dosages below can be given up to three times daily:

dried root (or as tea): 0.5–1 g

freeze-dried plant: 325–650 mg

juice of aerial portion of *E. purpurea* stabilized in 22% ethanol: 2–3 ml

tincture (1:5): 2–4 ml

fluid extract (1:1): 2–4 ml

solid (dry powdered) extract (6.5:1 or 3.5% echinacoside): 150–300 mg.

● **Physical medicine:** local application of heat often very helpful in reducing discomfort – apply as hot pack, with warm oil (mullein oil), or by blowing hot air into ear with straw and hair dryer; these help to reduce pressure in middle ear and promote fluid drainage.

Pelvic inflammatory disease

DIAGNOSTIC SUMMARY

- Dyspareunia, leukorrhea.
- Severe cramp-like, non-radiating lower abdominal pain; adnexal tenderness.
- Chills with moderately high, intermittent fever typical, but not invariably present.
- Cervical motion tenderness.
- WBC 20,000/µL, with marked leukocytosis and/or elevated sedimentation rate.
- *Neisseria gonorrhea* and *Chlamydia trachomatis* most common, followed by *Ureaplasma urealyticum*.
- *Mycoplasma hominis*, *Streptococcus* sp., *E. coli*, *H. influenzae*, *Peptostreptococcus*, and *Peptococcus*.

GENERAL CONSIDERATIONS

Pelvic inflammatory disease (PID) is a categorical name for a range of pelvic infections and inflammations; salpingitis is a particular condition under PID (adnexa always involved by definition); non-infectious states (pelvic adhesions and chronic salpingitis) also included; 2.5 million outpatient visits annually in US; 25% of patients suffer serious long-term sequelae with risk of recurrence; risk of ectopic pregnancy increases sixfold after one episode of PID; 13% risk of infertility after one infection, 70% after three.

Etiology

Organisms listed above are implicated in etiology of PID; asymptomatic chlamydial infections are a big cause of PID; higher proportion of PID ascribed to *Chlamydia trachomatis* than to *Neisseria gonorrhea*.

- ***Neisseria gonorrhea* (GC):** delicate and fastidious species but high infectivity, preferring human columnar and transitional epithelia; in < 1 h after intercourse, GC can establish itself on urethral mucosa, resisting flow of urine; favored sites in lower female genital tract are Bartholin's and Skene's glands, urethra, and endocervical canal; spreading occurs from endocervix across endometrium to tubal mucosa, or via migration through subendothelial vascular and lymphatic channels; most common method of spreading is vector – GC attached to spermatozoa are physically carried to fallopian tubes; retrograde menstruation or uterine contractions during intercourse are other modes of dissemination; acute state: GC and PMNs accumulate in subepithelial connective tissue, causing patchy destruction of overlying mucosa; consequent mucosal thinning may facilitate GC penetration into deeper tissue – GC survive only a short time in fallopian tubes; descent of microbe beyond surfaces being examined makes it difficult to detect; concomitant infections occur – primary role of GC is paving the way for secondary invaders from normal vaginal flora; *Chlamydia trachomatis* (CT) and anaerobic bacteria superinfections are possible.

- **_Chlamydia trachomatis_ (CT):** 20–30% of PID cases are caused by CT; acute chlamydial PID may be subclinical or silent in 66–75% of cases; lab diagnosis is difficult; frequently asymptomatic.

- **Anaerobes:** most commonly isolated from fallopian tubes or cul-de-sacs of PID patients; probably not chief causative agents, but opportunists; commonly found in immunocompromised hosts; generally of endogenous origin; cervices and vaginas of normal healthy women contain anaerobes and aerobes; anaerobic infections are more common in older patients and women with a history of prior PID.

- **Other organisms:** facultative aerobic organisms in tuboperitoneal fluids from women with salpingitis include coliforms, *Haemophilus influenzae*, streptococci, and *Mycoplasma hominis*; this last is a common agent of polymicrobial milieu of PID – in 81% of women patients with GC, and 64% of those without.

Ramifications

Sequelae of PID are abdominal pain, infertility, ectopic pregnancy, dyspareunia.

- **Death** from salpingitis is rare and generally due to rupture of tubo-ovarian abscess with subsequent peritonitis – mortality rate of 5.2–5.9% for tubo-ovarian abscesses.

- **Fitz-Hugh–Curtis syndrome:** perihepatitis complicating primary PID; characteristic violin-string adhesions attaching liver to abdominal wall; adhesions due to local peritonitis involving anterior liver surface and adjacent abdominal wall; historically, CT is a more frequent cause than GC.

- **Infertility:** PID puts woman at risk for recurrence – after fallopian tubes damaged by infection, normal defense mechanisms are impaired; reinfection is the most important cause of infertility after PID.

- **Ectopic pregnancy:** seven- to 10-fold increased risk

Risk factors

These include sexual contact, age, use or history of use of IUD, previous history of PID, earlier "sexual debut", especially with multiple sexual partners.

● Risk in sexually active 15-year-olds = 1 in 8; in average 24-year-old risk = 1 in 80; cervical mucus in younger woman may be estrogen-dominated, creating environment more accessible to pathogens.

● Women with multiple partners have 4.6-fold greater risk than monogamous women.

● IUDs increase risk; oral contraceptive (OC) users have less risk of GC but more risk for CT invasion; barrier methods of birth control decrease PID risk (women with vasectomized partners may have less risk).

● Iatrogenic: the following invasive procedures may introduce pathogens or disturb tract flora, and induce PID – cervical dilation, abortion, curettage, tubal insufflation, hysterosalpingography, insertion of IUD; PID may not be strictly an STD.

Pathogen access to upper female tract

Menstruation, sperm, and trichomonads help transport pathogens into salpinx.

● **Infections** occurring around menses tend to be GC rather than CT; menstrual regurgitation may carry sloughed endometrium with attached GC or intracellular CT that proliferate in tubal epithelium or on peritoneal surfaces.

● **Human sperm:** bacteriospermia is a cause of infertility in men – asymptomatic male carriers; 66–75% of men who tested positive for GC were asymptomatic; sperm are vectors; cervical mucus is an effective mechanical and immunologic barrier between flora of vagina and upper tract; organisms attached to sperm can easily traverse mucus column; sperm migrate through menstrual plasma, but not during luteal phase or through cervical mucus of pregnancy; sperm is intimately associated with cytomegalovirus, *Toxoplasma*, *Ureoplasma urealyticum*, and *Chlamydia*; motile trichomonads are another transporter, ascending from vagina to fallopian tubes, carrying additional invaders; trichomonads are never isolated from humans when heavy bacterial contamination is absent.

DIAGNOSIS

Pelvic or lower abdominal pain is the most dependable symptom of PID, but not specific; rebound tenderness not reliable; cervical motion tenderness and adnexal tenderness are much more common; clinical picture is misleading; many PID patients have atypical signs and symptoms; some have no signs and symptoms at all.

Common signs and symptoms in acute PID

Symptom	Incidence (%)
Lower abdominal pain	90
Adnexal tenderness on palpation	90
Pain on movement of the cervix	90
Vaginal discharge	55
Adnexal mass or swelling	50
Fever or chills	40
Irregular vaginal bleeding	35
Anorexia, nausea, and vomiting	25

- GC patients may appear more toxic and febrile with leukocytosis; CT-PID may give elevated sedimentation rate (ESR); most GC-PID occurs at or shortly after menses; GC-PID has a more severe clinical picture, but tissue damage and long-term sequelae can be more severe in CT; many infections mixed.

- Putrid discharge yields anaerobes – offensive odor is diagnostic of anaerobic infection and indicative of well-developed PID.

Differential diagnosis of PID

- Acute appendicitis
- Acute cholecystitis
- Acute pyelonephritis
- Ectopic pregnancy
- Endometriosis
- Hemorrhagic ovarian cysts
- Intrauterine pregnancy
- Mesenteric lymphadenitis
- Ovarian cyst with torsion
- Ovarian tumor
- Pelvic thrombophlebitis
- Septic abortion

- **Fitz-Hugh–Curtis syndrome:** symptoms from upper right quadrant in sexually active woman may be indirect sign of genital infection; pain – sudden onset overshadowing underlying PID.

- **Rupture of tubulo-ovarian abscess:** sudden severe exacerbation of pain; pain referred to side of rupture, followed by generalized peritonitis and collapse; shoulder pain is possible; pulse elevated out of proportion to fever, up to 170; surgery within 12 h required or mortality probable.

- **Careful history:** STDs, birth control methods, sexual activity, recent medical procedures, and nature and onset of symptoms.

Laboratory diagnosis

Lab findings during active PID are inconsistent; lack of correlation between organisms found in different sectors of female GU tract; pathogens in cervix are often not found in adnexa; GC from peritoneum not found in upper tract.

- **Invasive sampling of exudate and tissue** only warranted as last resort: diagnostic laparoscopies have death rate of 5.2/100,000 and major complications in 4.6/1,000 procedures.

- **Upper tract culture** via cervical entrance utilizing double-lumen, catheter-protected brush is the most recent and least invasive technique; poorly correlated and frequently compromised by lower tract contamination.

- **CBC and ESR** essential; ESR in pregnancy is elevated from increased plasma fibrinogen and globulin; ESR increased in anemia due to higher plasma-to-erythrocyte ratio; suspect infection with ESR > 35 in absence of pregnancy and anemia.

- **C-reactive protein (CRP):** local inflammatory reaction follows cell death in internal organs, inducing increased synthesis of series of plasma proteins; C-reactive protein is an acute-phase reactant that increases 1–2 days after any tissue injury affecting more than epithelial layer; increased CRP is quantitatively matched with degree of tissue injury; non-specific test – does not stand alone – evaluated with WBC and ESR.

- **Endocervical smears and cultures:** potentially misleading.

- **Urinalysis:** to help with differential diagnosis.

- **Serum human chorionic gonadotropin:** rule out pregnancy.

- **Abdominal ultrasound:** rule out ectopic pregnancy.

- **Liver enzymes** not elevated with chlamydial perihepatitis – parenchyma not involved.

- **Infections** polymicrobial.

THERAPEUTIC CONSIDERATIONS

Hospitalization recommended for pregnancy, pelvic abscess, adnexal masses, or peritoneal involvement; refer if diagnosis is uncertain or surgical emergency threatens; give antibiotic therapy plus supportive therapies if patient's clinical and lab status can be reassessed in 48–72 h; lab values and objective patient criteria should direct all acute-phase treatment.

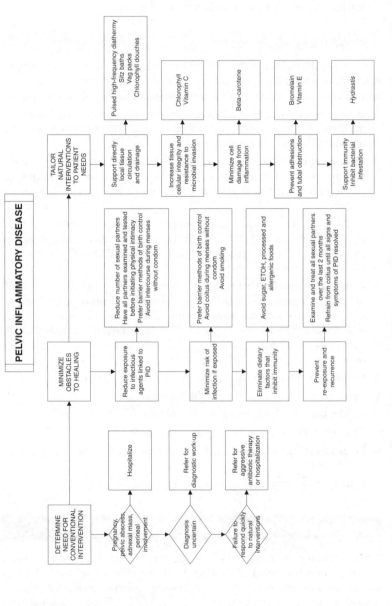

PELVIC INFLAMMATORY DISEASE

DETERMINE NEED FOR CONVENTIONAL INTERVENTION

Pregnancy, pelvic abscess, adnexal mass, perineal involvement → Hospitalize

Diagnosis uncertain → Refer for diagnostic work-up

Failure to respond quickly to natural interventions → Refer for aggressive antibiotic therapy or hospitalization

MINIMIZE OBSTACLES TO HEALING

Reduce exposure to infectious agents linked to PID → Reduce number of sexual partners. Have all partners examined and tested before initiating physical intimacy. Prefer barrier methods of birth control. Avoid intercourse during menses without condom

Minimize risk of infection if exposed → Prefer barrier methods of birth control. Avoid coitus during menses without condom. Avoid smoking

Eliminate dietary factors that inhibit immunity → Avoid sugar, ETOH, processed and allergenic foods

Prevent re-exposure and recurrence → Examine and treat all sexual partners over the last 2 months. Refrain from coitus until all signs and symptoms of PID resolved

TAILOR NATURAL INTERVENTIONS TO PATIENT NEEDS

Support directly local tissue circulation and drainage → Pulsed high-frequency diathermy. Sitz baths. Vag packs. Chlorophyll douches

Increase tissue cellular integrity and resistance to microbial invasion → Chlorophyll. Vitamin C

Minimize cell damage from inflammation → Beta-carotene

Prevent adhesions and tubal obstruction → Bromelain. Vitamin E

Support immunity. Inhibit bacterial infestation → *Hydrastis*

Antibiotics: not curative; antibiotic resistance increasing rapidly; 15% of women with PID fail to respond to primary antimicrobial treatment, 20% have at least one recurrence, and 15% are rendered infertile; more fundamental approach of combining immune enhancement and non-toxic therapies is more sound; antibiotics, herbal or pharmaceutical, can help in first phase of treatment, but are insufficient intervention for devastating sequelae.

Physical medicine

- **Diathermy:** Pulsed high-frequency diathermy is very beneficial in PID; pulsing electric energy of short duration (65 μs every 1600 μs) at high intensity achieves desired therapeutic result without hyperpyrexia associated with diathermy; local recovery is enhanced, reticuloendothelial system is stimulated, and gamma-globulin fractions increased.
- **Sitz baths:** contrast sitz bath increases pelvic circulation and drainage (*Textbook*, Ch. 42).

Nutritional supplements

- **Chlorophyll derivatives:** these are cell-stimulating agents that regenerate tissues; enhance production of hemoglobin and RBCs; non-toxic; increase resistance of cells so that enzymatic digestion of cell membrane by invading bacteria or their toxin is checked; theorized to break down carbon dioxide, resulting in liberation of oxygen which inhibits anaerobic bacteria; careful vaginal douching with chlorophyll is recommended in every case of PID to forestall or diminish anaerobes and to encourage cervical and possibly upper tract healing.
- **Vitamin C:** anti-inflammatory effects help to decrease tissue destruction; supports collagen tissue repair that helps prevent spread of infection (important in GC spread through subepithelial connective tissue, disorganizing collagen matrix); fibrinolytic activity helps prevent pelvic scarring.
- **Beta-carotene:** normal ovary has high beta-carotene; maintain optimal carotene to optimize defense against nearby inflammation; potentiates beneficial effects of interferon; enhances antibody response and WBC activity; it is an antioxidant, limiting cell damage from inflammation (*Textbook*, Ch. 67).
- **Bromelain:** adnexal exudate in PID frequently suppurates to form abscesses; alleviating tissue irritation during initial stages allows resorption of exudate with fewer adhesions; adhesions form as exudate lingers because structures are overwhelmed by inflammation; agglutination of villous fold in lumen of tube may cause scarring and tubal occlusion; bromelain activates fibrinolysis, diminishing sequelae of exudate; has antimicrobial properties; penetrates salpinx (*Textbook*, Ch. 69).

Botanical medicines

- **Vaginal depletion packs:** recommended to promote drainage of exudate from involved tissues (*Textbook*, App. 12).

- **Hydrastis canadensis:** immune-potentiating; specific anti-chlamydial properties; general antibacterial nature of goldenseal justifies its use in PID; trophorestorative to mucous membranes – use throughout rehabilitation period (*Textbook*, Ch. 91).

- **Symphytum officinale:** Comfrey is a soothing demulcent best used in second phase of treatment; allantoin content encourages cell regeneration. (Note: Only preparations from the aerial portion should be used.)

Prevention

Concern about asymptomatic male carriers of STDs; choice of birth control method is pivotal.

- **Oral contraceptives:** OCs inhibit GC; some suggest OC use after first episode of PID to prevent recurrence; estrogens create thicker cervical plug, protective against GC; OCs decrease length and volume of menstrual flow, thus decreasing exposure of GC to this culture medium; OCs may give higher risk of CT; progesterone induces hyperplasia and hypersecretion, producing cervical eversion, exposing endocervical columnar epithelium – target tissue of CT; estradiol may suppress endocervical antibodies necessary to resolve CT; estrogen-treated individuals may have higher number of infected cervical cells and longer duration of infection; OCs not recommended.

- **Intrauterine device:** IUD is an STD disaster; allows bacterial colonization on its surface while reducing local immunologic capacity; IUD not recommended.

- **Barrier methods:** excellent choices to prevent PID; condom preferred to cervical protectors – sperm reach vaginal vault more rarely.

- **Douching:** avoid haphazard douching – disturbs vaginal flora; douching with water-soluble chlorophyll solution is a good supportive measure if exposure to infection is suspected; used with caution; PID has been correlated to frequency of douching – those who douched 3+ times/month were 3.6 times more likely to get PID than those who douched < once/month.

- **Intercourse during menses:** not recommended unless condom used; GC risk increased by the loss of protective cervical mucus plug and prevalence of blood – medium of choice for GC; endometrium may offer local protection against bacteria – this layer sloughed off during menses.

- **Smoking:** current smokers, compared with those who have never smoked, have increased risk of PID; women who smoke 10+ cigarettes q.d. have higher risk than those who smoke less.

● **Education:** review signs and symptoms of PID with all sexually active women; encourage early intervention if clinical picture of PID appears.

THERAPEUTIC APPROACH

Two phases of treatment: (1) eliminate all pathogens and normalize adnexal microflora, and (2) rehabilitate damaged tissues; avoid intercourse until all signs and symptoms have resolved and male partners have been examined and treated; all partners during 2 months prior to illness must be examined; increase bedrest; *note*: referral for aggressive antibiotic treatment or hospitalization is mandatory if patient does not respond quickly.

● **Diet:** limit all dietary inhibitors of immunity (sugar, alcohol, processed and allergenic foods) during both phases of treatment.

● **Supplements:**
   — beta-carotene: 100,000 IU q.d. × 2+ months
   — vitamin E: 400 IU q.d. × 3 months
   — vitamin C: 500 mg q.i.d. during first week of treatment and then decrease over 3 days to 250 mg t.i.d.
   — chlorophyll: 10 mg of fat/oil soluble – four/day for 1 month
   — bromelain: 250 mg (1,800 mcu) q.i.d. for first week and t.i.d. for 6 weeks.

● **Botanical medicines:**
   — *Symphytum officinale* (aerial portion only and after the acute phase): 500 mg of freeze-dried herb three times/day
      1:1 fluid extract, 30 drops two times/day
   — *Hydrastis canadensis*: 400 mg of the solid extract three times/day during the acute phase; 200 mg three times/day during recovery
   — chlorophyll: douches alternating with vag packs
   — vag packs: daily during the acute phase until there is adequate clinical and laboratory response; after the acute phase, vag packs need to be used three times/week, alternating with chlorophyll douches, for 3 weeks.

● **Physical medicine:**
   — diathermy: pulsed, high-intensity diathermy for 10 min over the suprapubic area, 10 min over the liver, and 10 min in the area of the left adrenal (the right being presumably stimulated with the liver)
   — sitz baths: one to two times/day throughout the acute phase; contrast sitz baths are given in groups of three alterations of hot to cold; two separate tubs are necessary to facilitate this process – the hot is at 105–115°F, the cold at 55–85°F, with the temperatures dependent on the strength of the patient; standard treatment is 3 min hot and 30 s cold; the water level in the hot tub is set 2.5 cm higher than in the cold; adequate draping is necessary to prevent chilling; as with all hydrotherapy treatments, one always finishes with the cold.

Peptic ulcers

DIAGNOSTIC SUMMARY

- Epigastric distress 45–60 min after meals, or nocturnal pain; both relieved by food, antacids, or vomiting.
- Epigastric tenderness and guarding.
- Symptoms chronic and periodic.
- Gastric analysis shows acid in all cases, with hypersecretion in about half the patients with duodenal ulcers.
- Ulcer crater or deformity usually occurring at the duodenal bulb (duodenal ulcer) or pylorus (gastric ulcer) on X-ray or fiberoptic examination.
- Positive test for occult blood in stool.

GENERAL CONSIDERATIONS

Peptic ulcers (PUs) occur in stomach (gastric) and first portion of small intestine (duodenal); duodenal ulcers more common – prevalence = 6–12% in US; 10% of US population has clinical evidence of duodenal ulcer during lifetime; four times more common in men than women; four to five times more common than benign gastric ulcer.

- Most PUs are associated with abdominal discomfort 45–60 min after meals or during night – gnawing, burning, cramp-like, or aching, or "heartburn"; antacids usually give great relief.
- Duodenal ulcer (DuU) and gastric ulcer (GsU) result from similar mechanisms – specifically some influence damaging protective factors lining the stomach and duodenum.
- Gastric acid corrosive with pH = 1–3; lining of stomach and small intestine is protected by layer of mucin; constant renewing of intestinal cells and secretion of factors neutralizing acid contacting mucosa are also protective.
- Gastric ulcers – acid output normal or reduced; half of patients with duodenal ulcers have increased gastric acid output; increase may be due to increased number of parietal cells – duodenal ulcer patients have twice as many parietal cells as normal controls; problematic only when integrity of protective factors is impaired.
- Loss of integrity from *Helicobacter pylori*, NSAIDs, alcohol, nutrient deficiency, stress, etc; *H. pylori* and NSAIDs are most significant.

Helicobacter pylori: 90–100% of patients with DuUs, 70% with GsUs, and 50% of people over age 50 test positive for *H. pylori* – antibodies to *H. pylori* in blood or saliva, culturing material collected during endoscopy, measuring breath for urea; low gastric output and low antioxidant content in GI mucosa may predispose to *H. pylori* colonization that increases gastric pH, setting up positive feedback and increasing risk for colonization of other organisms.

Aspirin and other NSAIDs: linked to significant risk of PU; increased risk of GI bleeding due to PU at all dosages; 75 mg q.d. ASA associated with 40% less bleeding than 300 mg q.d., and 30% less bleeding than 150 mg q.d. – conventional prophylactic aspirin regimen not free of risk of peptic ulcer; combination of NSAIDs and smoking is particularly harmful.

THERAPEUTIC CONSIDERATIONS

PU complications are hemorrhage, perforation, and obstruction = MEDICAL EMERGENCIES requiring immediate hospitalization; identify cause and eliminate.

Lifestyle factors

- **Stress and emotions:** men and women with peptic ulcers have distinctly different psychological profiles; number of stressful life events is not significantly different in peptic ulcer patients compared with ulcer-free controls; patient's response to stress is a significant factor; people who perceive stress in their lives are at increased risk of developing peptic ulcers (*Textbook*, Ch. 60); psychological factors are important in some patients, but not in others; ulcer patients tend to repress emotions; encourage discovery of enjoyable outlets of self-expression and emotions.

- **Smoking:** increased frequency, decreased response to PU therapy, and increased mortality linked to smoking; three postulated mechanisms: (1) decreased pancreatic bicarbonate secretion, (2) increased reflux of bile salts into stomach, (3) acceleration of gastric emptying into duodenum; bile salts are very irritating to stomach and first portions of duodenum; bile salt reflux induced by smoking is the most likely factor; psychological aspects of smoking also important – chronic anxiety and psychological stress linked to smoking worsen ulceration.

Nutritional factors

- **Food allergy:** this is the prime etiological factor; PU lesions are histologically similar to Arthus reaction; 98% of PU patients had coexisting lower and upper respiratory tract allergic disease; elimination diet very successful treating and preventing recurrent ulcers; food allergy is consistent with high recurrence rate of PUs; milk should be avoided – the higher the milk consumption, the greater the likelihood of ulcer; milk significantly increases stomach acid production.

- **Fiber:** diet rich in fiber is linked to reduced rate of DuUs compared with low-fiber diet; high-fiber diet in patients with recently healed DuUs reduces recurrence rate by half; fiber delays gastric emptying of liquid phase, counteracting rapid movement into duodenum; supplemental fibers used: pectin, guar gum, psyllium, etc.; diet rich in plant foods is best.

- **Cabbage:** raw cabbage juice effective treating PUs; 1 L q.d. fresh juice in divided doses has induced total ulcer healing in only 10 days; high glutamine content of cabbage juice is a healing factor; 1.6 g q.d. glutamine is more effective than conventional treatment – almost all glutamine patients tested showed complete relief and healing within 4 weeks; glutamine involved in biosynthesis of hexosamine moiety in certain mucoproteins.

- **Bismuth subcitrate:** bismuth is a naturally occurring mineral antacid and inhibitor of *H. pylori*; bismuth subsalicylate (Pepto-Bismol) is the most popular form, but bismuth subcitrate produces best results against *H. pylori* and treating PUs; bismuth subcitrate is available through compounding pharmacies (International Academy of Compounding Pharmacists 1-800-927-4227); advantage of bismuth over standard antibiotics is the risk of developing bacterial resistance to antibiotics that is very unlikely relative to bismuth; dosage for bismuth subcitrate = 240 mg b.i.d. before meals; for bismuth subsalicylate, dosage = 500 mg q.i.d.; bismuth preparations are extremely safe at these dosages; bismuth subcitrate may cause temporary and harmless darkening of tongue and/or stool; avoid bismuth subsalicylate in children recovering from flu, chickenpox, or other viral infection – may mask nausea and vomiting of Reye's syndrome, a rare but serious illness.

- **Flavonoids**: counteract production and secretion of histamine (factor in ulcer formation); anti-allergy compounds indicated due to probable allergic etiology; catechin inhibits histidine decarboxylase; catechin displays significant anti-ulcer activity in various models; 1,000 mg catechin 5 times/day reduces histamine in gastric tissue of normal patients and those with GsU and DuU and acute gastritis; several flavonoids inhibit *H. pylori* in concentration-dependent manner; augment natural defense factors which prevent ulcer formation; flavone (most potent flavonoid studied in this context) has effect similar to bismuth subcitrate.

Miscellaneous

- **Vitamins A and E:** inhibit development of stress ulcers in rats; help maintain integrity of mucosal barrier.

PEPTIC ULCERS

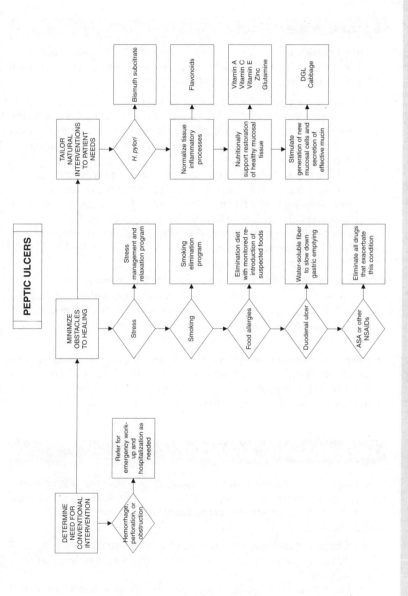

● **Zinc:** increases mucin production in vitro; has protective effect on PUs in animals and curative effect in humans.

Botanical medicines

● ***Glycyrrhiza glabra***: licorice used historically for PU; aldosterone-like side-effects of glycyrrhizinic acid (GA) avoided via removal of GA from licorice to form deglycyrrhizinated licorice (DGL).

— DGL is an anti-ulcer agent with no known side-effects (*Textbook*, Ch. 90); DGL stimulates differentiation to glandular cells, plus mucus formation and secretion; no significant differences in recurrence rates between cimitidine and DGL; prevents aspirin-induced ulceration and gastric bleeding

— DGL is composed of several flavonoids which inhibit *H. pylori*

— DGL must mix with saliva to be effective; may promote release of salivary compounds which stimulate growth and regeneration of stomach and intestinal cells; DGL in capsule not shown to be effective

— dosage = two to four 380 mg chewable DGL tablets between meals or 20 min before meals; continue at least 8–16 weeks after there is a full therapeutic/symptomatic response.

● **Rhubarb:** in cases of active intestinal bleeding, rhubarb (*Rheum* sp.) is extremely effective; more than 90% effective in clinical trials with bleeding GsUs and DuUs; time taken for stool occult blood test to change from positive to negative was 53–57 h; benefits due to astringent anthraquinones and flavonoids.

● **Plantain banana:** dried extract of unripe plantain banana antiulcerogenic against a variety of experimentally induced ulcers in rats; effect similar to that of DGL – stimulates mucosal cell growth rather than inhibition of gastric acid secretion.

THERAPEUTIC APPROACH

Peptic ulcer disease refers to heterogeneous group of disorders with common final pathway leading to ulcerative lesion in gastric or duodenal mucosa; determine which factors most relevant; more general approach may be easier to implement:

— identify and eliminate or reduce all factors implicated in etiology – food allergy, cigarette smoking, stress, drugs (especially aspirin and other NSAIDs)

— inhibit exacerbating factors (e.g. reducing excess acid secretion if present) and promote tissue resistance

— proper diet and lifestyle to prevent recurrence

— complications: hemorrhage, perforation, and obstruction are emergencies requiring immediate hospitalization.

● **Psychological:** stress reduction program – eliminate or control stressors, plus regular relaxation plan.

● **Diet:** eliminate allergenic foods; emphasize high-fiber foods; cabbage family vegetables.

● **Supplements:**

— vitamin A: 20,000 IU t.i.d.
— vitamin C: 500 mg t.i.d.
— vitamin E: 100 IU t.i.d.
— flavonoids: 500 mg t.i.d.
— zinc: 20 mg q.d.
— glutamine: 500 mg t.i.d.
— bismuth subcitrate: 240 mg b.i.d. before meals.

● **Botanical medicine:**

— deglycyrrhizinated licorice root (DGL): 380–760 mg dissolved in mouth 20 min before meals t.i.d.

Periodontal disease

DIAGNOSTIC SUMMARY

- Gingivitis – inflammation of the gingiva characterized by erythema, contour changes and bleeding.
- Periodontitis – localized pain, loose teeth, demonstration of dental pockets, erythema, swelling and/or suppuration; X-ray may reveal alveolar bone destruction.

GENERAL CONSIDERATIONS

Periodontal disease (PD) is an inclusive term for inflammatory condition of gingiva (gingivitis) and/or periodontium (periodontitis); disease process progresses from gingivitis to periodontitis; may be a manifestation of systemic condition (diabetes mellitus, collagen diseases, leukemia or other disorders of leukocyte function, anemia, or vitamin deficiency); linked to atherosclerosis.

- Alveolar bone loss may be non-inflammatory – our definition of periodontal disease excludes processes causing only tooth loss (due mainly to osteoporosis or endocrine imbalances); these conditions reflect systemic disease.
- Focus on underlying condition rather than "periodontal disease"; non-inflammatory alveolar bone loss is a separate entity which involves different etiology (see chapter on osteoporosis).
- Focus of this chapter is nutrition and lifestyle improvement as adjuncts to control and prevention of causes of inflammatory periodontal disease.
- Best treated with combined expertise – dentist or periodontist and nutritionally minded physician; oral hygiene is paramount but insufficient in many cases; host defense must be normalized; nutritional status determines status of host defense factors.

Prevalence and epidemiology: prevalence increases directly with age; 15% at age 10, 38% at 20, 46% at 35, 54% at 50; men have higher prevalence and severity than women; inversely related to increasing levels of education and income; rural inhabitants have higher severity and prevalence than urban counterparts.

Pathophysiology

Factors involved in host resistance include:

- **Gingival sulcus:** V-shaped crevice that surrounds each tooth, bounded by tooth on one side and epithelium lining free margin of gingiva on the other; ideal for bacteria – resistant to cleaning action of saliva; gingival fluid (sulcular fluid) is a rich nutrient source for microorganisms; depth of gingival sulcus = diagnostic parameter; PD patients should be monitored biannually by dentist.

- **Bacterial factors:** bacterial plaque is the etiological agent in PD; bacteria secrete compounds detrimental to host defenses: endotoxins and exotoxins, free radicals and collagen-destroying enzymes, leukotoxins, bacterial antigens, waste products, and toxic compounds.

- **Polymorphonuclear leukocytes:** neutrophils (PMNs) are the first line of defense against microbes; PMN functional defects are "catastrophic" to periodontium; PMNs are depressed in elderly, diabetes, Crohn's, Chediak–Higashi syndrome, Down's, and juvenile periodontitis – extremely high risk for rapidly progressing periodontal disease; transient neutropenia and PMN function defects may cause alternating quiescence and exacerbation in PD; PMNs release numerous free radicals, collagenases, hyaluronidases, inflammatory mediators, and osteoclast stimulator.

- **Macrophages and monocytes:** increased numbers in PD; phagocytize bacteria and debris; primary source of prostaglandins in diseased gingiva; release abundant enzymes involved in collagen destruction.

- **Lymphocytes:** produce lymphokines; role overshadowed by other immune components; promote PMN and monocyte chemotaxis, fibroblast destruction, and osteoclast activation.

- **Complement system:** 22 proteins (> 10% of total serum globulin) whose activation initiates cascade (classical or alternative pathway) triggering immunological and non-specific resistance to infection and pathogenesis of tissue injury; products of complement activation regulate: release of mediators from mast cells; promotion of smooth muscle contraction; chemotaxis of PMNs, monocytes, and eosinophils; and phagocytosis by immune adherence; net effect is increased gingival permeability, increased penetration of bacteria and by-products, and initiation of positive feedback cycle; other effects – solubilization of immune complexes, cell membrane lysis, neutralization of viruses, and killing of bacteria; in PD, activation of complement via alternative pathway in periodontal pocket is a major factor in tissue destruction.

- **Mast cells and IgE:** mast cell degranulation releases inflammatory mediators (histamine, prostaglandins, leukotrienes, kinins, serotonin, heparin, serine proteases); initiated by IgE complexes, complement components, mechanical trauma, endotoxins, and free radicals; increased IgE in gingiva of PD patients suggests allergic factor in progression of PD in some patients.

- **Amalgam restorations:** faulty dental restorations and prostheses are common causes of gingival inflammation and periodontal destruction; overhanging margins are ideal for plaque and bacteria; silver amalgam decreases activities of antioxidant enzymes; mercury accumulation depletes free radical-scavenging enzymes, glutathione peroxidase, superoxide dismutase, and catalase; proteoglycans and glycosaminoglycans (GAGs) of collagen are sensitive to free radicals.

- **Miscellaneous local factors:** food impaction, unreplaced missing teeth, malocclusion, tongue thrusting, bruxism, toothbrush trauma, mouth breathing, tobacco (see below).

- **Tobacco:** smoking is linked to increased susceptibility to severe PD and tooth loss; harmful effects are free radical damage to epithelial cells; smoking greatly reduces ascorbate, potentiating damaging effects; carotenes and flavonoids greatly reduce toxic effects of smoking.

- **Structure and integrity of collagen matrix:** collagen of periodontal membrane serves as periosteum to alveolar bone; allows dissipation of tremendous pressure exerted during mastication; collagen matrix of periodontium (specifically extracellular proteoglycans of gingival epithelium) determines rate of diffusion and permeability of inflammatory mediators, bacteria and by-products, and destructive enzymes; high rate of protein turnover in periodontal collagen – thus integrity of collagen is vulnerable to atrophy when cofactors needed for collagen synthesis (protein, vitamin C, B_6, A, Zn, Cu) are absent/deficient; collagen of periodontium rich in GAGs – heparin sulfate, dermatan sulfate, and chondroitin 4-sulfate; stabilizing collagen is the major treatment goal.

THERAPEUTIC CONSIDERATIONS

Therapeutic goals in treating PD from nutritional perspective:
- decrease wound healing time
- improve membrane and collagen integrity
- decrease inflammation and free radical damage
- enhance immune status.

Vitamin C (ascorbic acid): plays major role in preventing PD; classical symptom of gingivitis in scurvy shows ascorbate maintains membrane and collagen integrity and immunocompetence.

- Deficiency linked to defective collagen, ground substance, and intercellular cement substance in mesenchymal tissue; deficiency effects on bone are retardation/cessation of osteoid formation, impaired osteoblastic activity, and osteoporosis; subclinical deficiency also delays wound healing.

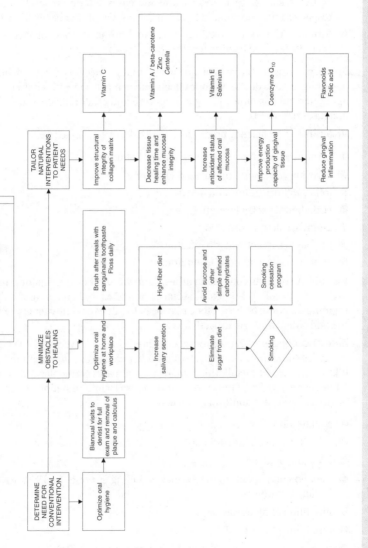

- Decreased vitamin C is linked to increased permeability of oral mucosa to endotoxin and bacterial by-products, and impaired leukocyte functions (PMNs).
- Increases chemotaxis and phagocytosis by PMNs, enhances lymphoproliferative response to mitogens and increases interferon levels, antibody response, immunoglobulin levels, and secretion of thymic hormones.
- Vitamin C has antioxidant and anti-inflammatory properties and decreases wound healing time.

Sucrose: sugar increases plaque accumulation; decreases PMN chemotaxis and phagocytosis due to osmotic effects and competition with vitamin C; average American consumes 175 g q.d. sucrose and other refined carbohydrates; increases risk for PD.

Vitamin A: deficiency predisposes to PD; deficiency linked to:

- keratinizing metaplasia of gingival epithelium
- early karyolysis of gingival epithelial cells
- inflammatory infiltration and degeneration
- periodontal pocket formation
- gingival calculus formation
- increased susceptibility to infection
- abnormal alveolar bone formation.

Vitamin A supports collagen synthesis and wound healing, maintains integrity of epithelial and mucosal surfaces and their secretions, and enhances immune function; beta-carotene may be better due to affinity for epithelial tissue and potent antioxidant activity.

Zinc and copper: Zn is synergist with vitamin A; severity of PD linked to increased Cu:Zn ratio – consistent with other causes of inflammation and signifies activation of metallothionein, which increases ceruloplasmin formation while increasing Zn sequestration in response to inflammation; Zn functions in gingiva and periodontium include:

- stabilization of membranes
- inhibition of calcium influxes
- antioxidant activity
- metallo-component in 40 enzymes including enzymes for DNA, RNA, and collagen synthesis
- inhibition of plaque growth
- inhibition of mast cell degranulation
- numerous immune activities, including increased PMN chemotaxis and phagocytosis.

Zinc reduces wound healing time; active in calcium- and calmodulin-mediated processes (mast cell degranulation, tissue damage induced by endotoxin, and increased vascular permeability); twice daily use of mouthwash with 5% zinc solution inhibits plaque growth.

Vitamin E and selenium: function synergistically in antioxidant mechanisms that deter PD; potentiate each other's effects; vitamin E decreases wound healing time; antioxidant effects of vitamin E are needed for silver amalgam – prevents toxic effects of Hg on antioxidant enzymes; Se and vitamin E prevent free radicals from damaging gingival proteo- and glycosaminoglycans.

Coenzyme Q: ubiquinone is a coenzyme in mitochondrial oxidative phosphorylation and an antioxidant; 70% of PD patients studied responded favorably to supplementation; superior to placebo in double-blind study.

Flavonoids: these are the most important components of anti-PD program; reduce inflammation and stabilize collagen:

● decrease membrane permeability, thereby decreasing load of inflammatory mediators and bacterial products
● prevent free radical damage via potent antioxidant properties
● inhibit enzymatic cleavage by hyaluronidases and collagenases
● inhibit mast cell degranulation
● cross-link with collagen fibers directly.

Supplement quercetin, catechin, anthocyanidins/proanthocyanidins; rutin has little collagen-stabilizing effect; 3-0-methyl-(+)-catechin retards plaque growth and alveolar bone resorption in animal models.

Folic acid: most common deficiency in the world; given either topically or systemically, reduces gingival inflammation – reduces color changes, bleeding tendency, exudate flow, and plaque scores; folate mouthwash (0.1% folic acid) is much more effective than oral supplement at 2 or 5 mg q.d., suggesting local mechanism; binds plaque-derived endotoxin; folate mouthwash is particularly indicated for pregnant women and oral contraceptive users, and in exaggerated gingival inflammatory response or folate anti-metabolites (phenytoin, methotrexate).

● Epithelium of cervix and oral mucosa suffer from "end-organ" folate deficiency under hormonal influences of pregnancy and oral contraceptives; cervical dysplasia of oral contraception also responds to pharmacological dose of folate (8–30 mg q.d.); sera and leukocytes of pregnant women and oral contraceptive users contain macromolecule that binds folate = major factor for "end-organ" folate deficiency.

Botanical medicines

● ***Sanguinaria canadensis:*** bloodroot contains benzophenanthridine alkaloids – sanguinarine in commercial toothpastes and mouth rinses; sanguinarine is antimicrobial and anti-inflammatory; inhibits bacterial adherence – bacteria aggregate and become morphologically irregular;

less effective than chlorhexidine mouthwash, but effective in many cases and is natural compound versus a synthetic.

- *Centella asiatica* **(gotu kola):** triterpenoids demonstrate impressive wound healing (*Textbook*, Ch. 74); useful in severe PD or if surgery required – speeds up recovery after laser surgery for severe PD.

THERAPEUTIC APPROACH

Control all relevant factors; general approach recommended; smoking greatly decreases success of any therapy for PD.

- **Hygiene:** periodic visits to dentist to eliminate plaque and calculus; brush after meals; daily flossing.

- **Diet:** high in dietary fiber – protective via increased salivary secretion; avoid sucrose and all refined carbohydrates.

- **Supplements:**
  — vitamin C: 3–5 g q.d. in divided doses
  — vitamin E: 400–800 IU q.d.
  — beta-carotenes: 250,000 IU q.d. (higher doses if indicated) for up to 6 months (instead of vitamin A due to similar effects and greater safety)
  — selenium: 400 µg q.d.
  — zinc: 30 mg q.d. of Zn picolinate (60 mg q.d. if another form); wash mouth with 15 ml of 5% solution b.i.d.
  — folic acid: 2 mg q.d.; wash mouth with 15 ml of 0.1% solution b.i.d.
  — quercetin: 500 mg t.i.d.

- **Botanical medicines:** high-flavonoid-containing extracts, such as those from bilberry (*Vaccinium myrtillus*), hawthorn (*Crataegus* sp.), grape seed (*Vitis vinifera*), or green tea (*Camellia sinensis*); green tea extract or liberal consumption of green tea is most cost-effective; green tea extract with 50% polyphenols – dosage = 200–300 mg b.i.d.
  — *Sanguinaria canadensis*: use toothpaste containing extract
  — *Centella asiatica* triterpenoids: 30 mg b.i.d. of pure triterpenoids.

Pneumonia: bacterial, mycoplasmal, and viral

GENERAL CONSIDERATIONS

Acute pneumonia is the fifth leading cause of death in US; particularly dangerous in elderly; usually in immunocompromised persons, especially drug/ETOH abusers; in healthy people, pneumonia follows insult to host defenses, viral infection (influenza), cigarette smoke and noxious fumes, impaired consciousness (which depresses gag reflex, allowing aspiration), neoplasms, and hospitalization.

- Airway distal to larynx normally sterile – mucus-covered ciliated epithelium propels sputum to larger bronchi and trachea, evoking cough reflex; respiratory secretions contain substances with non-specific antimicrobial actions: alpha-1-antitrypsin, lysozyme, and lactoferrin; alveolar defenses are alveolar macrophages, rich vasculature to rapidly deploy lymphocytes and granulocytes, and efficient lymphatic drainage network.

Immunoglobulin respiratory system defenses

- **IgA:** abundant in secretions of upper respiratory tract; protects against viruses; in lower tract, IgA helps:
  — agglutinate bacteria
  — neutralize microbial toxins
  — reduce bacterial attachment to mucosal surfaces
  — activate alternative complement pathway when complexed with an antigen.

- **IgG** present in lower respiratory tract; it:
  — serum agglutinates and opsonizes bacteria
  — activates complement
  — promotes chemotaxis of granulocytes and macrophages
  — neutralizes bacterial toxins and viruses
  — lyses Gram-negative bacteria.

THERAPEUTIC CONSIDERATIONS FOR ALL TYPES OF PNEUMONIA

- **Expectorants (botanical):** increase quantity, decrease viscosity, and promote expulsion of secretions of respiratory mucosa; many have antibacterial/antiviral activity; some are antitussives; *Lobelia inflata* helps promote cough reflex – much more effective clearing lungs than antitussive *Glycyrrhiza glabra* (licorice).
  - cough productive: use lobelia
  - cough non-productive: use licorice
  - other useful expectorants: balsam of Peru, senega root, grindelia, wild cherry bark, and horehound
  - bromelain is a mucolytic (discussed under "pneumococcal pneumonia").

- **Vitamin C:** effective, in large doses, only when started first or second day of infection; if started later, only lessens severity; in pneumonia WBCs uptake large amounts of vitamin C; value of vitamin C supplements in elderly patients – increased tissue vitamin C, even during acute respiratory infection; patients fare much better than those on placebo; most obvious benefit in patients with most severe illness.

- **Vitamin A:** valuable in pneumonia, especially in children with measles – increased rate of excretion of vitamin A during severe infections; study subjects with fever excreted much more retinol than those without fever; 400,000 IU (120 mg retinyl palmitate, half on admission and half a day later) given to children with measles, reduced death rate by > 50%, duration of pneumonia, diarrhea and hospital stay by 33%.

- **Vitamin E:** influenza complicated by pneumonia induces sharp rise in lipid peroxides (LPOs); alpha-tocopherol decreases LPO and improves clinical response.

- **Bromelain:** useful adjunct therapy – fibrinolytic, anti-inflammatory, and mucolytic actions; enhances antibiotic absorption; mucolysis responsible for efficacy in respiratory tract diseases – pneumonia, bronchitis, sinusitis.

THERAPEUTIC APPROACH FOR ALL TYPES OF PNEUMONIA

Enhance immune system (*Textbook*, Ch. 53); support respiratory tract drainage – local heat, massage, and expectorants.

- **Supplements:**
  - vitamin A: 50,000 IU q.d. for 1 week; OR beta-carotene: 200,000 IU q.d. (avoid vitamin A in women with reproductive capability due to teratogenic effect)

— vitamin C: 500 mg every 2 h

— vitamin E: 200 IU q.d.

— bioflavonoids: 1,000 mg q.d.

— zinc: 30 mg q.d.

— thymus extract: 120 mg pure polypeptides with molecular weights < 10,000 OR 500 mg crude polypeptide fraction.

● **Botanicals:**

— *Lobelia inflata*:
dried herb: 0.2–0.6 g t.i.d.
tincture: 15–30 drops t.i.d.
fluid extract: 8–10 drops t.i.d.

— *Echinacea* sp.:
dried root (or as tea): 0.5–1 g
freeze-dried plant: 325–650 mg
juice of aerial portion of *Echinacea purpurea* stabilized in 22% ethanol: 2–3 ml
tincture (1:5): 2–4 ml
fluid extract (1:1): 2–4 ml
solid (dry powdered) extract (6.5:1 or 3.5% echinacoside): 150–300 mg.

● **Physical therapy:**

— diathermy to chest and back: 30 min/day

— mustard poultice: once/day

— lymphatic massage: t.i.d.

— postural drainage: t.i.d.

For best results, use diathermy, then lymphatic massage, and finally postural drainage.

MYCOPLASMAL PNEUMONIA

DIAGNOSTIC SUMMARY

● Most commonly occurs in children or young adults.

● Insidious onset over several days.

● Non-productive cough, minimal physical findings, temperature generally less than 102°F.

● Headache and malaise are common early symptoms.

● WBC is normal or slightly elevated.

● X-ray pattern patchy or inhomogeneous.

THERAPEUTIC CONSIDERATIONS

Mycoplasma are bacteria that lack cell walls; *Mycoplasma pneumoniae* is the most frequent cause of community-acquired, non-pyogenic pneumonia; tracheobronchitis is more common than pneumonia; often with pharyngitis (children); slow recovery, but course variable; no specific natural medicine recommendations for mycoplasmal infections available; antibiotic (erythromycin) indicated; enhancement of general immunity recommended.

Additional therapies: *antibiotic* – erythromycin: 250– 500 mg q.i.d.

PNEUMOCOCCAL (STREPTOCOCCAL) PNEUMONIA

DIAGNOSTIC SUMMARY

- Pneumonia usually preceded by URI.
- Sudden onset of shaking, chills, fever, and chest pain.
- Sputum pinkish/blood-specked at first, rusty at height of infection, yellow/mucopurulent during resolution.
- Gram-positive diplococci in the sputum smear.
- Initially chest excursion diminished on involved side; breath sounds suppressed; fine inspiratory rales.
- Later classic signs of consolidation (bronchial breathing, crepitant rales, dullness).
- Leukocytosis.
- X-ray shows lobar or segmental consolidation.

THERAPEUTIC CONSIDERATIONS

Pneumococcal pneumonia (*Streptococcus pneumoniae*) is the most common bacterial pneumonia and most common cause of pneumonia requiring hospitalization; use careful clinical judgment to determine disease severity and patient's immune status – antibiotics/hospitalization may be needed; blood culture is more accurate than sputum culture – nasopharynx is the natural habitat of *Pneumococcus*.

- **Bovine spleen extracts:** most specific natural medicine for pneumococcal pneumonia (*Textbook*, Ch. 41); post-splenectomy syndrome – increased risk of pneumococcal pneumonia (2.5% of splenectomized patients die from pneumococcal pneumonia within 5 years); spleen extracts rich in tuftsin may be effective natural alternative to vaccines and prophylactic antibiotics in these patients; spleen extracts increase WBCs in patients with extreme WBC deficiencies and are beneficial in malaria and typhoid fever.

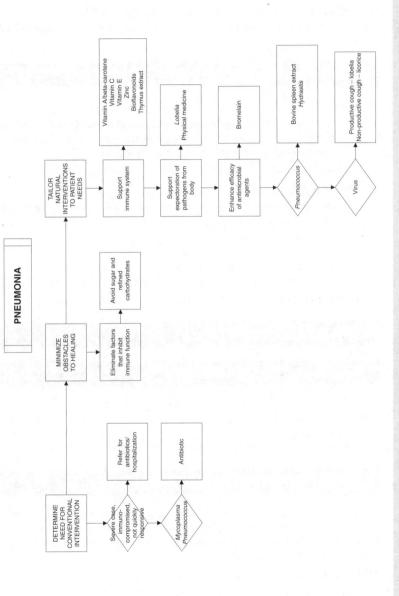

PNEUMONIA

DETERMINE NEED FOR CONVENTIONAL INTERVENTION

Severe case, immuno-compromised, not quickly responsive → Refer for antibiotics/hospitalization

Mycoplasma Pneumococcus → Antibiotic

MINIMIZE OBSTACLES TO HEALING

Eliminate factors that inhibit immune function → Avoid sugar and refined carbohydrates

TAILOR NATURAL INTERVENTIONS TO PATIENT NEEDS

Support immune system → Vitamin A/beta-carotene, Vitamin C, Vitamin E, Zinc, Bioflavonoids, Thymus extract

Support expectoration of pathogens from body → *Lobelia*, Physical medicine

Enhance efficacy of antimicrobial agents → Bromelain

Pneumococcus → Bovine spleen extract, *Hydrastis*

Virus → Productive cough – lobelia, Non-productive cough – licorice

- *Hydrastis canadensis*: berberine-containing botanicals are very important – berberine has documented antibiotic activity against pathogenic streptococci; spares normal GI microflora.
- **Antibiotics:** conventional antibiotics, typically penicillin G or V, are very beneficial; appropriately prescribed course of antibiotics gives substantial clinical improvement within a few days.

ADDITIONAL THERAPIES

- **Supplements:**
  - bovine spleen extracts: hydrolyzed (predigested) concentrated for tuftsin and splenopentin content preferred: 50 mg q.d. tuftsin and splenopentin or roughly 1.5 g q.d. of total spleen peptides
  - bromelain (1,200–1,800 mcu): 500–750 mg t.i.d. between meals.
- **Botanical medicines:**
  - *Hydrastis canadensis*: dosage based on berberine content; prefer standardized extracts; t.i.d. doses:
    dried root or as infusion (tea): 2–4 g
    tincture (1:5): 6–12 ml (1.5–3 tsp)
    fluid extract (1:1): 2–4 ml (0.5–1 tsp)
    solid (powdered dry) extract (4:1 or 8–12% alkaloid content): 250–500 mg.
- **Antibiotic:** penicillin V – 500 mg q.i.d. (for uncomplicated cases).

VIRAL PNEUMONIA

DIAGNOSTIC SUMMARY

- Onset typical of influenza: fever, myalgia, headache.
- Other symptoms, signs, and X-ray findings are similar to mycoplasmal pneumonia.

THERAPEUTIC CONSIDERATIONS

Treatment recommendations given under general discussion of pneumonia; *Glycyrrhiza glabra* (licorice) is antiviral, immune-enhancing, and expectorant (*Textbook*, Ch. 90), but it also has antitussive effect; unproductive cough – use licorice; productive cough – use lobelia.

Additional therapy: *Glycyrrhiza glabra* (licorice):

— powdered root: 1–2 g
— fluid extract (1:1): 2–4 ml
— solid (dry powdered) extract (4:1): 250–500 mg.

Diagnostic hierarchy

- Rule out hypothyroidism
  - determine basal body temperature
  - if temperature < 97.8°F, or if symptoms indicate, determine blood TSH and T_4.
- Rule out depression.
- If no improvement after 2 months, perform the following:
  - complete blood count (CBC)
  - chemistry panel
  - thyroid panel
  - T_3 uptake
  - thyroxin
  - free thyroxin index
  - ferritin
  - progesterone
  - estrogen
  - prolactin.
- If no apparent abnormalities in CBC, chemistry panel, or hormone levels, consider these tests in order of importance: liver detoxification, adrenal stress index, food allergy panel.

THERAPEUTIC CONSIDERATIONS

The primary causes of PMS

- Estrogen excess
- Progesterone deficiency
- Elevated prolactin levels
- Hypothyroidism
- Stress, endogenous opioid deficiency, and adrenal dysfunction
- Depression
- Nutritional abnormalities
  - macronutrient disturbances/excesses
  - micronutrient deficiency

Estrogen and progesterone

Common finding is elevated estrogen/progesterone ratio caused by mild estrogen elevation and mild progesterone deficiency; increased ratio contributes to PMS by inducing impaired liver function, reducing manufacture of serotonin, decreasing action of vitamin B_6, increasing aldosterone secretion, and increasing prolactin secretion.

- **Estrogen excess and liver function:** estrogen detox is a liver function requiring adequate B-vitamins; detox impaired by cholestasis arising from estrogen excess or birth control pills, pregnancy, gallstones, alcohol, endotoxins, hereditary disorders (e.g. Gilbert's syndrome), anabolic steroids, chemicals or drugs; cholestasis may be predisposing factor to PMS.

- **Effects of estrogen on neurotransmitters:** elevated estrogen/progesterone ratio impairs neurotransmitter synthesis; elevated ratio during luteal phase is also linked to decline in endorphins, adversely impacting mood; low endorphins are common in women with PMS.

- **Estrogen impairs vitamin B_6:** negative effects of estrogen excess on neurotransmitters may be a consequence of its effect on action of B_6; B_6 levels are low in depressed patients, especially those taking estrogens (birth control pills, Premarin); B_6 supplements have positive effects on all PMS symptoms, particularly depression.

- **Estrogen effects on aldosterone:** estrogen excess can increase aldosterone secretion 2–8 days prior to menses.

- **Estrogen and prolactin secretion:** endogenous and exogenous estrogens can increase prolactin secretion by pituitary; elevated prolactin linked to breast pain and fibrocystic breast disease; *Vitex agnus-castus* (chaste berry) may help elevated prolactin due to corpus luteum deficiency; B_6 and zinc supplements can lower prolactin; prolactin elevation can also be linked to low thyroid function.

Reducing estrogen/progesterone ratio

- **Dietary recommendations:** dietary factors can reduce circulating estrogens or block their attachment to receptors; increase plant foods (vegetables, fruits, legumes, whole grains, nuts, seeds); low to moderate meat and dairy; reduce fat and sugar intake; increase soy foods; reduce exposure to environmental estrogens – pesticides, herbicides, etc.

- **Establish proper gastrointestinal flora:** liver detoxifies hormones and carcinogenic compounds by binding them to glucuronic acid and excreting them in bile; undesirable colon bacteria produce enzyme beta-glucuronidase, which uncouples toxins from glucuronic acid, allowing toxins to be reabsorbed into circulation; establishing proper bacterial flora can reduce activity of this enzyme; probiotic supplements (*Lactobacillus acidophilus* and *Bifidobacterium bifidum*) can restore healthy flora.

- **Enhance liver detoxification:** protect liver by following dietary guidelines; use "lipotropic factors" (choline, methionine, betaine, folic acid, vitamin B_{12}, herbal cholagogues and choleretics) to reduce fat deposition in liver by improving fat metabolism; daily dosage of lipotropics: 1,000 mg choline and 500 mg methionine and/or cysteine.

- **Consider progesterone therapy:** clinical trials have failed to demonstrate consistent superiority of progesterone over placebo in PMS, which has a significant placebo response; positive studies used dosages (200–400 mg b.i.d. as vaginal or rectal suppository from 14 days before menses until onset) that far exceed normal progesterone levels and estrogen/progesterone ratio; mild side-effects are common: menstrual irregularity, vaginal itching, HA; philosophically preferable to address underlying causes (reduced estrogen detox and reduced corpus luteum function) rather than drastic artificial altering of estrogen/progesterone ratio.

Low thyroid function in PMS

Hypothyroidism affects large percentage of women with PMS; many women with PMS and confirmed hypothyroidism experience complete relief of symptoms when given thyroid hormone.

Stress, endorphins, and exercise in PMS

Extreme, unusual, or long-lasting stress can trigger brain changes arising from altered adrenal function and endorphin secretion; women in regular exercise programs do not suffer PMS nearly as often as sedentary women; exercise alleviates PMS by elevating endorphins and decreasing cortisol.

- **Coping style and PMS:** most women with PMS employ "negative" coping style, exemplified by feelings of helplessness, overeating, devoting too much time to television viewing, emotional outbursts, overspending, excessive behavior, dependence on chemicals (legal and illicit drugs, tobacco, alcohol); patients need to be counseled on more positive ways to cope.

- **Psychotherapy:** biofeedback and short-term individual counseling (especially cognitive therapy) have documented clinical efficacy; cognitive therapy has advantage over antidepressant drugs of producing excellent results that can be maintained over time.

- **Depression and low serotonin:** depression is a common feature of PMS; PMS symptoms are more severe in depressed women, seemingly because of decreased brain neurotransmitters: serotonin, gamma-amino-butyric acid; 80% of the 12 million Americans on Prozac are women aged 25–50.

Diet considerations

PMS women tend to eat diet even worse than standard North American diet; recommendations: predominantly vegetarian diet, reduce intake of fat, eliminate sugar, avoid environmental estrogens, increase soy foods, eliminate caffeine, keep salt intake low.

- **Vegetarian diet and estrogen metabolism:** vegetarian women excrete two to three times more estrogen in feces and have 50% lower free estrogen in blood compared with omnivores; these differences are consequences of lower fat, higher fiber in vegetarian diets and can explain lower incidence of breast cancer, heart disease, and menopausal symptoms among vegetarian women; minimal changes – reduce saturated fat and cholesterol by eating less animal products; increase fiber-rich plant food (fruits, vegetables, grains, legumes); limit animal protein to no more than 4–6 oz q.d., choosing fish, skinless poultry, lean meats; fiber promotes excretion of estrogens directly and indirectly by promoting favorable bacteria with lower levels of beta-glucuronidase.

- **Fat intake and estrogen metabolism:** reducing percentage of calories as fat (saturated) can dramatically reduce circulating estrogens; low-fat diet improves PMS symptoms; eliminate margarine and foods containing *trans* fatty acids and partially hydrogenated oils.

- **Eliminate sugar:** sugar is detrimental to organs involved in blood sugar control, especially in hypoglycemic and diabetic patients; sugar plus caffeine combination is detrimental to mood; most significant symptom-producing food in PMS is chocolate; high sugar intake may impair estrogen metabolism; women with high sugar intake have higher frequency of PMS; read food labels carefully to identify all forms of sugar.

- **Reducing exposure to environmental estrogens:** halogenated hydrocarbons group includes toxic pesticides (DDT, DDE, PCB, PCP, dieldrin, chlordane), which are not easily biodegraded, are stored in fat cells, and mimic estrogen in body; may be a major factor in epidemic of estrogen-related health problems (PMS, breast cancer, oligospermia); concentration of these compounds in fruits and vegetables is much lower than in animal fats, meat, cheese, whole milk, and eggs.

- **Increase soy foods:** soy contains "phytoestrogens" that bind to estrogen receptors; phytoestrogens are "anti-estrogens" with only 2% of potency of endogenous estrogens; balancing effect of phytoestrogens: low endogenous estrogen (menopause) augmented by mild estrogenic effect of phytoestrogens, while high endogenous estrogen effects (PMS) reduced by binding of less-potent phytoestrogens to estrogen receptors.

- **Caffeine and PMS:** avoid caffeine, especially if anxiety, depression, breast tenderness, or fibrocystic breast disease are major symptoms; caffeine is strongly linked to presence and severity of PMS; caffeine is particularly significant in psychological symptoms of PMS.

- **Salt and PMS:** excess NaCl intake, plus reduced intake of K^+, causes kidney stress which, in "salt-sensitive" people, leads to hypertension or water retention; patients with water retention during mid-luteal phase must reduce salt; increase K^+-rich foods; avoid processed foods high in Na; keep Na intake < 1,800 mg q.d.

Micronutrients in PMS

- **Vitamin B_6:** B_6 supplements alone benefit most patients; some women have impaired ability to convert B_6 to active form (pyridoxal-5-phosphate) due to deficiency in other nutrients (vitamin B_2); use broader-spectrum nutritional supplements or injectable pyridoxal-5-phosphate.

— dosage: therapeutic = 50–100 mg q.d. (safe long-term); daily intake above 50 mg divided into 50 mg doses due to limits on liver's capacity to convert B_6 to P5P

— safety of vitamin B_6: one-time dose > 2,000 mg q.d. can produce neurotoxicity in some patients – tingling sensations in feet, loss of muscle coordination, degeneration of nerve tissue; chronic dosing > 500 mg q.d. is toxic if taken for many months or years; toxicity has occurred in some people taking long-term doses as low as 150 mg q.d.; toxicity may arise from overwhelming liver conversion of B_6 to P5P – pyridoxine may itself be toxic to nerve cells or it may block receptors for P5P, leading to intracellular B_6 deficiency

— B_6 and magnesium: work together in many enzyme systems; B_6 may improve PMS symptoms by increasing intracellular Mg – B_6 is essential to transport of Mg into cell.

● **Magnesium and PMS:** RBC Mg in PMS patients is much lower than in normal subjects; Mg deficiency may account for wide range of PMS symptoms due to integral role in cell function; Mg supplements are effective treatment for PMS.

— plasma Mg in PMS patients and controls similar; no menstrual cycle effect on plasma Mg in either group; PMS patients have much lower RBC and MBC (mononuclear blood cell) Mg compared with controls; lower RBC/MBC Mg in PMS patients is consistent across menstrual cycle; Mg measures do not correlate with severity of PMS symptoms

— women with PMS are vulnerable to luteal phase mood destabilization – chronic intracellular Mg depletion is a major predisposing factor; PMS Mg deficiency is also characterized by nervous sensitivity, generalized aches and pains, and a lowered premenstrual pain threshold

— Mg is effective in itself but better combined with B_6 and other nutrients

— dosage: health maintenance = 6 mg/kg (2.2 lb) body weight; therapeutic for PMS: 12 mg/kg body weight

— prefer Mg bound to Krebs cycle intermediates (malate, succinate, fumarate, citrate) due to better absorption and fewer side-effects (laxative effects).

● **Calcium:** two-edged sword in PMS depending on form used; high milk intake is a causative factor, the combination of Ca, vitamin D, and phosphorus reducing Mg absorption; improved PMS symptoms (mood, concentration, behavior, water retention) are achieved with calcium supplements (1,000–1,336 mg q.d.); theory based on animal research: Ca improves hormonal patterns, neurotransmitter levels, and smooth muscle responsiveness; women with PMS have reduced bone mineral density (dual-photon absorptiometry).

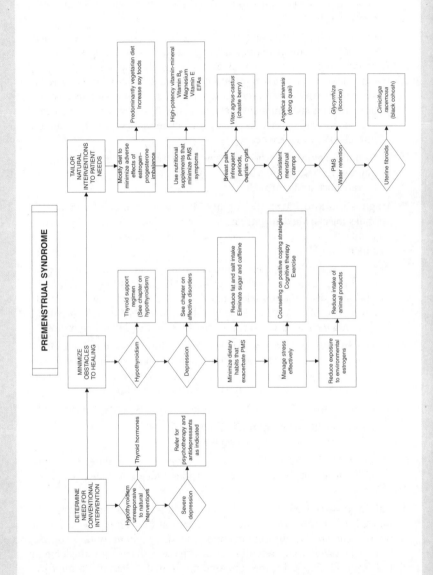

- **Zinc:** lower in women with PMS; serves as a control factor for prolactin secretion – low Zn promotes and high Zn inhibits prolactin release; zinc supplements essential in high prolactin states; dosage = 30–45 mg q.d.

- **Vitamin E:** significantly reduces a number of PMS symptoms: breast tenderness, nervous tension, HA, fatigue, depression, insomnia, craving for sweets; dosage: 400 IU q.d.

- **Essential fatty acids:** women with PMS exhibit EFA and prostaglandin abnormalities; chief abnormality is decreased gamma-linolenic acid (GLA); sources of GLA are borage oil, black currant, evening primrose; EPO alone is of little value for PMS; better approach is to provide broader range of nutrients necessary for EFA metabolism, plus good sources of EFAs.

- **Multiple vitamin-mineral supplements:** nutritional deficiency is relatively common among women with PMS; supplements produce significant benefits in PMS; supplements containing high doses of Mg and B_6 reduce (by 70%) pre- and post-menstrual symptoms.

Botanical medicines

Few have been specifically studied for their efficacy in alleviating PMS symptoms; tonic effects on female glandular system: improved hormonal balance (phytoestrogens) and blood flow to female organs; estrogenic activity of phytoestrogens = 2% of that of estrogen providing balancing influence.

- ***Angelica sinensis* (dong quai):** historical use – menopausal symptoms (hot flashes), dysmenorrhea, amenorrhea, metrorrhagia, to ensure healthy pregnancy and easy delivery; good uterine tonic – initial increase in uterine contraction followed by relaxation; increases uterine weight and glucose utilization by uterus and liver, indicating estrogenic activity; particularly helpful if patient also has dysmenorrhea; timing of administration: begin on day 14 of menstrual cycle and continue until menstruation; if dysmenorrhea, begin day 14 and continue until end of menstrual flow; dosage (t.i.d.): powdered root or as tea (1–2 g), tincture (1:5) (4 ml [1 tsp]), fluid extract (1 ml [1/4 tsp]).

- ***Glycyrrhiza glabra* (licorice):** traditional uses – female disorders, expectorant and antitussive (respiratory infections and asthma), peptic ulcers, malaria, abdominal pain, insomnia, infections; believed useful in PMS by lowering estrogen and elevating progesterone; raises progesterone by inhibiting enzyme that breaks it down; reduces water retention by blocking the hormone aldosterone; glycyrrhetinic acid binds to aldosterone receptors, competing with aldosterone for binding sites; lower activity of licorice constituents at these binding sites reduces water retention effect; long-term, large-dose ingestion of licorice by persons with normal aldosterone may cause Na^+ and water retention, elevating blood pressure; preventing this side-effect is possible with high-K^+, low-Na^+ diet; avoid if history of hypertension, renal failure, or current use of digitalis; timing of administration: start day 14 and continue until menstruation; dosage (t.i.d.): powdered root or as a tea (1–2 g); fluid extract (1:1) (4 ml [1 tsp]); solid (dry powdered) extract (4:1) (250–500 mg).

● *Cimicifuga racemosa* **(black cohosh):** historical use – menstrual cramps and menopause; concentrated, lab-standardized extract effective in reducing depression, anxiety, tension, mood swings; dosage (standardized extract containing 1 mg 27–deoxyactein per tablet): 1 tablet q.d. or b.i.d.

● *Vitex agnus-castus* **(chaste tree):** historical use – female complaints, to suppress libido; particularly useful for corpus luteum insufficiency or pro-lactin excess; profound effect on hypothalamus and pituitary, altering release of gonadotropin-releasing hormone (GnRH) and follicle-stimulating hormone-releasing hormone; normalizes secretion of hormones (pro-lactin) and reduces estrogen/progesterone ratio; may be useful in certain cases of amenorrhea due to prolactin excess (a frequent cause); may require 3 months of treatment to lower prolactin levels; dosage (q.d.): concentrated extract standardized to contain 0.5% agnuside (175–225 mg), liquid extract (2 ml).

THERAPEUTIC APPROACH

1. Evaluate PMS symptoms by having patient complete questionnaire (*Textbook*, App. 8).

2. Rule out hypothyroidism and/or depression.

3. Dietary recommendations:
   — predominantly vegetarian diet
   — reduce fat intake
   — eliminate sugar
   — reduce exposure to environmental estrogens
   — increase consumption of soy foods
   — eliminate caffeine
   — keep salt intake low.

4. Follow guidelines for nutritional supplements.

5. Use appropriate herbal support:
   — PMS-associated breast pain, infrequent periods, or history of ovarian cysts: chaste berry
   — consistent experience of menstrual cramps: *Angelica* (dong quai)
   — PMS water retention: licorice
   — uterine fibroids: black cohosh.

6. Reduce stress, use positive coping strategies, and exercise regularly.

7. Identify additional causative factors if significant improvement is not achieved after at least three complete menstrual cycles.

● **Nutritional supplements:**

— multivitamin and mineral
— vitamin B_6: 100 mg q.d.
— magnesium: 500 mg q.d.
— vitamin E: 400 IU q.d.

● **Botanical medicines:**

— *Angelica sinensis* (t.i.d.)
  powdered root or as tea: 1–2 g
  tincture (1:5): 4 ml (1 tsp)
  fluid extract: 1 ml (1/4 tsp)

— *Glycyrrhiza glabra* (t.i.d.)
  powdered root or as tea: 1–2 g
  fluid extract (1:1): 4 ml (1 tsp)
  solid (dry powdered) extract (4:1): 250–500 mg

— *Cimicifuga racemosa* (b.i.d.)
  standardized extract (4 mg 27-deoxyactein): 1 tablet (2 for menopausal women)

— *Vitex agnus-castus* (q.d.)
  standardized extract (0.5% agnuside): 175–225 mg
  liquid extract: 2 ml.

PREMENSTRUAL SYNDROME QUESTIONNAIRE

Grading of symptoms

1. None
2. Mild – present but does not interfere with activities
3. Moderate – present and interferes with activities, but not disabling
4. Severe – disabling (unable to function).

Grade your symptoms for last menstrual cycle only.

Subgroup	Symptoms	Week after period	Week before period
PMS-A	Anxiety	——	——
	Irritability	——	——
	Mood swings	——	——
	Nervous tension	——	——
	Total	——	——
PMS-C	Increased appetite	——	——
	Headache	——	——
	Fatigue	——	——
	Dizziness or fainting	——	——
	Palpitations	——	——
	Craving for sweets	——	——
	Total	——	——
PMS-D	Depression	——	——
	Crying	——	——
	Forgetfulness	——	——
	Confusion	——	——
	Insomnia	——	——
	Total	——	——
PMS-H	Weight gain > 3#	——	——
	Swollen extremities	——	——
	Breast tenderness	——	——
	Abdominal bloating	——	——
	Total	——	——
Total MSQ score		——	——

Subgroup	Symptoms	Week after period	Week before period
Other symptoms	Oily skin	——	——
	Acne	——	——
During first	Menstrual cramps	——	——
2 days of period	Menstrual backache	——	——

Psoriasis

DIAGNOSTIC SUMMARY

- Sharply bordered reddened rash or plaques covered with overlapping silvery scales.
- Characteristically involves the scalp, the extensor surfaces (backside of the wrists, elbows, knees, buttocks, and ankles), and sites of repeated trauma.
- Family history in 50% of cases.
- Nail involvement results in characteristic "oil drop" stippling.
- Possible arthritis.

GENERAL CONSIDERATIONS

Psoriasis is an extremely common skin disorder. US rate of occurrence = 2–4%; affects few Blacks in tropics, but more common among Blacks in temperate zones; common among Japanese, rare in American Indians; affects men and women equally; mean onset age = 27.8 years, but 2% onset by age 2 years.

- Classic hyperproliferative skin disorder – rate of cell division very high (1,000 times > normal skin), exceeding rate in squamous cell carcinoma; even uninvolved skin is 2.5 times greater than in nonpsoriatics.

- Basic defect is within skin cells; incidence increased in HLA-B_{13}, HLA-B_{16}, and HLA-B_{17} – genetic error in mitotic control; 36% of patients have family members with psoriasis; cell division rate controlled by delicate balance between cyclic AMP and cyclic GMP; increased cGMP is linked to increased proliferation; increased cAMP is linked to enhanced cell maturation and decreased proliferation; decreased cAMP and increased cGMP measured in skin of psoriatics.

THERAPEUTIC CONSIDERATIONS

Rebalancing cAMP:cGMP ratio achievable via natural medicine; controllable factors contributing to psoriasis are described below.

Incomplete protein digestion

Incomplete digestion or poor absorption increases amino acids/polypeptides in bowel – metabolized by bowel bacteria into toxins; toxic metabolites of arginine and ornithine are "polyamines" (putrescine, spermidine, cadaverine) – increased in psoriatics; polyamines inhibit formation of cAMP, inducing excess cell proliferation; lowered skin and urinary polyamines are linked to clinical improvement; natural compounds inhibit formation of polyamines – vitamin A and berberine alkaloids of *Hydrastis canadensis* (goldenseal) inhibit bacterial decarboxylase enzyme which converts amino acids into polyamines; evaluate digestive function with Heidelburg Gastric Analysis and/or Comprehensive Digestive Stool Analysis; reinforce digestion (HCl, pancreatic enzymes).

Bowel toxemia

Gut-derived toxins implicated – endotoxins (compounds from cell walls of Gram-negative bacteria), streptococci, *Candida albicans*, yeast, and IgE and IgA immune complexes); increase cGMP, promoting proliferation; chronic candidiasis may play major role in many cases.

● Low-fiber diet linked to increased gut-derived toxins; fiber of fruits, vegetables, whole grains, and legumes bind toxins and promote their excretion.

● Aqueous extract of *Smilax sarsaparilla* is effective in psoriasis, particularly chronic, large plaque-forming variety – improved psoriasis in 62% of patients and completely cleared another 18% (80% benefited); benefit due to sarsaparilla components binding and excretion endotoxins; severity and response correlate well with level of circulating endotoxins – control of gut-derived toxins is critical; support fecal excretion and proper handling of absorbed endotoxins by liver.

Liver function

Correcting abnormal liver function is beneficial; liver filters and detoxifies portal blood from bowels; if liver is overwhelmed by excess bowel toxins or if there is a decrease in liver's detox ability, systemic toxin level increases and psoriasis worsens; ETOH worsens psoriasis – increases toxin absorption by damaging gut mucosa and impairs liver function; eliminate ETOH; silymarin, flavonoid of *Silybum marianum*, is valuable in treating psoriasis by improving liver function, inhibiting inflammation, and reducing excess cellular proliferation.

Nutrition

Omega-3 fatty acids: EPA improves psoriasis due to competition for arachidonic acid binding sites, inhibiting synthesis of inflammatory leukotrienes from arachidonic acid, which is many times greater than normal in psoriatics; leukotrienes promote guanylate cyclase activity.

- Cellular free arachidonic acid and 12-HETE (product of lipoxygenase metabolism of arachidonic acid) are 250 and 810 times greater, respectively, than uninvolved epidermal tissue; tissue intrinsic unidentified inhibitor of cyclooxygenase is involved.

- Trauma releases free arachidonic acid – plaques at sites of repeated trauma; increased 12-HETE stimulates 5-lipoxygenase, promoting leukotriene formation; this pathway is inhibited by EPA and glutathione peroxidase – selenium deficiency may contribute (see below under nutritional considerations).

- Cyclooxygenase inhibitors (aspirin, NSAIDs) may exacerbate psoriasis; lipoxygenase inhibitors (benoxaprofen) may improve; natural substances (quercetin, ubiquitous plant flavonoid), vitamin E, onion, and garlic inhibit lipoxygenase.

- Arachidonic acid is found only in animal tissues; limit animal products – animal fats and dairy.

Diet, fasting, and food allergy control: psoriasis is positively linked to body mass index and inversely related to intake of carrots, tomatoes, fresh fruits, and index of beta-carotene intake; fasting and vegetarian regimens help psoriatics – probably due to decreased gut-derived toxins and polyamines; gluten-free and elimination diets are beneficial.

Individual nutrients:

- **Decreased vitamin A and zinc** is common in psoriasis; A and Zn are critical to skin health of skin.

- **Chromium** is indicated to increase insulin receptor sensitivity – psoriatics have increased serum insulin and glucose.

- **Glutathione peroxidase** (GP) low in psoriatics – possibly due to ETOH abuse, malnutrition, and excess skin loss of hyperproliferation; GP is normalized with oral Se and vitamin E; low serum concentrations in whole blood Se are common in psoriasis; lowest whole blood Se found in male patients with widespread disease of long duration requiring methotrexate and retinoids.

- **Active vitamin D** (1,25-dihydroxycholecalciferol) plays role in controlling cell proliferation/differentiation; topical 1,25-dihydroxycholecalciferol and oral 1alpha(OH)D_3 may be helpful; severe psoriasis patients have very low serum 1,25-dihydroxycholecalciferol which normalizes with oral 1alpha(OH)D_3.

- **Fumaric acid:** oral dimethylfumaric acid (240 mg q.d.) or monoethylfumaric acid (720 mg q.d.) and topical 1–3% of monoethylfumaric acid are useful, but side-effects (flushing of skin, nausea, diarrhea, malaise, gastric

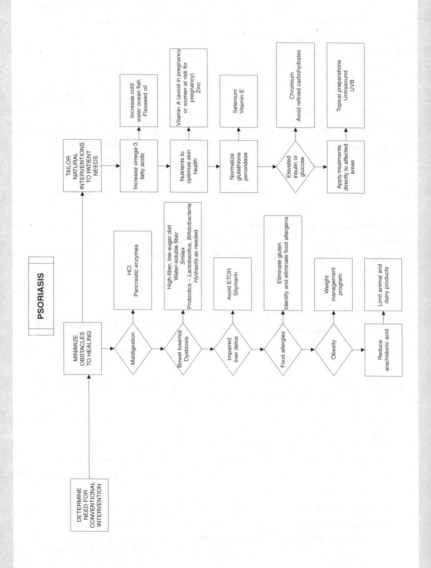

PSORIASIS

DETERMINE NEED FOR CONVENTIONAL INTERVENTION

MINIMIZE OBSTACLES TO HEALING

- Maldigestion
  - HCl
  - Pancreatic enzymes

- Bowel toxemia / Dysbiosis
  - High-fiber, low-sugar diet
  - Water-soluble fiber
  - *Smilax*
  - Probiotics – *Lactobacillus, Bifidobacteria*
  - *Hydrastis* as needed

- Impaired liver detox
  - Avoid ETOH
  - Silymarin

- Food allergies
  - Eliminate gluten
  - Identify and eliminate food allergens

- Obesity
  - Weight management program

- Reduce arachidonic acid
  - Limit animal and dairy products

TAILOR NATURAL INTERVENTIONS TO PATIENT NEEDS

- Increase omega-3 fatty acids
  - Increase cold water ocean fish
  - Flaxseed oil

- Nutrients to optimize skin health
  - Vitamin A (avoid in pregnancy or women at risk for pregnancy)
  - Zinc

- Normalize glutathione peroxidase
  - Selenium
  - Vitamin E

- Elevated insulin or glucose
  - Chromium
  - Avoid refined carbohydrates

- Apply treatments directly to affected areas
  - Topical preparations
  - Untrasound
  - UVB

pain, mild liver and kidney disturbances) can occur; use only if other natural therapies fail.

Psychological aspects

Thirty nine per cent of psoriatics report specific stressful event within 1 month prior to initial episode; such patients have better prognosis; a few cases are successfully treated with hypnosis and biofeedback alone.

Physical therapeutics

Sunlight (ultraviolet light) is extremely beneficial (standard medical treatment is drug psoralen plus ultraviolet A – PUVA therapy); ultraviolet B (UVB) alone inhibits cell proliferation and is as effective as PUVA with fewer side-effects; UV may benefit via induction of skin vitamin D synthesis; induction of localized elevation of temperature (42–45°C) in affected area by ultrasound and heating pads is effective.

Topical treatments

Botanical alternatives to hydrocortisone: glycyrrhetinic acid from licorice (*Glycyrrhiza glabra*), chamomile (*Matricaria chamomilla*), and capsaicin from cayenne pepper (*Capsicum frutescens*).

- *Glycyrrhiza glabra* **(licorice root):** glycyrrhetinic acid effect is similar to topical hydrocortisone; superior to topical cortisone, especially in chronic cases; can potentiate effects of topical hydrocortisone by inhibiting 11-beta-hydroxy-steroid dehydrogenase which catalyzes conversion of hydrocortisone to inactive form.

- *Matricaria chamomilla* **(chamomile):** flavonoid and essential oil components are anti-inflammatory and anti-allergic.

- *Capsicum frutescens* **(cayenne pepper):** capsaicin is the active component of cayenne pepper; topically applied, capsaicin stimulates and then blocks small-diameter pain fibers by depleting pain neurotransmitter substance P, which is elevated in the skin of psoriatics and activates inflammatory mediators in psoriasis; topical 0.025 or 0.075% capsaicin is effective in improving psoriasis – reduces scaling and redness; burning, stinging, itching, and skin redness noted by half of patients initially, but diminished or vanished with continued application; proven superior to placebo.

- *Aloe vera*: topical extract in hydrophilic cream is highly effective in psoriasis vulgaris; well tolerated by all patients studied, with no adverse drug-related symptoms and no drop-outs.

THERAPEUTIC APPROACH

Decrease bowel toxemia; rebalance fatty acid and inflammatory processes in skin; use therapeutic regimen to further balance abnormal cell proliferation.

- **Diet:** limit sugar, meat, animal fats, and alcohol; increase dietary fiber and cold-water fish; normalize weight; eliminate gluten; identify and address food allergies.

- **Supplements:**
  — high-potency multiple vitamin-mineral formula
  — flaxseed oil: 1 tbsp q.d.
  — vitamin A: 50,000 IU q.d. (avoid in pregnant or women at risk for pregnancy)
  — vitamin E: 400 IU q.d.
  — chromium: 400 µg q.d.
  — selenium: 200 µg q.d.
  — zinc: 30 mg q.d.
  — water-soluble fiber (psyllium, pectin, guar gum, etc.): 5 g at bedtime.

- **Botanical medicines:**
  — *Hydrastis canadensis* (goldenseal): dosage based on berberine content; prefer standardized extracts (t.i.d.):
  dried root or as infusion (tea): 2–4 g
  fluid extract (1:1): 2–4 ml (0.5–1 tsp)
  solid (powdered dry) extract (4:1 or 8–12% alkaloid content): 250–500 mg

  — *Smilax sarsaparilla* (t.i.d.):
  dried root or by decoction: 1–4 g
  liquid extract (1:1): 8–16 ml (2–4 tsp)
  solid extract (4:1): 250–500 mg

  — *Silybum marianum* (milk thistle):
  silymarin: 70–210 mg t.i.d.

- **Psychological:** evaluate stress levels and utilize stress reduction techniques as appropriate.

- **Physical medicines:**
  — ultrasound: 42–45°C, 20 min, three times/week
  — UVB: 295–305 nm, 2 mW/cm^2, 3 min, three times/week.

- **Topical treatment:** preparations containing one or more of the ingredients described above; apply to affected areas of skin b.i.d.–t.i.d.

Rheumatoid arthritis

DIAGNOSTIC SUMMARY

- Fatigue, low-grade fever, weakness, weight loss, joint stiffness, and vague joint pain preceding painful, swollen joints by several weeks.
- Severe joint pain with inflammation beginning insidiously in small joints and progressing to all joints.
- X-ray findings: soft tissue swelling, erosion of cartilage, and joint space narrowing.
- Rheumatoid factor in serum.
- Extra-articular manifestations: vasculitis, muscle atrophy, subcutaneous and systemic granulomas, pleurisy, pericarditis, pulmonary fibrosis, lymphadenopathy, splenomegaly, anemia, and leukopenia.

GENERAL CONSIDERATIONS

Rheumatoid arthritis (RA) is a chronic inflammatory condition affecting the entire body but especially synovial membranes of joints; joints involved: hands, feet, wrists, ankles, and knees; affects 1–3% of population; females outnumber males 3:1; age of onset is 20–40 years, but may begin at any age; onset gradual, but occasionally quite abrupt; several joints usually involved at onset in symmetrical pattern (both hands, wrists, or ankles); in one-third of cases, initially confined to one or a few joints; affected joints warm, tender, and swollen; overlying skin has ruddy purplish hue; disease progression – joint deformities in hands and feet ("swan neck", "boutonnière", and "cock-up toes").

Pathogenesis

Autoimmune reaction – antibodies against components of joint tissues; triggering mechanism unknown; factors are genetic susceptibility, abnormal bowel permeability, lifestyle and nutritional factors, food allergies, and microorganisms; classic multifactorial disease involving genetic and environmental factors.

- **Genetic factors:** histocompatibility antigen HLA-DRw$_4$ in 70% of RA patients vs. 28% of controls; severe RA at four times expected rate in first-degree relatives of those with seropositive disease; environmental factors are necessary for disease development – demonstrated in monozygotic twins.

● **Abnormal bowel permeability:** RA patients have increased intestinal permeability to dietary and bacterial antigens plus alterations in bowel flora; food allergies may contribute to increased permeability; NSAIDs implicated; permeability to gut-derived antigens increases endotoxins (lipopolysaccharide components of cell walls of Gram-negative bacteria) and immune complexes characteristic of RA; permeability and inappropriate bacterial flora can increase absorption of antigens similar to antigens in joint tissues; antibodies to microbial antigens may cross-react with joint tissue antigens – antibodies to *Campylobacter*, *Salmonella*, and *Shigella* cross-react with collagen, while antibodies to *Klebsiella pneumoniae*, *Proteus vulgaris* and *Yersinia enterocolitica* cross-react with other joint tissues.

● **Dysbiosis and small intestinal bacterial overgrowth:** many RA patients exhibit altered microbial flora and small intestinal bacterial overgrowth (SIBO); degree of SIBO is linked to severity of symptoms and disease activity (*Textbook*, Ch. 7).

● **Abnormal antibodies and immune complexes:** serum and joint fluid of nearly all RA patients contain rheumatoid factor (RF) = antibodies against Fc fragment of IgG; RF antibodies belong to IgM, IgG, and IgA classes, but only IgM RF is readily measured – by latex agglutination, bentonite flocculation, and sensitized sheep or human RBC test; most of RF formed locally in affected joints by infiltration of activated B-cells and plasma cells; serum titer of RF correlates with severity of symptoms; circulating immune complexes contribute to pathogenesis – cell-mediated, humoral, and non-specific immune responses to immune complexes lead to proliferative inflammation; abnormalities similar to Arthus reaction and serum sickness, immune complex-induced reactions dependent upon neutrophils, and complement activation; amount of circulating immune complexes is not correlated with disease activity, but immune complexes and abnormal antibodies plus sequelae are major factors in RA.

● **Microbial hypotheses:** not in themselves comprehensive enough to explain all events observed in RA; variety of suggested microbes: Epstein–Barr virus, rubella virus, amebic organisms, and *Mycoplasma*; no microbial agent consistently isolated in RA patients; attempts to isolate whole organisms from synovial fluids and antibodies to viable, whole organisms, and failure to isolate offending organisms, are suggestive, to some reseachers, of atypical viral-like agent(s); microbial factors (immune complexes) contribute, but a single causative microbe is unlikely.

● **Decreased DHEA levels:** defective androgen synthesis proposed as predisposing factor; dehydroepiandrosterone sulfate (DHEAS) levels are lower in postmenopausal women (aged 45–65) with RA than postmenopausal controls; supplemental DHEA (200 mg q.d.) is beneficial in systemic lupus erythematosus (SLE); may be beneficial for RA despite absence of double-blind clinical studies; can be used conservatively to correct physiological deficit; use 24-h urinary test; can be used aggressively to impact RA – dosage required > 50 mg q.d.; major side-effect is mild to severe acne and possibly increased androgenization in women.

DIAGNOSIS

Easily recognized in advanced and characteristic form; early diagnosis more difficult.

Classic RA: diagnosis requires seven of the following criteria; criteria 1–5: joint signs or symptoms must be continuous for 6 weeks; any one of exclusionary features exclude patient from this and other categories:

- Morning stiffness
- Pain on motion or tenderness in at least one joint
- Swelling (soft tissue thickening or fluid, not bony overgrowth alone) in at least one joint
- Swelling of at least one other joint with any interval free of joint symptoms between joint involvement may not be more than 3 months
- Bilateral joint swelling – proximal interphalangeal, metacarpophalangeal, or metatarsophalangeal joints – acceptable without absolute symmetry; terminal phalangeal joint involvement will not fulfill this criterion
- Subcutaneous nodules over bony prominences, on extensor surfaces, or in juxta-articular regions
- X-ray changes – bony decalcification localized to, or most marked adjacent to, involved joints and not just degenerative changes (which do not exclude patients from any RA group)
- Positive agglutination test – "rheumatoid factor" tested by acceptable method
- Poor mucin precipitate from synovial fluid or inflammatory synovial effusion with 2,000+ WBCs/mm^3 and without crystals
- Histologic changes in synovium with three or more of following: marked villous hypertrophy; proliferation of superficial synovial cells often with palisading; marked infiltration of chronic inflammatory cells with tendency to form lymphoid nodules; deposition of compact fibrin either on surface or interstitially; foci of necrosis
- Histologic changes in nodules – granulomatous foci with central zones of cell necrosis, surrounded by a palisade of proliferated mononuclear and peripheral fibrosis and chronic inflammatory cell infiltration.

Definite RA: requires five of the above criteria; criteria 1–5: joint signs must be continuous for 6+ weeks.

(continued over)

(continued)

> **Probable RA:** requires three of criteria; in at least one of criteria 1–5, joint signs/symptoms continuous for 6+ weeks.
>
> **Possible RA:** requires two of the following criteria and total duration of joint symptoms must be 3+ months:
>
> - morning stiffness
> - tenderness or pain on motion with history of recurrence or persistence of 3 weeks
> - history or observation of joint swelling
> - elevated sedimentation rate or C-reactive protein
> - iritis.

Laboratory and X-ray findings

- **Rheumatoid factor:** non-rheumatoid diseases elevate RF – diseases share common feature of chronic inflammation with persistent antigenic challenge and include other connective tissue diseases (SLE, Sjögren's syndrome, polymyositis, and scleroderma) and infectious diseases (TB, leprosy, syphilis, viral hepatitis, bacterial infections, infectious mononucleosis, and influenza); positive results in idiopathic pulmonary fibrosis, sarcoidosis, chronic active hepatitis and cirrhosis, lymphomas, cryoglobulinemia, and repeated blood transfusions; RF is transiently elevated after immunizations and other assaults to immune system; overall prevalence = 4%; persons over age 60 show prevalence > 40%; RF titers in elderly healthy persons are typically low (< 1:80).

- **Antinuclear antibodies (ANAs):** found in 20–60% of RA patients; titers specific for native DNA are typically normal; titers to single-stranded or denatured DNA are usually elevated; ANA titers are typically lower in RA than SLE.

- **EBV antibodies:** identified by immunodiffusion or by immunofluorescence in serum of most RA patients; called "anti-rheumatoid arthritis precipitin" (anti-RAP) and "anti-rheumatoid arthritis nuclear antigen" (anti-RANA); significance undetermined.

- **Other lab abnormalities:** anemia common – normocytic and normochromic or hypochromic; decreased erythropoiesis is common in chronic inflammatory conditions; serum Fe level and total iron binding capacity usually low – Fe supplements of no value, may actually promote free radical damage; Fe supplement is not indicated unless anemia is due to blood loss; serum ferritin levels are useful in determining appropriateness of Fe therapy – ferritin is elevated during acute inflammation and correlates with other indicators of disease activity (ESR and C-reactive protein); ESR is commonly elevated and useful as rough estimator of disease activity in patient monitoring – but occasionally it does not accurately reflect disease activity.

- **Synovial fluid:** reflects degree of inflammation; high fibrinogen may lead to spontaneous clotting of fluid; should not be confused with mucin clot; adding 1% acetic acid will dissolve fibrin; in RA, mucin clot is poor because of smaller-than-normal polymers of hyaluronic acid; neutrophils are primary cells in fluid with range of 10,000–50,000/mm^3; complement is generally low and neutrophils contain cytoplasmic inclusion bodies with ingested immune complexes.

- **X-ray findings:** soft tissue swelling, erosion of cartilage, and subtle joint space narrowing early in disease process; as disease progresses, erosion of joint spaces are more pronounced, as is diffuse osteoporosis.

THERAPEUTIC CONSIDERATIONS

Study of therapeutic efficacy requires 20 years follow-up; study of RA patients after 20 years of aggressive conventional treatment – only 18% able to lead normal lives; most patients (54%) were either dead (35%) or severely disabled (19%); most mortalities were directly related to RA; RA is a multifactorial condition requiring comprehensive approach focused on reducing contributing factors (gut permeability, circulating immune complexes, free radicals, immune dysfunction, etc.), controlling inflammation, and promoting joint regeneration; foremost in natural approach – use diet to control inflammation.

Diet

Strongly implicated in RA – cause and cure; RA not found in societies that eat "primitive" diet; found at relatively high rate in societies consuming "Western" diet; diet rich in whole foods, vegetables, and fiber, and low in sugar, meat, refined carbohydrate, and saturated fat is protective against RA; eliminate food allergens; follow vegetarian diet; change dietary fats and oils; increase antioxidant nutrients.

- **Food allergy:** eliminating allergic foods is very beneficial to some RA patients; any food can aggravate RA; most common offending foods are wheat, corn, milk and dairy, beef, and nightshade (tomato, potato, eggplant, peppers, and tobacco) plus food additives; short-term fasting (vegetable broth and juices) followed by vegetarian diet substantially reduces disease activity in many patients – eliminates food allergens, improves dietary fatty acids, and colon flora.

- **Colon microflora:** altered flora linked to RA and other autoimmune diseases; > 400 different species; there is significant alteration in intestinal flora when patients change from omnivorous to a vegetarian diet; positive changes in colon flora correlate with improvements in RA; total surface area of GI system = 300–400 m^2; only single epithelial layer separates host from enormous amounts of dietary and microbial antigens; gut-associated lymphoid tissue (largest lymphoid organ) is protective; alterations in intestinal flora change antigenic challenge, with significant impact on disease activity; gas-liquid chromatography of fatty acids in stool samples may be relatively quick and easy method of forecasting clinical improvement in RA.

● **Digestion:** incompletely digested food molecules can be inappropriately absorbed; many patients with RA are deficient in HCl and pancreatic enzymes – incomplete digestion may be a major factor; digestive aids are warranted; pancreatic enzymes offer additional benefits: proteases in pancreatin reduce circulating levels of immune complexes in autoimmune diseases (RA, SLE, periarteritis nodosa, scleroderma, ulcerative colitis, Crohn's disease, MS, AIDS); as clinical improvement corresponds with decreased immune complexes (use ESR as rough indicator), pancreatin or bromelain supplements are often warranted.

● **Dietary fats:** fatty acids are precursors of inflammatory prostaglandins, thromboxanes, and leukotrienes; altering dietary fatty acids can increase or decrease inflammation depending on preponderant type ingested; goals are to reduce arachidonic acid (AA) and increase DHGLA and EPA; vegetarian diets are beneficial, in part, by decreasing AA for conversion to inflammatory eicosanoids, while supplying linoleic and linolenic acids; cold-water fish (mackerel, herring, sardines, and salmon) are rich sources of EPA, which competes with AA for prostaglandin and leukotriene production; net effect is reduced inflammatory/allergic response; consumption of broiled or baked fish correlates with decreased risk of RA – dose-dependent response was noted: 2+ servings/week more protective than one serving/week; best diet for RA is vegetarian diet with exception of cold-water ocean fish; flaxseed oil is also useful.

Nutritional supplements

● **GLA:** evening primrose (EPO), black currant, and borage oil contain gamma-linolenic acid, an omega-6 fatty acid, precursor to anti-inflammatory prostaglandins of 1 series; although quite popular, research on GLA in RA is controversial and not as strong as research on omega-3 oils; long-term GLA supplementation increases tissue AA and decreases tissue EPA – contrary to treatment goal; key factor is whether or not subjects are allowed to take anti-inflammatory drugs – drugs inhibit formation of inflammatory prostaglandins – mask negative effects of altered tissue fatty acid profile produced by GLA; dosage for RA = 1.4 g q.d.; EPO is 9% GLA: 31–500 mg caps EPO required q.d. at cost of $100/month; omega-3 oils are better choice; GLA can be formed from linoleic acid – difficult to determine whether effects are due to GLA vs. linoleic acid; most sources of GLA are much richer in linoleic acid than GLA; (EPO contains 9% GLA, but 72% linoleic acid).

- **Omega-3 fatty acids:** fish oil EPA studies consistently show less morning stiffness and tender joints; reduces production of inflammatory compounds secreted by WBCs; many, but not all, commercially available fish oils have high levels of lipid peroxides; use cold-water fish and flaxseed oil or lab-certified fish oil; flaxseed oil is not as effective in increasing tissue EPA and lowering tissue AA as fish oils; for flax oil to be effective, patients must minimize dietary omega-6 fatty acids (other vegetable oils) while supplementing with 13 g (1 tbsp) flaxseed oil q.d.; flax can inhibit autoimmune reaction as well as EPA; conversion of alpha-linolenic acid to EPA requires adequate zinc nutriture; zinc deficiency is common in RA.

- **Dietary antioxidants:** fresh fruits and vegetables are the best sources of dietary antioxidants; vitamin C, beta-carotene, vitamin E, selenium, and zinc are well-recognized as antioxidants; flavonoids neutralize inflammation and support collagen structures; risk of RA is highest in people with lowest levels of nutrient antioxidants (serum alpha-tocopherol, beta-carotene, and vitamin C).

- **Selenium and vitamin E:** selenium levels are low in RA patients; Se is an antioxidant and cofactor in free radical scavenging enzyme glutathione peroxidase – reducing inflammatory prostaglandins and leukotrienes; selenium plus vitamin E have positive effect; food sources: Brazil nuts, fish, and whole grains; amount of Se in grains and other plant foods is related to amount of Se in soil.

- **Zinc:** antioxidant and cofactor in antioxidant enzyme superoxide dismutase (copper–zinc SOD); slight therapeutic effect alone; prefer zinc picolinate, monomethionine, or citrate forms; foods rich in zinc are oysters, whole grains, nuts, and seeds.

- **Manganese and superoxide dismutase:** manganese functions in different form of superoxide dismutase (manganese SOD); Mn-SOD is deficient in RA patients; injectable form of enzyme (available in Europe) is effective treating RA; not clear if oral SOD escapes digestion in GI tract to exert therapeutic effect; manganese supplements increase SOD activity; no clinical studies have been conducted to determine efficacy of manganese in RA; RA patients low in manganese; dietary sources are nuts, whole grains, dried fruits, and green leafy vegetables; meats, dairy, poultry, and seafood are poor sources of manganese.

- **Vitamin C:** antioxidant; WBC and plasma ascorbate significantly decreased in RA patients; vitamin C supplements increase SOD activity, decrease histamine levels, and provide some anti-inflammatory effects; food sources are broccoli, Brussels sprouts, cabbage, citrus fruits, tomatoes, and berries.

- **Pantothenic acid:** whole blood pantothenic acid is lower in RA patients vs. normal controls; disease activity is inversely correlated with pantothenic acid levels; correcting low pantothenic acid levels to normal improves duration of morning stiffness, degree of disability, and severity of pain; dietary sources: whole grains and legumes.

- **Copper:** copper aspirinate (salicylate) yields better results in reducing pain and inflammation than standard aspirin; wearing of copper bracelets is a long-time folk remedy; copper is absorbed through the skin and is chelated to another compound able to exert anti-inflammatory action; copper is a component (with zinc) in one type of SOD (copper–zinc SOD); deficiency may increase susceptibility to free radical damage; excess intake of copper is detrimental due to ability to combine with peroxides and damage joint tissues.

- **Sulfur:** sulfur (cysteine) content in fingernails of arthritics is lower than healthy controls; intragluteal colloidal sulfur alleviates pain and swelling; increased consumption of sulfur-rich foods (legumes, garlic, onions, Brussels sprouts, and cabbage) or supplements may be beneficial.

- **Niacinamide:** Kaufman and Hoffer – treatment of RA and osteoarthritis (OA) using high-dose niacinamide (900–4,000 mg in divided doses q.d.); confirmed in OA (*Textbook*, Ch. 176); not fully evaluated in clinical studies of RA; niacinamide impacts autoimmune process involved in insulin-dependent diabetes mellitus (*Textbook*, Ch. 147).

Botanical medicines

- ***Curcuma longa* (turmeric):** curcumin is a yellow pigment of *Curcuma longa*, which exerts excellent anti-inflammatory and antioxidant effects; curcumin is as effective as cortisone or phenylbutazone in models of acute inflammation, but without side-effects; inhibits formation of leukotrienes and other mediators of inflammation; in models of chronic inflammation, curcumin is much less active in adrenalectomized animals – enhances body's own anti-inflammatory mechanisms; beneficial effects in human studies comparable to standard drugs, but without side-effects at recommended doses; postoperative inflammation model for NSAIDs – curcumin has comparable anti-inflammatory action to phenylbutazone; does not possess direct analgesic action; turmeric or curcumin is beneficial in acute exacerbations of RA; dosage for curcumin = 400–600 mg t.i.d.; turmeric dosage = 8,000–60,000 mg; curcumin is formulated with bromelain to enhance absorption; bromelain is also anti-inflammatory; curcumin–bromelain combination is taken on an empty stomach 20 min before meals or between meals; lipid base (lecithin, fish oils, or EFAs) may increase absorption.

- **Bromelain:** mixture of enzymes in pineapple; reduces inflammation in RA; mechanisms – inhibits proinflammatory compounds and activates compounds which break down fibrin; fibrin forms matrix that isolates area of inflammation – results in blockage of blood vessels and inadequate tissue drainage and edema; bromelain blocks inflammatory production of kinin compounds that increase swelling and pain.

- **Zingiber officinalis (ginger):** antioxidant effects; inhibits prostaglandin, thromboxane, and leukotriene synthesis; fresh ginger may be more effective in RA than dried preparations – fresh contains protease with anti-inflammatory action similar to bromelain; substantially improves RA symptoms – pain relief, joint mobility, and decreased swelling and morning stiffness; recommended dosage = 500–1,000 mg q.d.; some patients have taken three to four times this amount with quicker and better relief; forms: 1 g of dry powdered ginger root; average daily dietary dose = 8–10 g in India; fresh (or freeze-dried) ginger root at equivalent dosage may be better – higher gingerol and active protease; daily dosage of 2–4 g of dry powdered ginger may be effective – equivalent to 20 g (2/3 oz) fresh ginger root (0.5 inch slice); incorporate into fresh fruit and vegetable juices; no apparent side-effects at these levels.

- **Bupleuri falcatum (Chinese thoroughwax), licorice and Panax:** *Bupleuri* root is component in Chinese traditional formulas for inflammatory conditions; now used in combination with corticosteroid drugs (prednisone); enhances activity of cortisone; active constituents are steroid-like "saikosaponins" – anti-inflammatory action: increase adrenal release of cortisone and other corticosteroids and potentiate their effects, prevent adrenal atrophy caused by corticosteroids; recommended for patients on corticosteroids to protect adrenals; *Glycyrrhiza glabra* (licorice) and *Panax ginseng* enhance action of *Bupleuri*; licorice and ginseng have anti-inflammatory constituents and improve adrenal function; licorice inhibits breakdown of adrenal hormones by liver; together *Bupleuri* and licorice increase corticosteroids in circulation; these plants are used to restore adrenal function in patients with a history of long-term or high-dosage corticosteroid use.

Physical medicine

Has a major role in managing RA; not curative, but improves comfort and preserves joint and muscle function; heat relieves stiffness and pain, relaxes muscles, and increases range of motion (ROM); moist heat (moist packs and hot baths) are more effective than dry heat (heating pad); paraffin baths used if skin irritation from water immersion develops; cold packs are valuable during acute flare-ups; strengthening and ROM exercises preserve joint function; well-developed disease and inflammation – begin with progressive, passive ROM and isometrics; as inflammation subsides – active ROM and isotonics exercises.

- **Balneotherapy:** therapeutic mineral baths and mud packs are a European tradition; confirmed by Israeli studies of Dead Sea spa therapy in conditions of high barometric pressures, low humidity, high temperatures, paucity of rainfall, and absence of air pollution; modalities are mud packs,

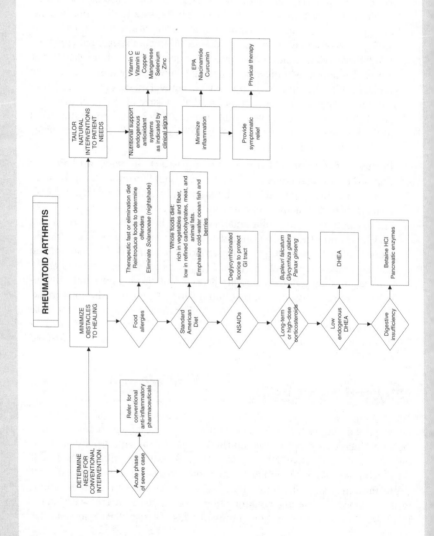

RHEUMATOID ARTHRITIS

DETERMINE NEED FOR CONVENTIONAL INTERVENTION

Acute phase of severe case → Refer for conventional anti-inflammatory pharmaceuticals

MINIMIZE OBSTACLES TO HEALING

Food allergies → Therapeutic fast or elimination diet
Reintroduce foods to determine offenders
Eliminate *Solanaceae* (nightshade)

Standard American Diet → Whole foods diet: rich in vegetables and fiber, low in refined carbohydrates, meat, and animal fats. Emphasize cold-water ocean fish and berries

NSAIDs → Deglycyrrhizinated licorice to protect GI tract

Long-term or high-dose corticosteroids → *Bupleuri falcatum*
Glycyrrhiza glabra
Panax ginseng

Low endogenous DHEA → DHEA

Digestive insufficiency → Betaine HCl
Pancreatic enzymes

TAILOR NATURAL INTERVENTIONS TO PATIENT NEEDS

Nutritional support endogenous antioxidant systems as indicated by clinical signs → Vitamin C
Vitamin E
Copper
Manganese
Selenium
Zinc

Minimize inflammation → EPA
Niacinamide
Curcumin

Provide symptomatic relief → Physical therapy

sulfur baths, and bathing in Dead Sea; provides significant improvement in duration of morning stiffness, 15 m walk time, grip strength, activities of daily living assessment, patient's assessment of disease activity, number of active joints, and Ritchie articular index; improvement noted with Dead Sea bathing superior to regular hot baths with table salt; trace elements (zinc and copper – components of superoxide dismutase – plus boron, selenium, rubidium, etc.) may be absorbed through skin; no side-effects or aggravation of disease noted.

THERAPEUTIC APPROACH

Effective treatment requires controlling as many contributing factors as possible; foremost – dietary measures to reduce causes and ameliorate symptoms; symptom relief through conventional physical therapy (exercise, heat, cold, massage, diathermy, lasers, and paraffin baths), anti-inflammatory botanicals and nutrients and, as appropriate, bowel detox; severe cases – NSAIDs may be necessary in acute phase; natural measures enhance efficacy of drugs – lower dosages required; when drugs given, prescribe deglycyrrhizinated licorice (DGL) to protect against peptic ulcers.

- **Diet:** therapeutic fast or elimination diet followed by careful reintroduction of foods to detect those which initiate symptoms; any food can aggravate RA; most common offenders are wheat, corn, milk and other, beef, nightshade (Solanum) family foods (tomato, potato, eggplants, peppers, and tobacco); after isolating and eliminating allergens, eat healthy diet rich in whole foods, vegetables, and fiber, and low in sugar, meat, refined carbohydrates, and animal fats; particularly beneficial – cold-water fish (mackerel, herring, sardines, and salmon) and flavonoid-rich berries (cherries, hawthorn berries, blueberries, blackberries, etc.) and their extracts.

- **Supplements:**
  - DHEA: 50–200 mg q.d.
  - EPA: 1.8 g q.d. (or flaxseed oil: 1 tbsp q.d.)
  - niacinamide: 500 mg q.i.d. (monitor liver enzymes)
  - pantothenic acid: 500 mg q.d.
  - quercetin: 250 mg between meals t.i.d.
  - tryptophan: 400 mg t.i.d.
  - vitamin C: 1–3 g q.d. in divided doses
  - vitamin E: 400 IU q.d.
  - copper: 1 mg q.d.
  - manganese: 15 mg q.d.
  - selenium: 200 μg q.d.
  - zinc: 45 mg q.d.
  - betaine HCl: 5–70 grains with meals (*Textbook*, App. 7)
  - pancreatin (10 × USP): 350–750 mg between meals t.i.d.; or bromelain: 250–750 mg (1,800–2,000 μu) between meals t.i.d.

- **Botanical medicines:** used alone or in combination; severe inflammation and joint destruction require more aggressive therapy; history of corticosteroid use and those weaning off corticosteroids – *Bupleuri falcatum*, *Glycyrrhiza glabra*, and *Panax ginseng* to prevent and/or reverse adrenal atrophy:

  — curcumin: 400 mg t.i.d. (or ginger: incorporate 8–10 g fresh ginger into diet q.d. or ginger extracts standardized to 20% gingerol and shogaol at dosage = 100–200 mg t.i.d.)

  — *Bupleuri falcatum*:
  dried root: 2–4 g
  tincture (1:5): 5–10 ml
  fluid extract (1:1): 2–4 ml
  solid extract (4:1): 200–400 mg

  — *Panax ginseng*:
  crude herb: 4.5–6 g q.d.
  standardized extract (5% ginsenosides): 100 mg q.d.–t.i.d.

  — *Glycyrrhiza glabra*:
  dried root: 2–4 g
  tincture (1:5): 10–20 ml
  fluid extract (1:1): 4–6 ml
  solid extract (4:1): 250–500 mg.

- **Physical medicine:**
  — heat (moist packs, hot baths, etc.): 20–30 min q.d.–t.i.d.
  — cold packs for acute flare-ups
  — paraffin baths (if skin irritation caused by hot water)
  — active (or in severe cases passive) ROM exercises: 3–10 repetitions q.d.–b.i.d.
  — progressive isometric (and isotonic as joints improve) exercise: 3–10 repetitions several times per day with generous periods of rest
  — massage: one to three times/week.

Rosacea

DIAGNOSTIC SUMMARY

- Chronic acneiform eruption on the face of middle-aged and older adults associated with facial flushing and telangiectasia.
- The acneiform component is characterized by papules, pustules, and seborrhea; the vascular component by erythema and telangiectasia; and the glandular component by hyperplasia of the soft tissue of the nose (rhinophyma).
- The primary involvement occurs over the flush areas of the cheeks and nose.

GENERAL CONSIDERATIONS

Rosacea is a chronic skin disorder – nose and cheeks are abnormally red and may be covered with pimples similar to acne (see acne chapter); relatively common in adults between ages 30 and 50; more common in women (3:1), but more severe in men.

- Many factors suspected: alcoholism, menopausal flushing, vasomotor neurosis, seborrheic diathesis, local infection, B-vitamin deficiencies, gastrointestinal disorders.
- Most cases – moderate to severe seborrhea, but sebum production is not increased in many; vasomotor lability is prevalent; migraine three times more common than in controls.

THERAPEUTIC CONSIDERATIONS

- **Hypochlorhydria:** Gastric analysis of rosacea patients indicates hypochlorhydria; psychological factors (worry, depression, stress) reduce gastric acidity; HCl supplements improve patients with achlorhydria or hypochlorhydria; decreased secretion of lipase (bicarbonate and chymotrypsin normal); pancreatic supplements benefit.
- *Helicobacter pylori:* high incidence of gastric *H. pylori* found in rosacea patients; flushing reaction in rosacea may be caused by gastrin or vasoactive intestinal peptides; some histologically positive patients are serologically

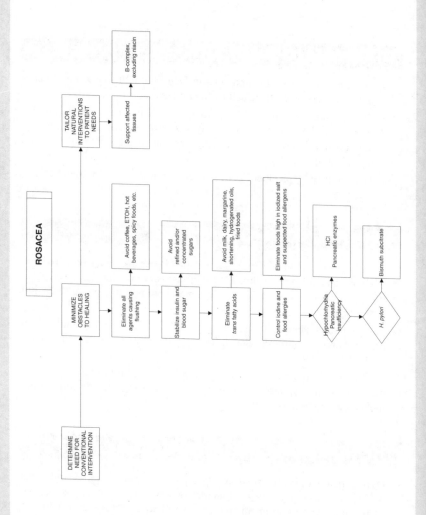

negative; clinical success in treating rosacea with metronidazole and abatement of *H. pylori* isolates and serology after treatment provide evidence connecting rosacea with *H. pylori*.

- **Food allergy:** migraine HAs accompanying rosacea point to food intolerance, as does reflex flushing by vasodilator substances.

- **B vitamins:** large doses of B vitamins are quite effective, with riboflavin (vitamin B_2) as key factor.

  — Mite *Demodex folliculorum* is considered a factor, but is a normal inhabitant of follicles; may account for more granulomatous response of some patients (researchers able to infect skin of B_2-deficient rats with Demodex, but not skin of normal rats).

  — Some patients' rosacea may be aggravated by large doses of these nutrients; inflammation and exacerbations of acne related to B_2, B_6, and B_{12} are reported in European literature.

THERAPEUTIC APPROACH

Cause(s) undetermined; adequate treatment possible for most patients; control hypochlorhydria and food intolerance; support with B-complex and avoidance of vasodilating foods.

- **General recommendations:** see acne chapter.
- **Diet:** avoid coffee, alcohol, hot beverages, spicy foods, and any other food/drink causing flush; eliminate refined and/or concentrated sugars, *trans* fatty acids (milk, milk products, margarine, shortening, synthetically hydrogenated vegetable oils, fried foods); avoid foods high in iodized salt.
- **Supplements:**
  — B-complex: 100 mg q.d. (avoid niacin)
  — pancreas extract (8–10 × USP): 350–500 mg before meals
  — hydrochloric acid (*Textbook*, App. 6).

Seborrheic dermatitis

DIAGNOSTIC SUMMARY

- Superficial erythematous papules and scaly eruptions on scalp, cheeks, and intertrigo of axilla, groin, and neck.
- Usually non-pruritic.
- Seasonal, worse in winter.

GENERAL CONSIDERATIONS

Seborrheic dermatitis (SD) is a common papulosquamous condition with appearance similar to eczema; may be associated with excessive oiliness (seborrhea) and dandruff; scale is yellowish and either dry or greasy; erythematous, follicular, scaly papules may coalesce into large plaques or circinate patches; flexural involvement is often complicated with *Candida* infection:

- Occurs in infancy (between 2 and 12 weeks of age) or in the middle-aged and elderly; prognosis = lifelong recurrence.
- Cause unknown; genetic predisposition, emotional stress, diet, hormones, and infection with yeast-like organisms are implicated.
- Common manifestation of AIDS, affecting 83% – gives increased credence to infection theory of SD.

THERAPEUTIC CONSIDERATIONS

Food allergy: SD begins as "cradle cap"; not primarily allergic disease, but linked to food allergy (67% develop some form of allergy by age 10).

Biotin: underlying factor in infants is biotin deficiency; syndrome is clinically similar to SD induced in rats fed a diet high in raw egg white (high in avidin, a glycoprotein that binds biotin, making it bio-unavailable).

- Large portion of human biotin supply is provided by intestinal bacteria – dysbiosis may cause biotin deficiency in infants; SD successfully treated with biotin in nursing mothers and infants.
- In adults, biotin alone is ineffective; long-chain fatty acid synthesis may be impaired in SD lesions; B vitamins (biotin, pyridoxine, pantothenic acid, niacin, thiamin and lipotropics) are vital for fatty acid metabolism.

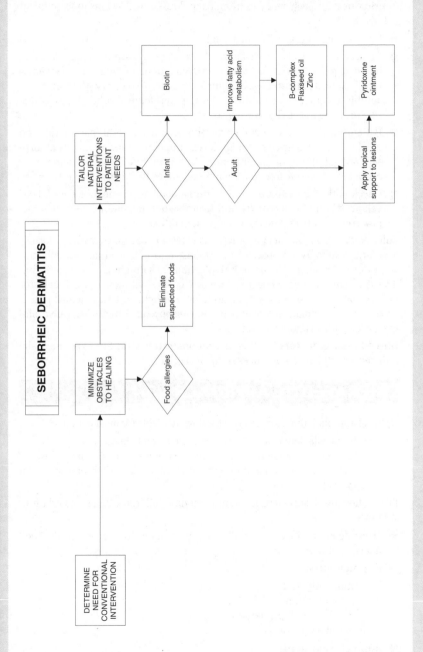

SEBORRHEIC DERMATITIS

DETERMINE NEED FOR CONVENTIONAL INTERVENTION

MINIMIZE OBSTACLES TO HEALING

Food allergies → Eliminate suspected foods

TAILOR NATURAL INTERVENTIONS TO PATIENT NEEDS

Infant → Biotin

Adult → Improve fatty acid metabolism → B-complex / Flaxseed oil / Zinc

Apply topical support to lesions → Pyridoxine ointment

Pyridoxine: B_6 deficiency in humans and rats cause lesions indistinguishable from SD.

- Oral and parenteral B_6 unsuccessful.
- In sicca form of disorder (scalp – dandruff – brow, nasolabial folds, and bearded area with varying degrees of greasy adherent scales on erythematous base), all patients cleared completely within 10 days with local water-soluble ointment containing 50 mg/g pyridoxine; other types of SD (flexural and infected) unresponsive
- Patients with elevated urinary xanthurenic acid – oral, parenteral, and local B_6 all normalized excretion levels, implying transcutaneous absorption of B_6; but improvement from topical B_6 may be due to reducing sebaceous secretion rate from ointment itself, added B_6 having no effect.
- Check patient for exposure to B_5 antimetabolites – hydrazine dyes (FD&C yellow #5) and drugs (INH and hydralazine), dopamine, penicillamine, oral contraceptives, and excessive protein intake.

Folic acid: oral folic acid is only moderately successful (tetrahydro form – dramatic results for one patient unresponsive to folic acid after childbirth); sicca form unresponsive; parenteral injections of vitamin B_{12} (synthetic and liver-extracted) are very effective in many cases – vitamin B_{12} is a cofactor (with choline) in 5-methyl-tetrahydrofolate methyltransferase, which regenerates tetrahydrofolate; folate may become trapped as 5-methyl-tetrahydrofolate by lack of B_{12} and/or choline.

Miscellaneous factors: other B vitamins involved in SD; experimentally induced ariboflavinosis produces sicca form of SD.

THERAPEUTIC APPROACH

Optimal approach unclear; effective therapy available for most patients:

— infants: alleviate biotin deficiency; control food allergies
— adults: correct impaired long-chain fatty acid synthesis – large doses of vitamin B complex; maximize therapeutic results with broad-spectrum approach.

(The following dosages are for adults; modify children's doses according to weight.)

- **Diet:** detect and treat food allergies; in nursing infants – consider food allergies of mother.
- **Supplements:**
  — biotin: 3 mg b.i.d.
  — B-complex: 50 mg b.i.d.
  — zinc: 25 mg q.d.(picolinate)
  — flaxseed oil: 1 tbsp q.d.
- **Topical treatment:**
  — pyridoxine ointment: 50 mg/g (in water-soluble base).

Senile (aging-related) cataracts

DIAGNOSTIC SUMMARY

- Clouding or opacity in the crystalline lens of the eye.
- Absence or altered red reflex (small cataracts stand out as dark defects).
- Gradual loss of vision.

GENERAL CONSIDERATIONS

Leading cause of impaired vision and blindness in US: 4 million people have vision-impairing cataract; 40,000 people in US are blind due to cataracts; cataract surgery is the most common major surgical procedure in US; classified by location and appearance of lens opacities, by cause or significant contributing factor, and by age of onset.

- **Causes and contributing factors:** ocular disease, injury, surgery, systemic diseases (diabetes mellitus, galactosemia), toxin, UV and near-UV light, radiation exposure, and hereditary disease.

Transparency of lens decreases with age; most elderly people display some degree of cataract formation – progressive increase in size, weight, and density of lens throughout life.

- **Histopathology of cataract:**
  — fibrous metaplasia of epithelium
  — liquefaction of fibers resulting in Morgagnian globule formation (drops of fluid beneath capsule and between lens fibers)
  — sclerosis (melding of fibers)
  — posterior migration and swelling of epithelium.

- **Topoanatomic classification of cataracts:**
  — *anterior subcapsular cataract*: fibrous metaplasia of lens epithelium (following iritis and adherence of iris to lens – posterior synechia)
  — *anterior cortical cataract*: liquefaction of lens fibers and Morgagnian globules in cortex anteriorly
  — *nuclear cataract*: exaggeration of normal, aging-related, melding of fibers in nucleus

— *posterior cortical cataract*: liquefaction and globular degeneration of posterior lens cortex

— *posterior subcapsular cataract*: epithelial cells migrate posteriorly under capsule and form large irregular nucleated cells.

Seventy-five per cent of senile cataracts are cortical; 25% nuclear; cortical cataracts take three forms:

- spoke wheel, beginning in periphery and coursing anteriorly and posteriorly to nucleus

- perinuclear punctate opacities

- granular opacities under posterior capsule (subcapsular cataracts).

THERAPEUTIC CONSIDERATIONS

Etiology of cataract: inability to maintain normal homeostatic concentrations of Na^+, K^+, and Ca^{2+} within lens, the result of decreased Na^+, K^+-ATPase activity – defect due to free radical damage to sulfhydryl proteins in lens, including Na^+, K^+-ATPase that contains sulfhydryl component.

- Normal protective mechanisms are unable to prevent free radical damage – lens is dependent on superoxide dismutase (SOD), catalase, glutathione (GSH), and accessory antioxidants vitamins E and C and selenium to prevent free radical damage.

- People with higher intake of vitamin C and E, Se, and carotenes have much lower risk for cataracts.

Antioxidants

- **Vitamin C:** supplements can halt cataract progression and, in some cases, improve vision; supplements reduced cataract development and number of surgeries required among cataract patients over a period of 11 years; dosage necessary to increase vitamin C content of lens = 1,000 mg; vitamin C in blood = 0.5 mg/dl, but in adrenal and pituitary glands, level is 100 times this and in liver, spleen, and lens of eye, it is 20 times; enormous amounts of energy are required to pull vitamin C out of blood against tremendous gradient; keeping blood vitamin C elevated with high dosing reduces the gradient.

- **Glutathione (GSH):** this is a tripeptide composed of glycine, glutamic acid, and cysteine; very high concentrations in lens; key protective factor against intra- and extralenticular toxins; antioxidant; maintains reduced sulfhydryl bonds within lens proteins; coenzyme of various enzyme systems; participates in amino acid transport with gamma-glutamyl transpeptidase; involved in cation transport; GSH diminished in virtually all forms of cataracts.

- **Ascorbic acid (AA) and glutathione interactions:** work in close conjunction; most important of all host protective factors against induction of cataracts; enzymatic and non-enzymatic scavenging of free radicals occurs as follows:

  $$AA + superoxide \rightarrow dehydroascorbate + H_2O_2$$

  Light may also cause oxidation of AA, leading to hydrogen peroxide formation:

  $$AA + light \rightarrow dehydroascorbate + H_2O_2$$

  Dehydroascorbate and hydrogen peroxide produced are reduced by Se-containing glutathione peroxidase:

  $$2\,GSH + dehydroascorbate \rightarrow GSSG + AA$$

  $$2\,GSH + H_2O_2 \rightarrow GSSG + 2\,H_2O$$

  Oxidized glutathione (GSSG) is an inducer of hexose monophosphate shunt, which provides NADPH to reduce GSSG via riboflavin-dependent glutathione reductase:

  $$GSSG + 2\,NADPH \rightarrow 2\,GSH + 2\,NADP$$

  NADP is reduced by hexose monophosphate dehydrogenase as follows:

  $$NADP + glucose\text{-}6\text{--}(P) \rightarrow NADPH + ribulose\ 5\text{--}(P) + CO_2$$

- **Selenium and vitamin E:** these are antioxidants functioning synergistically; glutathione peroxidase is Se-dependent; Se content in lens with cataract = 15% of normal; Se in serum and aqueous humor is much lower in cataract patients than in normals, but Se in lens itself did not differ much in cataract patients and normal controls; decreased Se in aqueous humor is a major finding; excess H_2O_2 (25 times normal) in aqueous humor in cataract patients – associated with increased lipid peroxidation and altered lens permeability from damaged sodium–potassium pump; lens left unprotected against free radical and sun damage; Se-dependent glutathione peroxidase breaks down H_2O_2.

- **Superoxide dismutase (SOD):** activity in human lens is lower than in other tissues due to increased ascorbate and GSH; progressive SOD decrease parallels cataract progression; oral SOD supplements do not affect tissue SOD activity; prefer trace mineral cofactors of SOD that are greatly reduced in cataractous lens (Cu, 90%; Mn, 50%; Zn, 90%).

- **Catalase:** concentrated in epithelial portion of lens (anterior surface); very low levels in rest of lens; primary function – to reduce (to water and oxygen) hydrogen peroxide formed from oxidation of ascorbate.

- **Tetrahydrobiopterin:** pteridine compounds protect against cataract formation by preventing oxidation and damage by UV light – prevents formation of high-molecular-weight proteins in lens; tetrahydrobiopterin is a coenzyme in hydroxylation of monoamines (phenylalanine hydroxylase, tyrosine hydroxylase, tryptophan hydroxylase); decreased pteridine-synthesizing enzymes and tetrahydrobiopterin in senile cataracts; supplemental folic acid may help to compensate.

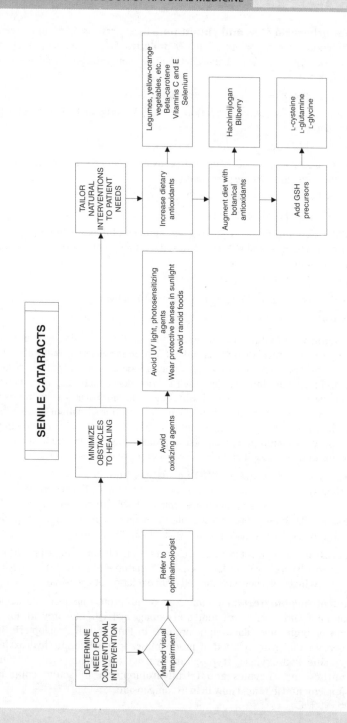

SENILE CATARACTS

Other nutritional factors

- **Riboflavin:** lenticular GSH requires flavin adenine dinucleotide (FAD) as coenzyme for GSH reductase; B_2 is a precursor of FAD; B_2 deficiency may enhance cataract formation via depressed GSH reductase activity; B_2 deficiency is common in elderly (33%); riboflavin status can be determined via RBC GSH reductase activity before and after FAD stimulation; correction of the deficiency is warranted, but no more than 10 mg q.d. B_2 should be prescribed for cataract patients – photosensitizing effect – superoxide radicals generated by interaction of light, ambient oxygen, and riboflavin/FAD; B_2 and light (at physiological levels) were used experimentally to induce cataracts; excess B_2 does more harm than good in cataract patients.

- **Amino acids:** methionine is a component of lens antioxidant enzyme methionine sulfoxide reductase; precursor of cysteine, component of GSH; cysteine and other amino acid precursors of GSH are helpful in cataract treatment.

- **Zinc, vitamin A and beta-carotenes:** antioxidants are vital for normal epithelial integrity; beta-carotene may act as filter, protecting against light-induced damage to fiber portion of lens; beta-carotene is the most significant singlet oxygen free radical scavenger and is used to treat photosensitive disorders.

- **Melatonin:** efficient free radical scavenger and antioxidant; neutralizes hydroxyl and peroxyl radicals; enhances endogenous and exogenous antioxidant efficiency; inhibits DNA damage, lipid peroxidation and cataract formation in animals; present at significant levels in cell nucleus, aqueous cytosol, and lipid-rich cell membranes.

Diet

Protective action from some vegetables, fruit, calcium, folic acid, and vitamin E; increased incidence with elevated salt and fat intake.

- **Dairy products:** cataracts often develop in infants with homozygous deficiency of either galactokinase or galactose-1-phosphate uridyl transferase; also in lab animals fed high-galactose diet; abnormalities of galactose metabolism identified by measuring activity of these enzymes in RBCs; important mechanism in 30% of cataract patients; mechanism of cataract formation is only significant in diabetic cataracts and probably not relevant to senile cataract (see chapter on diabetes).

Heavy metals

Increased concentrations in aging lens and cataractous lens; levels higher in cataracts, but significance unknown.

- **Cadmium:** concentration in cataractous lens is 2–3 times higher than controls; Cd displaces Zn from binding in enyzmes by binding to sulfhydryl groups; contributes to deactivation of free radical quenching and other protective/repair mechanisms.

- **Other elevated elements** of unknown significance include bromine, cobalt, iridium, and nickel.

Botanical medicines

- **Flavonoid-rich extracts:** *Vaccinium myrtillus* (bilberry), *Vitis vinifera* (grape seed), *Pinus maritima* (pine bark), and curcumin from *Curcuma longa*; flavonoid components in well-defined diets may be protective; bilberry anthocyanosides may offer greatest protection – bilberry plus vitamin E stopped progression of cataract in 97% of patients with senile cortical cataracts.

- **Hachimijiogan:** ancient Chinese formula that increases antioxidant level of lens; used in treating cataracts for hundreds of years; therapeutic effect is impressive in early stages; 60% of subjects noted significant improvement, 20% showed no progression, and only 20% displayed progression of cataract; contains the following eight herbs (per 24 g):

  — *Rehmania glutinosa*: 6,000 mg
  — *Poria cocos sclerotium*: 3,000 mg
  — *Dioscorea opposita*: 3,000 mg
  — *Cormus officinalis*: 3,000 mg
  — *Epimedium grandiflorum*: 3,000 mg
  — *Alisma plantago*: 3,000 mg
  — *Astragalus membranaceus*: 2,000 mg
  — *Cinnamonum cassia*: 1,000 mg.

THERAPEUTIC APPROACH

Marked vision impairment – cataract removal and lens implant; prevention or treatment at early stage most effective; free radical damage is the primary inducing factor – avoid oxidizing agents and promote free radical scavenging; avoid direct UV light, bright light, and photosensitizing substances; wear protective lenses outdoors; greatly increase antioxidant nutrients; progression can be stopped and early lesions can be reversed; significant reversal of well-developed cataracts unlikely; elderly are especially susceptible to nutrient deficiencies – ensure they are ingesting and assimilating adequate macro- and micronutrients.

- **Diet:** avoid rancid foods and other sources of free radicals; increase legumes (sulfur-containing amino acids), yellow vegetables (carotenes), and vitamin E- and C-rich foods.

- **Supplements:**
  — vitamin C: 1 g t.i.d.
  — vitamin E: 600–800 IU q.d.

— selenium: 400 µg q.d.
— beta-carotene: 200,000 IU q.d.
— L-cysteine: 400 mg q.d.
— L-glutamine: 200 mg q.d.
— L-glycine: 200 mg q.d.

● **Botanical medicines:**
— bilberry extract (25% anthocyanidin): 80 mg t.i.d.
— Hachimijiogan formula: 150 mg t.i.d.

Streptococcal pharyngitis

DIAGNOSTIC SUMMARY

- Abrupt onset of sore throat, fever, malaise, nausea, and headache.
- Throat red and edematous, with or without exudation.
- Tender cervical lymph nodes.
- Positive rapid detection of streptococcal antigen.
- Group A streptococci on throat culture.

GENERAL CONSIDERATIONS

Throat cultures yield group A beta-hemolytic streptococci in 10% of patients presenting with sore throat; signs and symptoms of "strep throat" resemble viral pharyngitis, requiring culture for definitive diagnosis; 10–25% of general, asymptomatic population are carriers for group A *Streptococcus*.

- Rapid strep screens detect group A strep antigens; definitive positive culture takes 2 days; antibiotics during this period lead to unnecessary developing of antibiotic-resistant organisms and patient to antibiotics; "second-generation" rapid strep screens (Strep A OIA test) have excellent sensitivity and specificity.

- Even if positive, antibiotics may not be necessary; strep throat is usually self-limiting; clinical recovery similar in cases treated with antibiotics and those that were not.

- Concern with not using antibiotics = "non-suppurative post-streptococcal syndromes" (rheumatic fever, post-streptococcal glomerulonephritis, etc.); but antibiotics do not significantly reduce incidence of sequelae; most cases of sequelae are result of afflicted not consulting a physician.

- Reserve antibiotics for patients suffering from severe infection, unresponsive to therapy (unresponse after 1 week of immune support), and those with history of rheumatic fever (RF) or glomerulonephritis (GN); even then, antibiotics like penicillin fail to eradicate strep in over 20% of patients – beta-lactase-positive organisms (*Staphylococcus aureus* and *Bacteroides* sp.) deactivate penicillin.

- Dramatic decrease in incidence of RF began before advent of antibiotics; improved socioeconomic, hygienic, and nutritional conditions are more

STREPTOCOCCAL PHARYNGITIS

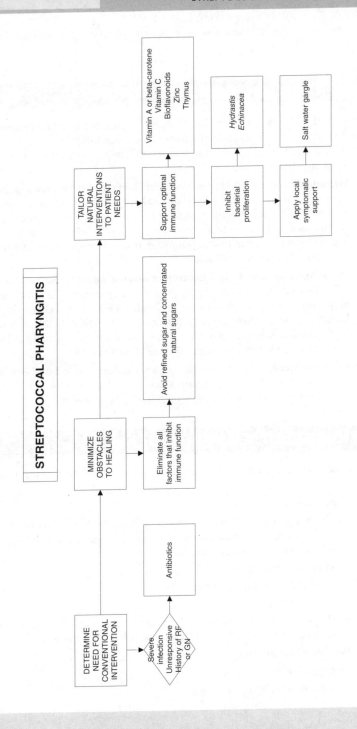

important; present attack rates after strep infection = 0.4–2.8% for RF and 0.2–20% for GN.

THERAPEUTIC CONSIDERATIONS

Primary therapeutic consideration is status of patient's immune system; if good function, illness short-lived; enhance immune function (*Textbook*, Ch. 53) to shorten course; poor immune function – make every effort to strengthen immune system.

- **Vitamin C:** correlation between vitamin C deficiency and strep sequelae; RF is virtually non-existent in tropics, where vitamin C intake is higher; 18% of children in high-risk groups have subnormal serum vitamin C; preventive against RF in animals; very positive results when children given orange juice supplementation; promising research dropped due to advent of supposedly effective antibiotics.

- ***Hydrastis canadensis* and *Echinacea angustifolia*:** berberine alkaloid of hydrastis exerts antibiotic activity against strep and inhibits attachment of group A strep to pharyngeal epithelial cells; streptococci secrete hyaluronidase to colonize tissue; this enzyme is inhibited by *Echinacea* and bioflavonoids; *Echinacea* promotes increased phagocytosis, natural killer cell activity, and properdin levels (*Textbook*, Chs 82 and 91).

- **Bacteriotherapy:** colonizing throat with group A non-beta-hemolytic strep may prevent recurrent group A beta-hemolytic streptococci pharyngitis; spray used for at least 5 days; no side-effects were reported.

THERAPEUTIC APPROACH (*Textbook*, Ch. 53)

If antibiotics used, follow recommendations for *Lactobacillus acidophilus* (*Textbook*, Ch. 105).

- **Supplements:**
  — vitamin A: 50,000 IU q.d. for 1 week; or beta-carotene: 200,000 IU q.d. (avoid vitamin A in menstruating women or women at risk for pregnancy, due to its teratogenic effect)
  — vitamin C: 500 mg every 2 h
  — bioflavonoids: 1,000 mg q.d.
  — zinc: 30 mg q.d.
  — thymus extract: equivalent of 120 mg pure polypeptides with molecular weights < 10,000 OR 500 mg crude polypeptide fraction.
- **Botanical medicines:**
  — *Echinacea* sp.:
   dried root (or as tea): 0.5–1 g

freeze-dried plant: 325–650 mg

juice of aerial portion of *E. purpurea* stabilized in 22% ethanol: 2–3 ml

tincture (1:5): 2–4 ml

fluid extract (1:1): 2–4 ml

solid (dry powdered) extract (6.5:1 or 3.5% echinacoside): 150–300 mg

— *Hydrastis canadensis* (dosage based on berberine content; prefer standardized extracts) (t.i.d.):

dried root or as infusion (tea): 2–4 g

tincture (1:5): 6–12 ml (1.5–3 tsp)

fluid extract (1:1): 2–4 ml (0.5–1 tsp)

solid (powdered dry) extract (4:1 or 8–12% alkaloid content): 250–500 mg.

● **Local treatment:** gargle with salt water b.i.d.: 1 tbsp salt/240 ml of warm water.

Trichomoniasis

DIAGNOSTIC SUMMARY

- Profuse, malodorous, white to green colored discharge from vagina.
- Discharge usually has a pH greater than 4.5, a weak amine odor, and large numbers of WBCs and trichomonads on wet mount.
- Vulvovaginal pruritus, burning, and/or irritation.
- Vulva and introitus usually show erythema.
- Cervix may or may not have a mottled erythema "strawberry cervix" (less than 5%).
- Dysuria and/or dyspareunia may be present.
- R/O trichomoniasis in males exhibiting signs of prostatitis, urethritis, or epididymitis.

GENERAL CONSIDERATIONS

Trichomoniasis (trich) is a common disease: 1 in 5 women in US during lifetime; 2.5 million women annually; present in 3–15% of asymptomatic women treated at ob/gyn clinics and 20–50% of women treated at STD clinics.

- GC and trich commonly coexist – 40% of women with trich have GC and vice versa.
- Trich frequently causes (90%) cervical erosion, a factor in malignancy.
- Trich may complicate interpretation of Pap smears, increasing number of false-positives.
- Trich increases sterility in females (salpingitis) and males (toxins decrease motility of spermatozoa).
- Increased postpartum fever and discharge in women with *T. vaginalis* at delivery.
- Neonates infected via birth canal may manifest serious illness (rare).
- Prostatitis and epididymitis are common in infected males.
- Infection may confuse and/or complicate other GU tract problems.
- Metronidazole (Flagyl) (most common anti-trich agent) is carcinogenic and teratogenic in rodents.

DIAGNOSIS

Trichomonas vaginalis is flagellate 15–18 μm long; shaped like a turnip, with three to four anterior and one posterior flagella mounted in undulating membrane; transmission via sexual intercourse; men and women are reservoirs; diagnosis via signs and symptoms (above), saline wet mount, and culture; trich cultures (Feinberg Trichomonas medium) increase diagnostic sensitivity; 50% of women with Trichomonas (defined by positive culture) have organism identified by microscopic wet mount; organism can be cultured from vagina and para-urethral glands in 98%, urethra in 82%, and endocervix in 13%; in 65%, T. vaginalis seen on Pap smear.

Trichomonal vaginitis

In women, T. vaginalis infests vagina and urethra, but may involve endocervix, Bartholin's glands, Skene's glands, and bladder.

● Vagina is a good reservoir – estrogen causes walls to be glycogenated; prepubescent and postmenopausal women seldom have trich symptoms.

● Elevated pH increases susceptibility; normal adult vaginal pH = 3.5–4.5 via Lactobacillus acidophilus converting free glucose into lactic acid; decreased lactobacilli increases pH; Trichomonas grows optimally at pH = 5.5–5.8; other conditions increasing vaginal pH are progesterone (latter half of menstrual cycle and during pregnancy), excess intravaginal secretions (cervical mucus), and bacterial overgrowth (Streptococcus, Proteus).

Trichomonas in the male

Incidence lower in men, but 5–15% of NGU caused by Trichomonas; often asymptomatic, yet mild urethritis, prostatitis, and epididymitis reported; identified in semen, urethral discharge, and urine, plus prostatic fluid, prostatic secretions and semen of 23% of men with chronic non-GC prostatitis; persists in male GU tract; reinfection of sexually active treated females is well-documented; sexual partners must be treated.

THERAPEUTIC CONSIDERATIONS

Diet: affects body defenses; it is not pathogenicity of microbe, but "fertility of the soil" that allows microbe to flourish; well-balanced diet high in natural fiber (vegetable, fruits), low in fat, sugar, and refined carbohydrates.

Lifestyle: depression and anxiety are linked to exacerbations of trich infections; reduce stress – exercise and meditation; safe sex or abstinence (while infected) lowers incidence of infection/reinfection; 66% of prostitutes not practicing safe sex have trich infection.

Nutritional supplements

● **B-complex:** pyridoxine, pantothenic acid, vitamin B_{12}, and folate aid phagocytic and bactericidal effects of neutrophils and B- and T-cell activity.

● **Ascorbic acid:** aids phagocytic cell migration and killing functions; vitamin C preserves cell integrity by inactivating free radicals and oxidants produced during phagocytosis.

● **Vitamin A:** secretory IgA production is impaired in vitamin A-deficient humans; modest increases in vitamin A enhance resistance to infection; vitamin A maintains composition of external cell membranes and surface glycoproteins, decreasing susceptibility to infectious organisms; high-dose vitamin A is teratogenic and toxic; avoid in pregnant women and women at risk for pregnancy; caution in children and elderly (*Textbook*, Ch. 121).

● **Vitamin E:** doses two to 10-fold greater than RDA enhance antibody responses, accelerate clearance of particulate matter by reticuloendothelial system (RES), and enhance host resistance; megadose vitamin E in healthy volunteer inhibits multiple immune functions.

● **Calcium and magnesium:** bivalent cations regulate external membrane functions of body cells; Ca and Mg ions also help activate complement pathway – *Trichomonas* activates alternate complement pathway (ACP) leading to parasite lysis; unlike classical complement pathway (requiring both Ca and Mg), ACP requires only Mg.

● **Zinc:** broad antimicrobial spectrum – GU pathogens: Gram-positive and -negative bacteria, *T. vaginalis*, *Candida albicans*, *Chlamydia trachomatis*, viruses; trichomonads readily killed by Zn at concentration of 0.042% (6.4 mmol/L) – Zn concentration in prostatic fluid ranges from 0.015 to 0.10% (2.3–15.3 mmol/L), suggesting persistent trichomonal infections in men may be due to Zn deficiency; Zn sulfate (220 mg b.i.d. for 3 weeks) is a possible treatment for trich infections refractory to metronidazole; for women with drug-resistant trich, Zn douches plus metronidazole may relieve.

● **Iron:** deficiency too small to lower hemoglobin values, can cause immune dysfunctions; Fe-deficient humans have defective macrophage and neutrophil functions; iron excess increases growth of pathogen.

Botanical medicines

Trichomonas activates ACP that lyses *T. vaginalis*; botanicals that activate ACP are *Angelica* sp. and *Echinacea purpura*; *Angelica* spp. contain coumarin compounds which activate both classical and alternate pathways (*Textbook*, Ch. 65); inulin (constituent of *Echinacea*) activates complement and promotes chemotaxis of neutrophils, monocytes, and eosinophils (*Textbook*, Ch. 82).

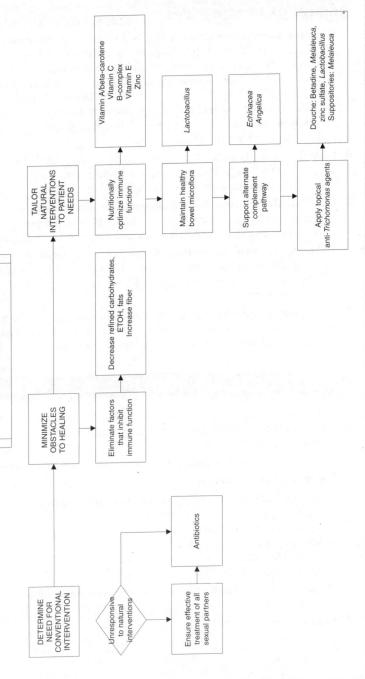

Topical trichomonacides

- **Betadine (povidone-iodine):** iodine is a potent trichomonacide; povidone-iodine (PVP) is a broad-spectrum antimicrobial for vaginal pathogens; PVP (iodine absorbed into polyvinyl pyrrolidone) has advantages over iodine – little sensitizing potential, does not sting, water-soluble, washes out of clothing; success rate = 98.1% in intractable trichomonal, monolial, non-specific, and mixed vaginitis with 2-week regimen using Betadine preparations; 28-day course of Betadine pessaries indicated if patient using oral contraceptives.

- **Propolis:** ethanol extract of propolis (150 µg/ml) is 100% lethal in vitro on protozoans *T. vaginalis* and *Toxoplasma gondii* after 24 h of contact; decreases the inflammation associated with trichomonal vaginitis.

- **Essential oils:** diverse antimicrobial action of essential oils demonstrated; strong antitrichomonal properties – *Mentha piperita* (peppermint) and *Lavandula angustifolia* (lavender) have fastest killing effects (15–20 min).

- ***Melaleuca alternifolia*** (tea tree) oil: powerful topical antimicrobial agent (*Textbook*, Ch. 96); 40% solution very effective with no irritation, burning, or other side-effects; daily douches (0.4% solution melaleuca oil in 1 L water) also effective.

- **Berberine botanicals:** plant alkaloid, berberine sulphate; inhibit in vitro several protozoa – *Entamoeba histolytica*, *Giardia lamblia* and *T. vaginalis*; no clinical trials reported in trichomoniasis (*Textbook*, Ch. 91).

THERAPEUTIC APPROACH

Trichomonas is a sexually transmitted disease (STD) – treatment of sexual partner(s) necessary to prevent reinfection; during treatment, avoid sexual intercourse; use condom otherwise.

- **Diet:** decrease refined carbohydrates, alcohol, and fats; increase fiber.
- **Nutritional supplements:**
  - vitamin A: 25,000 IU q.d. (or beta carotene: 200,000 IU q.d.)
  - vitamin C: 500–1,000 mg every 4 h
  - B-complex: 20–50 mg q.d.
  - zinc (picolinate): 10–15 mg q.d.
  - vitamin E: 200 IU q.d.
  - *Lactobacillus acidophilus*: 2 caps q.d.

  If effective, *L. acidophilus* changes quantity and quality of stool; if this change does not occur, check quality of product (*Textbook*, Ch. 105).
- **Botanical medicines (t.i.d.):**
  - *Hydrastis canadensis*
    dried root: 0.5–1.0 g

tincture (1:10): 6–12 ml
fluid extract (1:1): 1–2 ml
solid extract (4:1): 250 mg

— *Echinacea angustifolia*
dried root: 1–2 g
tincture (1:10): 8–12 ml
fluid extract: 1.5–3.0 ml
solid extract (6.5:1): 250 mg

— *Angelica* sp.
dried root or rhizome: 1–2 g
tincture (1:5): 3–5 ml
fluid extract (1:1): 0.5–2 ml

● **Topical treatment:**

— Betadine douche, pessary, or saturated tampon b.i.d. for 14 days

— *Melaleuca alternifolia* oil (40% solution): swab on affected area b.i.d., or
douche: 1 L of a 0.4% solution b.i.d.
suppository: one at night

— zinc sulfate douche: 1% solution b.i.d.

— *Lactobacillus* culture yogurt douches daily, preferably in the morning.

Urticaria

DIAGNOSTIC SUMMARY

- **Urticaria (hives):** well-circumscribed erythematous wheals with raised serpiginous borders and blanched centers which may coalesce to become giant wheals; limited to the superficial portion of the dermis.
- **Angioedema:** similar eruptions to urticaria, but with larger well-demarcated edematous areas that involve subcutaneous structures as well as the dermis.
- **Chronic versus acute:** recurrent episodes of urticaria and/or angioedema of less than 6 weeks' duration are considered acute, while attacks persisting beyond this period are designated chronic.
- **Special forms:** special forms have characteristic features – dermographism, cholinergic urticaria, solar urticaria, cold urticaria.

Introduction: 15–20% of general population; young adults (post-adolescence through third decade) most often affected.

PATHOPHYSIOLOGY

Release of inflammatory mediators from mast cells or basophilic leukocytes; mechanisms other than IgE-antigen complexes; incidence of IgE-mediated urticaria is probably low compared with non-immunologic urticaria; signs and symptoms are consistent despite diverse etiologic and initiating factors, yet pathogenesis not ascribed to any one mechanism; mast cells and mast cell-dependent mediators play most prominent role.

Three distinct sources of mediators:

- *preformed mediators* – contained in granules and released immediately
- *secondarily formed mediators* – generated immediately or within minutes by interaction of primary mediators and nearby cells and tissues
- *granule matrix-derived mediators* – preformed but slowly dissociate from granule after discharge and remain in tissues for hours.

Most common immunological mechanism mediated by IgE.

- Early vascular changes arise from mast cells – histamine and end-products of arachidonic acid; wheal and flare occur within minutes of initiation and last 30–60 min.

- Prolonged and delayed reactions represent leukocytic infiltration in response to mast cell chemotactic factors; develop over time – erythema, edema, and induration beginning within 2 h and lasting 12–24 h; leukocyte infiltration may induce second wave of mast-cell activation, or release toxic lysosomal enzymes and mediators.

- Events triggered by mediators depend on type of mediator and tissues where they are released.

CAUSES OF URTICARIA

Physical

Urticaria can result from reactions to physical stimuli; most common forms of physical urticarias are dermographic, cholinergic, and cold urticarias; less common types of physical urticarias/angioedema are contact, solar, pressure, heat contact, aquagenic, vibratory, and exercise-induced.

Dermographism: readily elicited whealing of skin evolving rapidly after moderate pressure; simple contact with furniture, garters, bracelets, watch bands, towels, or bedding; incidence of dermographism = 1.5–5%; most frequent physical urticaria; female:male raio = 2:1; average age of onset in third decade; incidence much greater among obese wearing tight clothing.

- Lesions start within 1–2 min of contact – erythema, replaced within 3–5 min by edema and surrounding reflex urticaria; maximal edema within 10–15 min; erythema regresses within an hour, edema persists up to 3 h.

- Associated with other diseases: parasitosis, insect bites, neuropsychiatric disorders, hormonal changes, thyroid disorders, pregnancy, menopause, diabetes, immunological alterations, other urticarias, during or following drug therapy, *Candida albicans*, angioedema, hypereosinophilia.

Cholinergic urticaria: heat reflex urticaria is the second most frequent physical urticaria; these lesions involve stimulation of sweat gland via cholinergic afferent fibers; lesions are pinpoint wheals surrounded by reflex erythema; wheals arise at or between follicles preferentially on upper trunk and arms.

- Three basic types of stimuli – passive overheating, physical exercise, and emotional stress.

- Eliciting activities – physical exercise, warm bath or sauna, eating hot spices, drinking ETOH.

- Lesions arise within 2–10 min and last 30–50 min.

- Systemic symptoms suggest generalized mast cell release beyond skin – HA, periorbital edema, lacrimation and burning of eyes; also N&V,

abdominal cramps, diarrhea, dizziness, hypotension, and asthmatic attacks.

Cold urticaria: urticarial and/or angioedematous reaction of skin contacting cold objects, water, or air; lesions restricted to area of exposure; develop within a few seconds to minutes after removal of cold object and rewarming of skin; the colder the object/element, the faster the reaction; widespread local exposure and generalized urticaria accompanied by: flushing, HAs, chills, dizziness, tachycardia, abdominal pain, nausea, vomiting, myalgia, SOB, wheezing, unconsciousness.

- Cold urticaria accompanies a variety of clinical conditions, including: viral infections, parasitic infestations, syphilis, multiple insect bites, penicillin injections, dietary changes, stress.

- Associated with infectious mononucleosis, cryoglobulinemia and myeloma where cold urticaria may precede diagnosis by several years.

Drugs

Leading cause of urticaria in adults; in children – due to foods, food additives, or infections; most drugs are small molecules incapable of inducing antigenic/allergenic activity of themselves; typically act as haptens binding to endogenous macromolecules, inducing hapten-specific antibodies; alternatively, interact directly with mast cells, inducing degranulation; many drugs produce urticaria; most common are penicillin and aspirin.

- **Penicillin:** antibiotics are most common cause of drug-induced urticaria; population rate of allergenicity of penicillin = 10%, with 25% of these displaying urticaria, angioedema, or anaphylaxis; penicillin cannot be destroyed by boiling or steam distillation – undetected in foods; penicillin in milk more allergenic than in meat – penicillin can be degraded into more allergenic compounds in presence of carbohydrate and metals.

- **Aspirin:** urticaria is a more common indicator of ASA sensitivity than asthma (*Textbook*, Ch. 132); incidence of ASA sensitivity in patients with chronic urticaria 20 times > normal controls; 2–67% of patients with chronic urticaria are sensitive to ASA; aspirin inhibits cyclooxygenase – shunts eicosanoids towards leukotriene synthesis, increasing smooth muscle contraction and vascular permeability; ASA and other NSAIDs increase gut permeability and may alter normal handling of antigens; 650 mg ASA q.d. for 3 weeks may desensitize patients and reduce responsiveness to foods to which they usually react; effect also in patients with asthma, but effect disappears within 9 days after stopping treatment – loss of effect or possible placebo response.

Food allergy

IgE-mediated urticaria occurs upon ingestion of specific reaginic antigen; most common are milk, fish, meat, eggs, beans, and nuts; atopic patient experiences urticaria due to IgE mechanisms; basic requirement for food allergy is absorption of allergen through intestinal mucosa.

● Factors increasing gut permeability – vasoactive amines in foods or produced by bacterial action on amino acids, ETOH, NSAIDs, and food additives (*Textbook*, Ch. 21).

● Alterations in gastric acidity, intestinal motility, and function of small intestine and biliary tract in 85% of patients with chronic urticaria – selective IgA deficiency, gastroenteritis, hypochlorhydria, achlorhydria, etc. may alter barrier and immune function of gut wall.

● IgG reactions may cause most adverse food reactions (*Textbook*, Ch. 51); IgG antigen–antibody complexes can promote complement activation and anaphylatoxins triggering mast cell degranulation.

Food additives

Food colorants: food additives are a major factor in chronic urticaria in children; colorants (azo dyes), flavorings (salicylates, aspartame), preservatives (benzoates, nitrites, sorbic acid), antioxidants (hydroxytoluene, sulfite, gallate), and emulsifiers/stabilizers (polysorbates, vegetable gums) produce urticaria in sensitive people.

● **Tartrazine (azo dye FD&C yellow #5):** first food dye reported to induce urticaria; average daily per capita consumption of certified dyes in US =15 mg – 85% is tartrazine; children consume much more; tartrazine sensitivity in 0.1% of population, 20–50% in persons sensitive to ASA; tartrazine is a cyclooxygenase inhibitor, inducer of asthma, and urticaria in children; tartrazine, benzoate and ASA increase lymphokine leukocyte inhibitory factor, increasing perivascular mast cells and mononuclear cells – 95% of urticaria patients have increased perivascular mast cells and mononuclear cells; eliminating food dyes from diet is very beneficial.

Food flavorings:

● **Salicylates:** salicylic acid esters are used to flavor foods – cake mixes, puddings, ice cream, chewing gum, and soft drinks; mechanism of action similar to ASA; daily salicylate intake from foods = 10–200 mg – level of salicylate used in clinical testing = 300 mg; dietary sources are fruit (berries, dried fruits) – raisins and prunes have highest amounts; also licorice and peppermint candies; moderate levels – nuts and seeds; salicylate is very high in some herbs and condiments – curry powder, paprika, thyme, dill, oregano, and turmeric.

● **Other flavoring agents:** cinnamon, vanilla, menthol, and other volatile compounds may produce urticaria; also artificial sweetener aspartame.

Food preservatives:

- **Benzoates:** benzoic acid and benzoates are the most common food preservatives; incidence of adverse reactions overall is < 1%, but positive challenges in chronic urticaria patients varies from 4 to 44%; fish and shrimp may have very high levels of benzoates – common adverse reactions to these foods in urticaria patients.

- **Butylated hydroxytoluene (BHT) and butylated hydroxyanisol (BHA):** primary antioxidants in prepared and packaged foods; 15% of chronic urticaria patients test positive to oral challenge with BHT.

- **Sulfites:** induce asthma, urticaria, and angioedema in sensitive persons; ubiquitous in foods and drugs; prevent microbial spoilage, browning and changing color; sprayed on fresh foods (shrimp, fruits, vegetables); antioxidants and preservatives in pharmaceuticals; average per capita intake = 2–3 mg/day sulfites; wine and beer drinkers ingest up to 10 mg/day; persons relying on restaurant meals ingest up to 150 mg/day; enzyme sulfite oxidase metabolizes sulfites to safer sulfates excreted in urine; those with poorly functioning sulfoxidation system have increased urine sulfite:sulfate ratio; sulfite oxidase is dependent on trace mineral molybdenum.

- **Food emulsifiers and stabilizers:** most foods containing these also contain antioxidants, preservatives, and dyes; polysorbate in ice cream induces urticaria; vegetable gums (acacia, gum arabic, tragacanth, quince, carrageenin) induce urticaria in susceptible individuals.

Infections

Major cause of urticaria in children; in adults, immune tolerance occurs to many microbes – repeated exposure.

- **Bacterial infections:** contribute to urticaria in two settings:
  — acute strep tonsillitis in children: acute urticaria predominates
  — chronic dental infections in adults: chronic urticaria predominates.

- **Viruses:** hepatitis B is the most frequent cause of viral-induced urticaria; study – 15.3% of patients with chronic urticaria had anti-hepatitis B surface antibodies; also linked to infectious mononucleosis (5%) and may develop several weeks before clinical manifestation.

- ***Candida albicans:*** 19–81% of patients with chronic urticaria react positively to immediate skin test with *Candida* antigens; sensitivity to *Candida* is an important factor in 25% of patients with chronic urticaria; 70% of patients with positive skin reaction also react to oral provocation using foods prepared with yeasts; elimination of organism can cure some individuals with positive skin tests, but more patients responded to "yeast-free" diet than to elimination of organism; yeast-free diet excludes bread, buns, sausage, wine, beer, cider, grapes, sultanas, Marmite, Bovril, vinegar, tomato, ketchup, pickles, and prepared foods containing food yeasts; use

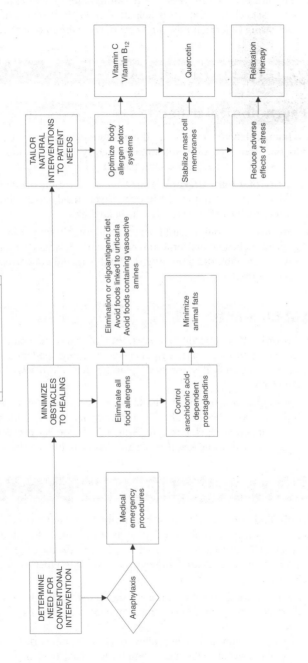

URTICARIA

DETERMINE NEED FOR CONVENTIONAL INTERVENTION

Anaphylaxis

Medical emergency procedures

MINIMIZE OBSTACLES TO HEALING

Eliminate all food allergens

Elimination or oligoantigenic diet
Avoid foods linked to urticaria
Avoid foods containing vasoactive amines

Control arachidonic acid-dependent prostaglandins

Minimize animal fats

TAILOR NATURAL INTERVENTIONS TO PATIENT NEEDS

Optimize body allergen detox systems

Vitamin C
Vitamin B₁₂

Stabilize mast cell membranes

Quercetin

Reduce adverse effects of stress

Relaxation therapy

diet plus eliminating yeast via nystatin; desensitizing patients to *Candida* via yeast cell wall extract is helpful in some, but treatment also included increasing GI fermentation and acidity, plus elimination of yeast.

OTHER CONSIDERATIONS

Psychological aspects

Psychological factors (stress) are the most frequent primary cause in chronic urticaria; stress decreases intestinal secretory IgA; relaxation therapy and hypnosis may be beneficial for some patients.

- **Ultraviolet light therapy:** some benefit in chronic urticaria; both ultraviolet A (UVA) and B (UVB) have been used; cold, cholinergic, and dermographic urticaria respond most favorably.
- **Thyroid:** thyroid hormone replacement therapy has dramatically improved chronic urticaria in patients with normal thyroid function but thyroid autoimmunity; antithyroid antibodies did not correlate with clinical response.

Supplements

- **Vitamin B_{12}:** anecdotal reports are of value in acute and chronic urticaria; although serum B_{12} is normal in most patients, additional B_{12} helpful; injectable B_{12} was used – placebo effect (*Textbook*, Ch. 4) cannot be ruled out.
- **Quercetin:** in vitro, mast cell stabilizer and inhibitor of many pathways of inflammation (*Textbook*, Ch. 87); sodium cromoglycate (200–400 mg q.i.d.) is a compound similar to quercetin, which confers excellent protection against urticaria and angioedema in response to ingested food allergens.

THERAPEUTIC APPROACH

Identify and control all factors that promote patient's urticarial response; thorough history is paramount; acute urticaria is usually self-limiting, especially after eliciting agent is removed or reduced; chronic urticaria responds to removal of eliciting agent(s); in severe anaphylaxis, emergency measures are imperative.

- **Diet:** elimination or oligoantigenic diet is paramount in chronic urticaria (*Textbook*, Chs 15 and 51) – eliminate suspected allergens and all food additives:
  — strictest elimination diets allow only water, lamb, rice, pears, and vegetables; avoid foods most commonly linked to urticaria (milk, eggs,

chicken, fruits, nuts, additives); avoid foods containing vasoactive amines even if no direct allergy to them is noted; primary foods to eliminate are cured meat, ETOH, cheese, chocolate, citrus fruits, and shellfish

— control arachidonic acid-dependent prostaglandins via low animal fat diet.

- **Supplements:**
  - vitamin C: 1 g t.i.d.
  - vitamin B_{12}: 1,000 µg i.m. per week
  - quercetin: 250 mg 20 min before meals.
- **Psychological:** relaxation techniques daily; audiotaped relaxation programs.

Vaginitis and vulvovaginitis

DIAGNOSTIC SUMMARY

- Increased volume of vaginal secretions.
- Abnormal color, consistency, or odor of vaginal secretions.
- Vulvovaginal itching, burning, or irritation.
- Introitus may show patchy erythema, and vaginal mucosa may exhibit congestion, or petechiae.
- Dysuria or dyspareunia may be present.

GENERAL CONSIDERATIONS

Vaginitis is a common female complaint – 7% of all visits to gynecologists; 72% of young sexually active females have one or more forms of vulvo-vaginitis; vaginal infections six times more common than UTIs – dysuria more likely caused by vaginitis than UTI; most women can distinguish "internal" dysuria of UTI from "external" dysuria felt when urine passes over inflamed labial tissues – question dysuria patients more specifically about symptoms of vaginal discharge or irritation; medical importance of vaginitis as follows:

- Symptom perhaps overlying serious problem (chronic cervicitis or STD); if infectious, agent may ascend genital tract, leading to endometritis, salpingitis, and PID – leading to tubal scarring, infertility or ectopic pregnancies.
- Implicated in recurrent UTIs by acting as reservoir of infectious agents.
- Some vaginal infections during pregnancy increase the risk of miscarriage, and, if present at delivery, cause neonatal infections.
- Some forms of vaginitis are linked to cervical cellular abnormalities and increased risk of cervical dysplasia.

TYPES OF VAGINITIS

Hormonal, irritant, and infectious – each divided into subgroups based on etiology.

Hormonal vaginitis

- **Atrophic vaginitis:** postmenopausal women and post-oophorectomy; vaginal epithelium atrophies due to lack of estrogenic stimulation – may cause adhesions, dyspareunia, and increased susceptibility to infection; most common symptoms are itching or burning and thin watery discharge, occasionally blood-tinged (any vaginal bleeding in post-menopausal woman requires complete work-up to rule out carcinoma) (see chapter on menopause).

- **Increased vaginal discharge:** increased normal secretions in absence of other symptoms, diagnosis of "physiological vaginitis" often applied – inappropriate, as no inflammation actually exists; increased discharge often reflects increased hormonal stimulation (pregnancy or some stages of menstrual cycle); primarily diagnosis of exclusion after ruling out other causes; usually no further treatment required other than reassurance; overly zealous douching/washing briefly alleviates symptoms, but may aggravate by causing irritant vaginitis.

Irritant vaginitis

Caused by physical or chemical agents damaging delicate vaginal membranes; cause identified by careful history and examination.

- **Chemical vaginitis:** medications or hygiene products can irritate vaginal mucosa; "allergic vaginitis" – damage elicited by immunologic reaction to product rather than direct toxic reaction.

- **Traumatic vaginitis:** injury caused by physical agents or sexual activity.

- **Foreign body vaginitis:** foul discharge may indicate foreign body in vagina; most common is a forgotten tampon; also contraceptive devices, pessaries, etc.

Infectious vaginitis

May be sexually transmitted or disturbance of delicate ecosystem of healthy vagina; often involves common organisms found in cervices and vaginas of healthy, asymptomatic women.

- Unifying factor in pathogenesis of pelvic infections – not which microbes present but rather cause of patient susceptibility.

- Factors influencing vaginal environment are pH, glycogen content, glucose level, presence of other microbes (lactobacilli), natural flushing action of vaginal secretions, presence of blood, and presence of antibodies and other compounds in vaginal secretions – affected by woman's internal milieu and general health.

- Immune dysfunction predisposes increased vaginal infections – nutritional deficiencies, medicines (e.g. steroids), pregnancy, or serious illness.

Diagnostic differentiation of common causes of infectious vaginitis

	Candida	NSV	Trichomonas	Gonorrhea	Herpes	Chlamydia
Keynote symptoms	Itching	Odor	Odor and itching	Asymptomatic or cervicitis	Vesicles or ulcers	Asymptomatic
Discharge						
pH	<4.5	>4.5	>5.0	<4.5	<4.5	<4.5
Odor	None	Fishy/amines	May be fishy	None	None	None
Appearance	Curdy, adherent, scant to thick	Gray, homogeneous	Greenish-yellow, frothy	Mucopurulent cervicitis	None	None
Pelvic examination	Adherent white patches with an erythematous border	Unremarkable	May show petechial lesion on cervix or vaginamucosa, a "strawberry cervix"	Cervical discharge, may have adnexal tenderness	Small, multiple vesicles or ulcers on cervix or vulva	Unremarkable or may show signs of PID
Microscopic examination	Mycelia (10% KOH)	"Clue cells", few WBCs	Motile, flagellated organisms, few WBCs	Many WBCs with Gram-negative intracellular diplococci	Unremarkable	Unremarkable
Culture media	Sauerbaud's	CNAF	Diamond's	Thayer–Martin	Live cell	Live cell or antibody test

- Other predisposing factors are diabetes mellitus, synthetic pantyhose (retain moisture), and suspected but unproven link between birth control pills and *Candida* infections.

- Risk factors for STDs – increased number of sexual partners, unusual sexual practices, and type of birth control (barriers reduce risk).

- 90% of vulvovaginitis associated with three organisms – *Trichomonas vaginalis*, *Gardnerella vaginalis*, or *Candida albicans*; relative frequency of each varies with population and sexual activity levels; less frequent causes are *Neisseria gonorrhea*, herpes simplex, and *Chlamydia*.

Trichomonas vaginalis: flagellated protozoan in lower GU tract of men and women; humans are the only host; sexual intercourse is the primary mode of dissemination; *Trichomonas* does not invade tissues; rarely causes serious complications.

- Most frequent symptoms are leukorrhea, itching and burning; discharge malodorous, greenish yellow, and frothy.

- "Strawberry cervix" with punctate hemorrhages – only small percentage of *Trichomonas* cases.

- Grows optimally at pH = 5.5–5.8; conditions elevating pH (increased progesterone) favor *Trichomonas*; vaginal pH = 4.5 in woman with vaginitis suggests agent other than *Trichomonas*.

- Saline wet mount of fresh vaginal fluid shows small motile organisms, confirming diagnosis in 80–90% of symptomatic carriers.

Candida albicans: 2.5-fold increase in candidal vaginitis in past 20 years – parallels declining incidence of GC and *Trichomonas*; contributing factors – increased use of antibiotics, changing vaginal ecosystem to favor *Candida*.

- 100% correlation between genital and GI *Candida* cultures – significant intestinal colonization with *Candida* may be single most significant predisposing factor in vulvovaginal candidiasis.

- Steroids, oral contraceptives, and diabetes mellitus contribute; candidiasis 10–20 times more frequent during pregnancy – elevated vaginal pH, increased vaginal epithelial glycogen, elevated blood glucose, and intermittent glycosuria.

- Candidiasis is three times more prevalent in women wearing pantyhose than those wearing cotton underwear – prevents drying of area.

- Recurrent candidal vaginitis due to autoinoculation from GI tract or failure to recognize and treat predisposing factors – allergies, antibiotics, DM, elevated vaginal pH, GI candidiasis, oral contraceptives, pantyhose, pregnancy, steroids.

- Extremely persistent cases – examine and treat sexual partners.

- Allergies can cause recurrent candidiasis, resolving after allergies treated.

- Primary symptom of candidiasis is vulvar itching (sometimes severe); also thick, curdy or "cottage cheese" discharge, which may reveal pinpoint bleeding when removed; such discharge is strong evidence of yeast infection, but absence does not rule out *Candida*; < 20% of symptomatic candidiasis displays classic thrush patches.

● Other clues – brightly erythematous satellite patches, vaginal pH near 4.5, and absence of foul odor.

● Neither character of discharge nor symptoms are sufficient alone for diagnosis of *Candida*; wet mount in saline or 10% KOH – mycelia confirmatory; budding forms of yeast found in normal and symptomatic vaginas, but mycelial stage only found in symptomatic women.

Non-specific vaginitis (NSV): vaginitis not due to *Trichomonas*, GC, or *Candida*.

● Discharge and odor are keynotes to NSV; odor – fishy, foul, rotten from production of amines putrescine and cadaverine by anaerobic bacteria.

● Discharge non-irritating, grey, homogeneous; may be frothy, or thick and pasty; pH elevated to 5.0–5.5; correlation between elevated pH and presence of odor; saline wet mounts reveal "clue cells" (epithelial cells covered with bacteria which obliterate the edges); application of 10% KOH to another slide or to speculum accentuates characteristic amine odor.

● Organism often associated is *Gardnerella vaginalis* (formerly *Haemophilus vaginalis*); recovered from 95% of women with NSV, but also 40% of asymptomatic women; *Gardnerella* is a saprophyte, prospering in conditions of NSV; responsible organism may be anaerobic microbes or combination of *Gardnerella* and vaginal anaerobes; *Gardnerella* lacks enzymes to produce amines characteristic of NSV, but anaerobes have them; antibiotic most effective treating NSV is more active against anaerobes than *Gardnerella*.

Neisseria gonorrhea: uncommon cause of vaginitis, responsible for < 4% of cases; GC vaginitis more common in young girls because vaginal epithelium is thinner prepubertally.

● Mucopurulent cervicitis is primary symptom; spread of infection causes urethritis, bartholinitis or salpingitis.

● GC, alone or with other microbes, is cultured in 40–60% of PID cases, which are a major cause of infertility.

● 80% of GC infections in women are asymptomatic – GC cultures imperative; any purulent discharge from cervical os – culture and examine microscopically; 3+ PMNs with Gram-negative intracellular diplococci per HPF are highly suggestive of GC, with less than 2% false-positives.

Herpes simplex: most common cause of genital ulcers in US; other causes to be ruled out are syphilis, chancroid, lymphogranuloma venereum, and granuloma inguinale (see chapter on herpes simplex).

Chlamydia trachomatis: an obligate intracellular parasite rarely causing vaginitis but frequently found with other common etiologic agents; infects 5–10% of women.

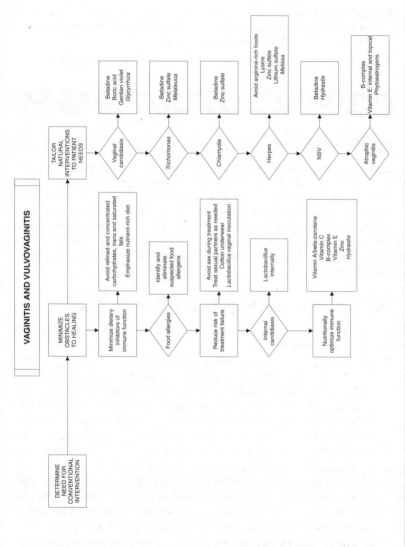

VAGINITIS AND VULVOVAGINITIS

DETERMINE NEED FOR CONVENTIONAL INTERVENTION

MINIMIZE OBSTACLES TO HEALING

Minimize dietary inhibitors of immune function → Avoid refined and concentrated carbohydrates, *trans* and saturated fats
Emphasize nutrient-rich diet

Food allergies → Identify and eliminate suspected food allergens

Reduce risk of treatment failure → Avoid sex during treatment
Treat sexual partners as needed
Cotton underwear
Lactobacillus vaginal inoculation

Internal candidiasis → *Lactobacillus* internally

Nutritionally optimize immune function → Vitamin A/beta-carotene
Vitamin C
B-complex
Vitamin E
Zinc
Hydrastis

TAILOR NATURAL INTERVENTIONS TO PATIENT NEEDS

Vaginal candidiasis → Betadine
Boric acid
Gentian violet
Glycyrrhiza

Trichomonas → Betadine
Zinc sulfate
Melaleuca

Chlamydia → Betadine
Zinc sulfate

Herpes → Avoid arginine-rich foods
Lysine
Zinc sulfate
Lithium sulfate
Melissa

NSV → Betadine
Hydrastis

Atrophic vaginitis → B-complex
Vitamin E: internal and topical
Phytoestrogens

- Usually asymptomatic until complications – cervicitis, salpingitis, or urethritis.
- Organism most frequently recovered from PID patients; tubal scarring more frequent after *Chlamydia* than GC – *Chlamydia* is a more important cause of infertility and ectopic pregnancy.
- Infection during pregnancy increases risk of prematurity and neonatal death; 50% chance that healthy, full-term baby will develop chlamydial conjunctivitis and 10% chance of pneumonia.
- Test for this agent in all vaginitis patients, particularly if pregnant.

THERAPEUTIC CONSIDERATIONS

Dietary considerations

Vaginal secretions are continuously released, and contain water, nutrients, electrolytes, and proteins (secretory IgA) – altered by hormonal and dietary factors; well-balanced diet low in fats, sugars, and refined foods; nutrients for proper immune function are zinc, vitamin A, vitamin C, vitamin E, manganese, and B-complex; diet high in lysine and low in arginine reduces number and severity of herpetic outbreaks; but many foods high in lysine are animal products high in fats; low-arginine diet plus lysine supplements is a viable alternative.

Nutritional supplements

High-quality multivitamin–multimineral supplement is a low-cost compensation for dietary inadequacies.

- **Vitamin A and beta-carotene:** necessary for epithelial tissues of vaginal mucosa; vitamin A is needed for adequate immune response and resistance to infection; secretory IgA is a major factor in resistance to infection; beta-carotene is a non-toxic vitamin A precursor that enhances T-cell number and ratio; excessive vitamin A is toxic and teratogenic – caution in females of reproductive age; limit total vitamin A intake to 5,000 IU q.d.; use mixed carotenoids rather than synthetic beta-carotene.

- **B vitamins:** needed for carbohydrate metabolism, protein catabolism and synthesis, cell replication, and immune function; B_2 and B_6 have estrogen-like effects and act synergistically with estradiol; B_1 and pantothenic acid enhance estradiol activity, without estrogenic activity themselves; useful in estrogen deficiency (atrophic vaginiti), especially if combined with phytoestrogens.

- **Vitamin C and bioflavonoids:** vitamin C deficiency reduces phagocytic activity of leukocytes; vitamin C and bioflavonoids improve connective tissue integrity, reducing spread of infection and frequency and severity of herpetic outbreaks.

- **Vitamin E:** supplemental vitamin E increases resistance to *Chlamydia*; regulates retinol in humans – inadequacy of vitamin E hinders utilization of vitamin A; used to treat atrophic vaginitis; has beneficial effects upon symptoms of menopause without risks of estrogen therapy; symptoms improved – hot flashes, vaginal atrophy, chills, HAs, vaginal infection rates, and diabetic vulvovaginitis; reduces oxidative breakdown of progesterone, favoring its transformation into pregnanediol; topical plus oral doses may offer best results; excess vitamin E intake may be immunosuppressive (>1200 IU q.d.) and transiently elevate BP; improves glycogen storage and tone of heart muscle; need extra caution in patients with diabetes, hypoglycemia, hypertension, or heart disease; in high-risk patients, begin with daily dose of 100 IU; monitoring blood sugar or BP, increase dosage slowly over time (e.g. 50 IU q.d.).

- **Zinc:** all DNA and RNA polymerases and repair and replication enzymes require zinc; enhances PGE_1 synthesis, normalizes lymphocyte activity, and enhances epithelial growth; zinc deficiency is linked to depressed immunity and thymic atrophy – corrected when zinc replenished; essential for utilization of vitamin A; topical and oral zinc reduce duration and severity of herpes outbreaks – due to antiviral activity; high levels are toxic to *Chlamydia* and *Trichomonas*, and effective in some cases unresponsive to antibiotic.

- **Lysine:** decreases frequency and severity of herpes outbreaks; may not shorten healing time; becomes incorporated into virus capsule in place of arginine, generating inactive virus; taken at low doses prophylactically and higher doses at first sign of prodrome, the time of greatest viral replication; efficacy is dose-related; best when combined with low-arginine diet.

- **Lithium:** lithium ointment interferes with replication of DNA viruses without affecting host cells; lithium succinate (8% solution) may be combined with Zn in topical ointment, or used alone.

Botanical medicines

- ***Glycyrrhiza glabra:*** licorice is antiviral against RNA and DNA viruses; effective in treating herpes; number and severity of recurrences reduced by the repeated applications of gel to active lesions; isoflavonoids in licorice effective against *Candida* (*Textbook*, Ch. 90).

- **Chlorophyll:** bacteriostatic and soothing action; water-soluble chlorophyll added to douching solutions offers symptomatic relief.

- ***Allium sativum:*** garlic is antibacterial, antiviral, and antifungal; effective against some antibiotic-resistant organisms; add to douching solutions or wrap in gauze and place as tampon/suppository for most forms of infectious vaginitis.

- ***Hydrastis canadensis*** **and** ***Berberis vulgaris:*** goldenseal and Oregon grape contain berberine, a broad-range antibacterial; berberine enhances immune

function taken internally and offers symptomatic relief used in douching solutions – soothes inflamed mucous membranes (*Textbook*, Ch. 91).

● **Estrogenic plants:** atrophic vaginitis due to lack of estrogen is treatable with phytoestrogens – molecular structure similar to estrogen but weaker effects; phytoestrogen plants include: soy, black cohosh, fennel, anise, ginseng, dong quai, alfalfa, red clover, licorice; use as teas, in salads, or in capsules; simultaneous advantage and disadvantage of phytoestrogens is that they lack the potency of synthetic estrogens – benefits slower to be noticed, but less likely to produce side-effects (*Textbook*, Chs 75, 123, 170, 183).

● *Melaleuca alternifolia*: alcoholic extract of tea tree oil diluted to 1% in water – strong antibacterial and antifungal; effective in treating trichomoniasis, candidiasis, and cervicitis; daily douching plus saturated tampons weekly; no adverse reactions reported; soothing effect (*Textbook*, Ch. 96).

● *Melissa officinalis*: member of mint family; effective in controlling herpetic symptoms and reducing frequency and severity of oral and genital herpes; taken orally as water extract or applied topically as creams.

● **Botanical mixture:** cream containing *Azadirachta indica* (neem) seed oil, *Sapindus mukerossi* (reetha) saponin extract and quinine – effective and better than placebo; applied intravaginally at bedtime for 14 days, for *Chlamydia trachomatis* vaginitis and bacterial vaginosis; no benefit for candidal or trichomonal infections.

Other agents

● *Lactobacillus acidophilus*: helps maintain healthy vaginal ecosystem by preventing overgrowth of undesirable species; produces lactic acid, natural antibiotic substances, and peroxides; competes with other bacteria by consuming glucose; insert live *Lactobacillus* culture unflavored yogurt (read labels carefully); more efficient and less messy method is to insert 1 capsule *Lactobacillus* into vagina b.i.d. for 1–2 weeks; use whenever antibiotics are used to reduce risk of complications (*Candida*) (*Textbook*, Ch. 105).

● **Iodine:** used as douche – effective against many organisms (*Trichomonas*, *Candida*, *Chlamydia*), and non-specific vaginitis; povidone-iodine (Betadine) does not sting or stain; effective in treating 100% of cases of candidal vaginitis, 80% of *Trichomonas*, and 93% of combination infections; douching solution diluted to 1 part iodine to 100 parts water (1.5–3 tsp Betadine to 1 quart water) used b.i.d. for 14 days.

● **Boric acid:** capsules of boric acid treat candidiasis almost as well as nystatin; inexpensive, accessible.

● **Gentian violet:** swabbing vagina with gentian violet is "as close to a specific treatment for *Candida* as exists".

DIAGNOSTIC APPROACH

Question women directly regarding pruritus, vaginal discharge, dysuria, etc.

- Complete gynecological and sexual history – sexual activity and practices of patient and partner(s), method of contraception, personal hygiene, self-medication; rule out associated symptoms suggesting PID or systemic infection; previous occurrences – diagnosis, treatment, and resolution.

- Identify causative agent – avoid douching, intercourse, and vaginal medications for 1–2 days prior to office visit.

- Determine by speculum exam whether discharge emanates from vagina or cervix, condition of vaginal mucosa, and character of discharge; collect specimens and place on slides for saline and KOH exam.

- Culture if diagnosis remains in question, or if screening for GC or *Chlamydia*.

- Best time to test for low-level persistent infection (*Candida*) is just before menstrual period.

THERAPEUTIC APPROACH

Focus of this protocol is on *Candida*, *Trichomonas*, and *Gardnerella*; for atrophic vaginitis, see chapter on menopause; for herpes simplex, see herpes chapter; for *Chlamydia*, see chapter on chlamydial infections.

- **Diet:** nutrient-dense diet – avoid refined foods and simple carbohydrates; minimize *trans* and saturated fats; determine and eliminate suspected food allergens.

- **Supplements:**
  — vitamin A: 5,000 IU q.d.; or beta-carotene: 50,000 IU q.d.
  — vitamin C: 500–1000 mg every 4 h
  — B-complex: balanced B-complex averaging 20–50 mg of each of major components
  — zinc: 10–15 mg q.d. (picolinate is best; 30–50 mg if using other forms)
  — vitamin E: 200 IU q.d. of D-alpha-tocopherol
  — *Lactobacillus* sp.: 0.5 tsp b.i.d.

- **Botanical medicines:**
  — *Hydrastis* + *Echinacea* + *Phytolacca* (2:2:1):
    tincture: 20–60 drops every 2–4 h
    tea: 1 tsp/cup every 2–4 h.

- **Topical treatment – douches and saturated tampons:** choose one or more of agents below; do not try to include all at once; variety provides alternatives for resistant cases.
  — Betadine: 1:100 dilution in retention douche kills most organisms within 30 s.

— boric acid: 600 mg in capsules (repeated use may irritate; use >7 days – problems from systemic absorption).

— *Allium sativum*: chopped fresh garlic added to douching solution or 1 clove peeled, wrapped in gauze, inserted as suppository; if irritation, remove immediately.

— gentian violet swab: sensitivity reactions common; stains clothes if pad not used.

— *Hydrastis canadensis*: decoction of 2 tsp/cup of hot water for douching.

— *Lactobacillus* sp: 1/2 tsp or 1/4 cup of yogurt in 1 cup warm water.

— *Glycyrrhiza glabra*: decoction in douches or apply gel locally.

— lithium sulfate: 8% solution.

— *Melaleuca alternifolia*: 1% dilution as douche, plus insertion of saturated tampon for 24 h once a week (repeated use may result in sensitivity in some women).

— white vinegar: 1–2 tbsp white vinegar and 2 tbsp green clay plus pint of water – douche.

— zinc sulfate: 1 tbsp of 2% solution in 1 pint water – douche or combined with galvanic therapy.

— other botanicals: traditional texts and modern practitioners find efficacy in treating vaginitis with the following herbs, used alone or with other agents in douching solutions: *Abies canadensis* (hemlock); *Hydrastis canadensis* (goldenseal); *Eucalyptus*; *Calendula officinalis* (marigold – use succus); chlorophyll.

General recommendations

● **Lactobacillus** capsules or yogurt with active cultures – use daily to reinoculate vagina.

● **Treatment failures** – incorrect diagnosis, reinfection, untreated predisposing factors, resistance to treatment.

● **Sexual activity:** avoid during treatment – to avoid reinfection and reduce trauma; at least use condoms.

● **Recurrent cases** – consider treating sexual partners.

● **Prefer cotton underwear** – especially with candidal vaginitis.

● **Early symptomatic relief of pruritus** and burning – warm sitz baths, plain or with herbs or Epsom salts.

● **Severe cases** – cleanse vagina of microbe-infested discharge with calendula succus-soaked cotton swabs.

● **Constant uterine discharge** alkalinizes vagina, decreasing natural resistance; identify and treat cause of discharge; vaginal depletion pack very useful (*Textbook*, App. 12).

Specific recommendations

- **Candida:** treat internal candidiasis simultaneously to prevent recurrences; continue *Candida* treatment for at least one full menstrual cycle; some suggest therapy 3–4 months thereafter during week preceding menses:
  - Betadine: b.i.d.
  - boric acid caps: inserted daily for 14 days
  - gentian violet swab: use daily for 14 days or longer
  - *Glycyrrhiza glabra*: daily.
- **Trichomonas:**
  - Betadine: b.i.d.
  - zinc sulfate: daily
  - *Melaleuca alternifolia* oil: daily.
- **Chlamydia:**
  - Betadine: daily
  - zinc sulfate: daily.
- **Herpes:**
  - avoid arginine-rich foods
  - lysine: 1,000–2,000 mg/day maintenance dose, double during outbreak
  - zinc sulfate: daily
  - lithium sulfate: add to the zinc sulfate douching solution
  - *Melissa officinalis*: ointment or cream t.i.d.
- **NSV:**
  - Betadine: daily
  - *Hyrastis canadensis*: daily.
- **Atrophic vaginitis:**
  - B-complex: 100 mg/day
  - vitamin E: 400 IU/day
  - topical application: vitamin E cream.

Varicose veins

DIAGNOSTIC SUMMARY

- Dilated, tortuous, superficial veins in the lower extremities.
- May be asymptomatic or associated with fatigue, aching discomfort, feeling of heaviness, or pain.
- Edema, pigmentation, and ulceration of the skin of the distal leg may develop.
- Women are affected four times as frequently as men.

GENERAL DISCUSSION

Veins are frail structures; defects in venous wall allow dilation of vein and damage to valves; valve damage increases static pressure, causing bulging known as varicose vein.

- 50% of middle-aged adults affected.
- Subcutaneous veins of legs most commonly affected – gravitational pressure that standing exerts on veins; standing for long periods increases pressure up to 10 times; occupations requiring long periods of standing are greatest risk for varicose veins.
- Women affected four times as frequently as men; obesity greatly increases risk; risk increases with age – due to loss of tissue tone and muscle mass, weakening vein walls; pregnancy increases risk by increasing venous pressure in legs.
- Pose little harm if involved vein is near surface, but cosmetically unappealing; significant symptoms uncommon, but legs may feel heavy, tight, and tired.
- Serious varicosities involve obstruction and valve defects of deeper veins of leg; can lead to thrombophlebitis, pulmonary embolism, MI, and stroke; phlebography and Doppler ultrasonography are most accurate methods of diagnosing deep vein involvement.

Cause of varicose veins

- Genetic weakness of veins or venous valves.
- Excess venous pressure due to low-fiber-induced increase in straining during defecation.

- Long periods of standing, and/or heavy lifting.
- Damage to veins or venous valves secondary to thrombophlebitis.
- Weakness of vascular walls due to either abnormalities in proteoglycans of interendothelial cement substance or excessive release of lysosomal enzymes which break down ground substance, increasing capillary permeability and loss of integrity of venous structure.

THERAPEUTIC CONSIDERATIONS

Dietary factors

- **Fiber:** varicose veins are rarely seen in parts of world with high-fiber, unrefined diets; low-fiber diet contributes to development of varicose veins – need to strain more during BMs (smaller, harder stools more difficult to pass); straining increases abdominal pressure, obstructing return of blood through legs; long-term increased pressure may weaken vein wall, causing varicosities or hemorrhoids, or may weaken wall of large intestine, producing diverticuli; high-fiber diet is the most important treatment and prevention of varicose veins (and hemorrhoids).
- **Bulking agents:** psyllium seed, pectin, and guar gum have mild laxative action – attract water and form gelatinous mass, keeping feces soft, promoting peristalsis, and reducing straining during defecation.

Physical measures

Exercise and avoiding standing for long periods reduce risk; walking, riding a bike, and jogging are particularly beneficial; contraction of leg muscles pushes pooled blood back into circulation; elastic compression stockings are occasionally beneficial; surgical stripping of vein is performed in severe cases.

Botanical medicines

Centella asiatica: extract containing 70% triterpenic acids (asiatic acid, madecassic acid, asiatoside) is impressive in treating cellulite, venous insufficiency of lower limbs, and varicose veins; exerts normalizing action on metabolism of connective tissue – enhances tissue integrity by stimulating glycosaminoglycan (GAG) synthesis without promoting excessive collagen synthesis or cell growth; GAGs are major components of amorphous intercellular matrix (ground substance) in which collagen fibers are embedded; net effect is normal tissue; effect in venous insufficiency and varicose veins is to enhance connective tissue structure, reducing sclerosis and improving blood flow through affected limbs.

Escin: compound isolated from seeds of *Aesculus hippocastanum* (horse chestnut); anti-edema and anti-inflammatory properties; decreases capillary permeability by reducing number and size of small pores of capillary walls; inhibits lysosomal enzymes that break down proteoglycans of ground substance; has venotonic activity.

● Venotonic = substance improving venous tone by increasing contractile potential of elastic fibers in vein wall; escin's venotonic activity confirmed in treatment of varicose veins and thrombophlebitis.

● Extracts of horse-chestnut seed standardized for escin are as effective as compression stockings without the nuisance.

● Can be given orally, or escin/cholesterol complex can be applied topically; topical formula is beneficial in treatment of bruises by decreasing capillary fragility and swelling.

***Ruscus aculeatus*:**   Butcher's broom is a subshrub of the lily family native to Mediterranean region; active ingredients are ruscogenins – anti-inflammatory and vasoconstrictive effects; extracts are used internally and externally in Europe for treating varicose veins and hemorrhoids.

Flavonoid-rich extracts:

● Berries (hawthorn berries, cherries, blueberries, blackberries) are beneficial in preventing and treating varicose veins; berries are rich sources of proanthocyanidins and anthocyanidins; bioflavonoids give berries blue-red color; proanthocyanidins and anthocyanidins improve integrity of ground substance and vascular system.

● Buckwheat (*Fagopyrum esculentum*) is high in rutin; tea standardized to 5% total flavonoids, yielding daily dosage of 270 mg of rutin, decreased total leg volume from edema of chronic venous insufficiency.

● Efficacy of these extracts is related to their ability to:
— reduce capillary fragility
— increase the integrity of the venous wall
— inhibit the breakdown of the compounds composing ground substance
— increase the muscular tone of the vein.

Bromelain and other fibrinolytic compounds: persons with varicose veins have decreased ability to break down fibrin; fibrin deposited in tissue near varicosity; skin then becomes hard and "lumpy" from fibrin and fat; decreased fibrinolysis increases risk of thrombi and thrombophlebitis, MI, pulmonary embolism, or stroke; herbs increasing fibrinolytic activity of blood indicated are capsicum (cayenne), garlic, onion, ginger – all increase fibrin breakdown, use liberally in food; bromelain (proteolytic enzyme from pineapple) is also indicated; vein walls are an important source of plasminogen activator, which promotes breakdown of fibrin; varicosed veins have decreased plasminogen activator; bromelain acts in similar manner to

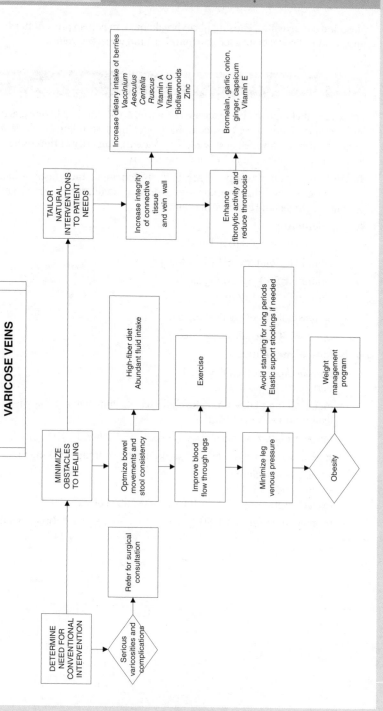

plasminogen activator, causing fibrin breakdown; may help prevent hard and lumpy skin ((lipodermatosclerosis) found around varicosed veins.

THERAPEUTIC APPROACH

Consume a diet high in fiber; exercise regularly; avoid standing in one place for long periods of time (use elastic support stocking if standing is necessary); avoid obesity; employ measures which increase the integrity of the connective tissue and vein wall; enhance fibrinolytic activity.

- **Diet:** high-complex carbohydrate diet rich in dietary fiber – liberal amounts of proanthocyanidin- and anthocyanidin-rich berries; garlic, onions, ginger, and cayenne liberally.
- **Supplements:**
  - vitamin A: 10,000 IU q.d.
  - vitamin B: complex – 10–100 mg q.d.
  - vitamin C: 500–3,000 mg q.d.
  - vitamin E: 200–600 IU q.d.
  - bioflavonoids: 100–1,000 mg q.d.
  - zinc: 15–30 mg q.d.
- **Botanical medicines:**
  - *Aesculus hippocastanum*:
    bark of root: 500 mg t.i.d.
  - escin: 10 mg t.i.d. – an escin/cholesterol complex may be applied topically in a 1% concentration
  - *Centella asiatica* extract (70% triterpenic acid content): 30 mg t.i.d.
  - *Ruscus aculeatus* extract (9–11% ruscogenin content): 100 mg t.i.d.
  - *Vaccinium myrtillus*:
    fresh berries: 55–110 g t.i.d.
    extract containing 25% anthocyanoside: 80–160 mg t.i.d.
  - bromelain (minimum 1,500 mcu): 500–750 mg t.i.d. between meals.

Viral pharyngitis

DIAGNOSTIC SUMMARY

- Sore throat with pain on swallowing.
- Throat infected, with edematous tonsils and fauces.
- Throat culture negative for group A beta-hemolytic streptococci.
- Fever, malaise, cervical lymphadenopathy, and leukocytosis.

GENERAL CONSIDERATIONS

In adults, 90% of "sore throats" are viral; but rule out "strep throat" (group A beta-hemolytic streptococci pharyngotonsillitis) – physical findings in viral and strep pharyngitis are indistinguishable.

THERAPEUTIC CONSIDERATIONS

Many plants and constituents are antiviral; but general, patient-oriented, approach is indicated – consider all factors affecting resistance status of host: past infection, fatigue, stress (physical, emotional, mental), environmental pollution, nutritional status, current medications; self-limiting condition – support natural defenses to shorten illness and reduce morbidity (*Textbook*, Ch. 53).

- **Antiviral botanicals:**
  — *Echinacea* sp.
  — *Glycyrrhiza glabra* (licorice root)
  — *Melissa officinalis* (lemon balm)
  — *Aloe vera*
  — *Astragalus membranaceus*
  — *Allium sativum* (garlic).

- *Zingiber officinale* **(ginger):** not a particularly strong antiviral; analgesic properties useful for relieving pharyngeal irritation.

- **Zinc lozenges:** provide relief of pharyngitis; prevent progression when utilized at first signs of pharyngeal discomfort presaging common cold; shortens duration of symptoms – cough, HA, hoarseness, muscle ache, nasal drainage, nasal congestion, scratchy throat, sore throat, sneezing,

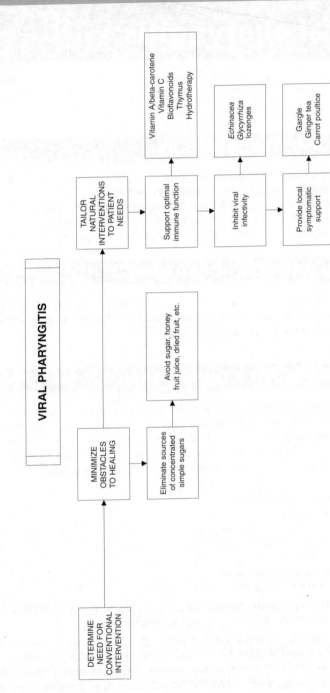

VIRAL PHARYNGITIS

DETERMINE NEED FOR CONVENTIONAL INTERVENTION

MINIMIZE OBSTACLES TO HEALING

→ Eliminate sources of concentrated simple sugars

→ Avoid sugar, honey fruit juice, dried fruit, etc.

TAILOR NATURAL INTERVENTIONS TO PATIENT NEEDS

Support optimal immune function

→ Vitamin A/beta-carotene
Vitamin C
Bioflavonoids
Thymus
Hydrotherapy

→ Inhibit viral infectivity

→ *Echinacea*
Glycyrrhiza
lozenges

→ Provide local symptomatic support

→ Gargle
Ginger tea
Carrot poultice

and fever; mild side-effects – nausea and bad-taste reactions; hard candy lozenges containing zinc gluconate and citric acid deliver insignificant amount of Zn^{2+}; saliva completely suppresses ionization of zinc salts to free Zn^{2+} in presence of citric acid or 30-fold molar excess of mannitol plus sorbitol; with excess glycine under same conditions, no interference with ionization; even large excesses of glycine do not interfere, with > 90% of zinc from zinc gluconate released as free Zn^{2+}.

- *Echinacea*: 20 drops every 2 h on first day of symptoms followed by 20 drops t.i.d. until cured reduces number of colds by 50% and duration by 50% (4 days) in patients with frequent URIs; decreases duration and symptoms by 30% in patients symptomatic for 1–3 days; significantly more effective at first stage than waiting until symptoms fully develop.

- **Other considerations:** chronic pharyngitis – consider other factors, e.g. microbes residing in toothbrush, food allergy; upper respiratory tract symptoms of chronic delayed food allergy: chronic rhinitis, sinusitis, pharyngitis, lateral and lingual tonsil hypertrophy, chronic laryngitis, glossitis, face and neck rashes, eczema.

THERAPEUTIC APPROACH

Drink plenty of fluids, restrict food intake, plenty of rest should be instituted; eliminate concentrated sugars that suppress immune function; avoid suspected allergens; do not suppress fever unless temperature approaches 104°F; hydrotherapy, diaphoretics, and "drainage remedies" (*Textbook*, Ch. 42).

- **Diet:** eliminate all sources of concentrated simple sugars: sugar, honey, fruit juice, dried fruit, etc; restrict food intake to < 1,000 calories q.d.; increase fluids to 8 oz/h – water and herbal teas listed below.

- **Supplements:**

  — vitamin A: 50,000 IU q.d. for 1 week; or beta-carotene: 200,000 IU q.d. (avoid vitamin A in menstruating women due to teratogenic effect)

  — vitamin C: 500 mg every 2 h

  — bioflavonoids: 1,000 mg q.d.

  — zinc: use lozenges supplying 15–25 mg of elemental zinc (gluconate without citrate mannitol or sorbitol); dissolve in mouth every two waking hours after initial double dose; continue up to 3 days

  — thymus extract: equivalent of 120 mg pure polypeptides with molecular weights < 10,000, or 500 mg crude polypeptide fraction.

- **Botanicals:**

  — *Echinacea* sp.:
    dried root (or as tea): 0.5–1 g
    freeze-dried plant: 325–650 mg
    juice of aerial portion of *E. purpurea* stabilized in 22% ethanol: 2–3 ml

tincture (1:5): 2–4 ml
fluid extract (1:1): 2–4 ml
solid (dry powdered) extract (6.5:1 or 3.5% echinacoside): 150–300 mg

— *Glycyrrhiza glabra*:
powdered root: 1–2 g
fluid extract (1:1): 2–4 ml
solid (dry powdered) extract (4:1): 250–500 mg.

● **Local treatment:**

— gargle with salt water b.i.d.: 1 tbsp salt/240 ml of warm water

— *Zingiber officinalis* (ginger): strong tea with fresh root or chew fresh root.

● **Physical therapy:**

— carrot poultice around neck

— hydrotherapy (*Textbook*, Ch. 42).

Index